Precision Medicine in Diabetes

Rita Basu
Editor

Precision Medicine in Diabetes

A Multidisciplinary Approach to an Emerging Paradigm

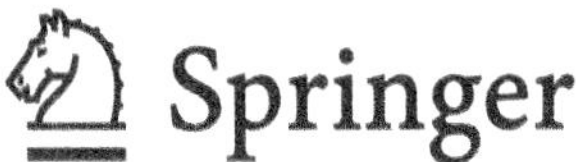

Editor
Rita Basu
Division of Endocrinology
University of Virginia
Charlottesville, VA, USA

ISBN 978-3-030-98929-3 ISBN 978-3-030-98927-9 (eBook)
https://doi.org/10.1007/978-3-030-98927-9

This Springer imprint is published by the registered company Springer Nature Switzerland AG
The registered company address is: Gewerbestrasse 11, 6330 Cham, Switzerland

Foreword

Precision medicine is gaining a lot of attention in clinical practice, particularly with the development of drugs in some disease states such as cancer, where compared to previous toxic chemotherapy, the use of targeted treatments based on genetic mutations in the tumors has led to considerable success with fewer side effects. However, such an approach has so far been elusive in the management of diabetes. Nevertheless, the availability of new drugs and the wealth of data in clinical trials as well as new developments in technology have led to the development of approaches to be more precise in our treatment of people with type 2 diabetes, in particular, so that good control of glucose and prevention of complications may be achieved. This book, *Precision Medicine in Diabetes*, is therefore a useful summary of the current state of knowledge in this field.

The book begins with a discussion of current therapeutics and a call for tailoring the metabolic derangement, pointing out that one size does not fit all. This is followed by discussions about diabetes and the heart, with considerable new data in this aspect of diabetes management derived from large cardiovascular outcome trials. This focuses not only on glucose-lowering but also on lipid management and leads to an approach for implementation of precision medicine in both type 1 and type 2 diabetes.

The most classic area where precision medicine can be applied in diabetes is the recognition that a small but significant proportion of people with what appears to be type 2 diabetes actually have the monogenic form previously called variants of maturity-onset diabetes in the young [MODY]. Recent advances have pointed out the huge therapeutic advantages of recognition of monogenic diabetes leading to better treatments from what appears miraculous in patients with mutations of the potassium channel, who respond to sulfonylurea drugs rather than insulin, which can be stopped in many cases, as well as successful treatment of other forms of monogenic diabetes with either sulfonylureas or, importantly, no treatment at all in the case of mutations of the glucokinase gene.

Novel approaches in the management of diabetes due to precise therapy have led to better management of patients in the hospital, better diets have led to remission of diabetes in some cases, and surgical approaches have also led to remission along with weight loss. Ultimately, we hope to understand nutrition and exercise better so that those treatments can be tailored to individuals, leading to better outcomes.

Finally, technology has led to dramatic improvements in the management of type 1 diabetes with the ability to use glucose sensors in a closed-loop system with insulin pumps, leading to less glucose variability and a substantial reduction in the risk of hypoglycemia while achieving better control.

Thus, precision medicine has come of age for both type 1 and type 2 diabetes and will surely lead to better outcomes. This book summarizes the current state of knowledge, and understanding of these advances will help us refine our research to deliver better and more precise therapies and manage the millions of people living with diabetes.

Vivian Fonseca, MD
Professor of Medicine and Pharmacology
Assistant Dean for Clinical Research
Tullis Tulane Alumni Chair in Diabetes
Chief, Section of Endocrinology
Tulane University Health Sciences Center
New Orleans, LA, USA

Preface

President Barack Obama, in his State of the Union address on January 20, 2015, had announced "Tonight, I'm launching a new Precision Medicine Initiative to bring us closer to curing diseases like cancer and diabetes — and to give all of us access to the personalized information we need to keep ourselves and our families healthier." Following the announcement, the National Institute of Health's director Dr. Francis Collins advocated, "What is needed now is a broad research program to encourage creative approaches to precision medicine, test them rigorously, and ultimately use them to build the evidence base needed to guide clinical practice."

The concept of precision or personalized medicine is not new. Precision medicine, like its precursor, evidence-based medicine, aims at diagnostic specificity. In terms of precision diabetes management, one aims at identifying the underlying pattern of dysglycemia, determining whether the cause is genetic, physiologic, behavioral, and/or pharmacologic; identifying concurrent comorbidities; and matching appropriate management strategies by proper initiation, adjustment, and assessment of clinical response to avoid metabolic and other complications.

I had the honor of organizing a symposium related to precision diabetes management at the American Diabetes Association scientific sessions in June 2018, after which the idea of bringing together world-renowned physician scientists working in diabetes to write a book about this topic came to mind.

However, as I began to give shape to this idea in early 2020, our lives changed forever with a pandemic that one had previously only read about in medical textbooks and journals but had not faced. I am grateful to my colleagues for continuing their patient care through the COVID-19 crisis and still finding time to write the chapters presented to you.

For many of us working in the field of diabetes, there are often personal stories to share why we chose this career. I began my journey in diabetes research back in the mid-1990s and soon realized that if we want to make change happen, then there is a need to conduct translational research and advance science so that newer and better management strategies can be brought to patients. We hope that this collection of topics encourages you to consider precision diabetes approaches when providing care to your patients.

Lastly, I wish to dedicate this book to my father, a dedicated physician himself whom I lost during the lockdown in 2020; my mother, who encouraged me to be independent and freethinking; and to my loving family, my husband and two daughters, who have always inspired me to do better.

Charlottesville, VA, USA Rita Basu

Contents

Contributors

Ethan Alexander Divisions of Endocrinology, Metabolism and Genetics, University of Kansas School of Medicine, Kansas City, KS, USA

Rita Basu Division of Endocrinology, University of Virginia, Charlottesville, VA, USA

Orly Ben-Yacov Department of Computer Science and Applied Mathematics and Department of Molecular Cell Biology, Weizmann Institute of Science, Rehovot, Israel

Saif M. Borgan Endocrinology and Metabolism Institute, Cleveland Clinic Foundation, Cleveland, OH, USA

Normand G. Boulé Faculty of Kinesiology, Sport, and Recreation, University of Alberta, Edmonton, AB, Canada

Alberta Diabetes Institute, Edmonton, AB, Canada

M. Luiza Caramori Division of Diabetes, Endocrinology and Metabolism, Department of Medicine, Division of Pediatric Nephrology, Department of Pediatrics, University of Minnesota, Minneapolis, MN, USA

Juliana C. N. Chan Department of Medicine and Therapeutics, The Chinese University of Hong Kong, Hong Kong, China

Hong Kong Institute of Diabetes and Obesity, The Chinese University of Hong Kong, Hong Kong, China

Li Ka Shing Institute of Health Sciences, The Chinese University of Hong Kong, Hong Kong, China

David Chen Monash School of Medicine, Monash University, Melbourne, VIC, Australia

NHMRC Clinical Trials Centre, University of Sydney, Sydney, NSW, Australia

Horng H. Chen Department of Cardiovascular Diseases, Mayo Clinic, Rochester, MN, USA

Claudio Cobelli Department of Woman and Child's Health, University of Padova, Padova, Italy

Maria Collazo-Clavell Division of Endocrinology, Diabetes, Metabolism, and Nutrition, Department of Medicine, Mayo Clinic, Rochester, MN, USA

Elizabeth Cristiano Divisions of Endocrinology, Metabolism and Genetics, University of Kansas School of Medicine, Kansas City, KS, USA

Long Davalos Department of Neurology, University of Michigan, Ann Arbor, MI, USA

Georgia Davis Division of Endocrinology, Department of Medicine, Emory University School of Medicine, Atlanta, GA, USA

Eva L. Feldman Department of Neurology, University of Michigan, Ann Arbor, MI, USA

Jordan Fulcher NHMRC Clinical Trials Centre, University of Sydney, Sydney, NSW, Australia

Austin and Repatriation General Hospital, Melbourne, VIC, Australia

A. Maria Daniela Hurtado Division of Endocrinology, Diabetes, Metabolism, and Nutrition, Department of Medicine, Mayo Clinic Health System, La Crosse, WI, USA

Division of Endocrinology, Diabetes, Metabolism, and Nutrition, Department of Medicine, Mayo Clinic, Rochester, MN, USA

Alicia J. Jenkins NHMRC Clinical Trials Centre, University of Sydney, Sydney, NSW, Australia

Department of Medicine, University of Melbourne, Melbourne, VIC, Australia

Department of Endocrinology, St. Vincent's Hospital, Melbourne, VIC, Australia

Sangeetha R. Kashyap Cleveland Clinic Lerner College of Medicine, Cleveland, OH, USA

Alice Pik Shan Kong Chinese University of Hong Kong, Hong Kong, PRC, China

Lee-Ling Lim Hong Kong Institute of Diabetes and Obesity, The Chinese University of Hong Kong, Hong Kong, SAR, China

Department of Medicine, University of Malaya, Kuala Lumpur, Malaysia

Andrea O. Y. Luk Department of Medicine and Therapeutics, The Chinese University of Hong Kong, Hong Kong, SAR, China

Hong Kong Institute of Diabetes and Obesity, The Chinese University of Hong Kong, Hong Kong, SAR, China

Ronald C. W. Ma Department of Medicine and Therapeutics, The Chinese University of Hong Kong, Hong Kong, China

Hong Kong Institute of Diabetes and Obesity, The Chinese University of Hong Kong, Hong Kong, China

Li Ka Shing Institute of Health Sciences, The Chinese University of Hong Kong, Hong Kong, China

Lalo Magni Department of Civil and Architecture Engineering, University of Pavia, Pavia, Italy

Roger S. Mazze AGP Clinical Academy, Portsmouth, UK

John M. Miles Divisions of Endocrinology, Metabolism and Genetics, University of Kansas School of Medicine, Kansas City, KS, USA

Francisco J. Pasquel Division of Endocrinology, Department of Medicine, Emory University School of Medicine, Atlanta, GA, USA

Goran Petrovski Cornell University/Sidra Medicine, Doha, Qatar

Michal Rein Department of Computer Science and Applied Mathematics and Department of Molecular Cell Biology, Weizmann Institute of Science, Rehovot, Israel

School of Public Health, Faculty of Social Welfare and Health Sciences, University of Haifa, Haifa, Israel

Michael Roden Department of Endocrinology and Diabetology, Medical Faculty and University Hospital Düsseldorf, Heinrich-Heine-University Düsseldorf, Düsseldorf, Germany

Institute for Clinical Diabetology, German Diabetes Center, Leibniz Institute for Diabetes Research at Heinrich-Heine-University, Düsseldorf, Germany

German Center for Diabetes Research, Partner Düsseldorf, München-Neuherberg, Germany

Peter Rossing Steno Diabetes Center Copenhagen, Herlev, Denmark

Department of Clinical Medicine, University of Copenhagen, Copenhagen, Denmark

Stacey A. Sakowski Department of Neurology, University of Michigan, Ann Arbor, MI, USA

Vera B. Schrauwen-Hinderling Institute for Clinical Diabetology, German Diabetes Center, Leibniz Institute for Diabetes Research at Heinrich-Heine-University, Düsseldorf, Germany

German Center for Diabetes Research, Partner Düsseldorf, München-Neuherberg, Germany

Department of Radiology and Nuclear Medicine/Nutrition and Movement Sciences, NUTRIM School of Nutrition and Translational Research in Metabolism Maastricht University Medical Center, Maastricht, The Netherlands

Emma S. Scott NHMRC Clinical Trials Centre, University of Sydney, Sydney, NSW, Australia

Royal North Shore Hospital, Sydney, NSW, Australia

Dinesh Selvarajah Department of Oncology and Metabolism, Medical School, University of Sheffield, Sheffield, UK

Jay S. Skyler Diabetes Research Institute, University of Miami Miller School of Medicine, Miami, FL, USA

Amro M. Stino Department of Neurology, University of Michigan, Ann Arbor, MI, USA

Solomon Tesfaye Diabetes Research Unit, Sheffield Teaching Hospital, Sheffield, UK

Chiara Toffanin Department of Electrical, Computer and Biomedical Engineering, University of Pavia, Pavia, Italy

Guillermo E. Umpierrez Division of Endocrinology, Department of Medicine, Emory University School of Medicine, Atlanta, GA, USA

Siu-Hin Wan Minneapolis Heart Institute, United Hospital, Saint Paul, MN, USA

Jane E. Yardley Faculty of Kinesiology, Sport, and Recreation, University of Alberta, Edmonton, AB, Canada

Alberta Diabetes Institute, Edmonton, AB, Canada

Augustana Faculty, University of Alberta, Edmonton, AB, Canada

Women's and Children's Health Research Institute, Edmonton, AB, Canada

Oana Patricia Zaharia Department of Endocrinology and Diabetology, Medical Faculty and University Hospital Düsseldorf, Heinrich-Heine-University Düsseldorf, Düsseldorf, Germany

Institute for Clinical Diabetology, German Diabetes Center, Leibniz Institute for Diabetes Research at Heinrich-Heine-University, Düsseldorf, Germany

German Center for Diabetes Research, Partner Düsseldorf, München-Neuherberg, Germany

Introduction

Precision Medicine in Diabetes describes solid approaches to diagnosing and treating diabetes in various divisions of medicine.

Alicia Jenkins, David Chen, Jordan Fulcher, and Emma S. Scott write the first chapter, "Precision Medicine Approaches for Management of type 2 Diabetes." It summarizes the relevant evidence base from the literature and major guidelines for type 2 diabetes care, including the prevention and treatment of diabetes and its associated complications. Dr. Jenkins uses mnemonics, flowcharts, and summary tables to guide the busy clinician in type 2 diabetes care. She reviews some ongoing research that will likely enhance the application of precision medicine in diabetes, and notes that "efforts must be made to ensure equitable access for all people with diabetes as per locally available resources."

Horng H. Chen and Siu-Hin Wan author the second chapter, "Precision Medicine for Diabetes and Cardiovascular Disease." They describe how diabetes is a definite risk factor for the development and progression of coronary heart disease and heart failure. Evidence shows that patients with both cardiovascular risk and diabetes are at increased risk of myocardial infarctions, strokes, heart failure, and death compared to the general population. To manage the conditions of diabetes and heart failure, patients must incorporate both lifestyle modifications as well as glycemic control. Some additional cardiovascular benefits may come from newer pharmacologic agents such as SGLT2 inhibitors and GLP1 agonists.

In "Precision Medicine for Diabetes and Dyslipidemia," Chap. 3, John Miles, Ethan Alexander, and Elizabeth Cristiano discuss several classes of medications that primarily target LDL cholesterol and have been shown to reduce cardiovascular events. Medication classes include the statins, ezetimibe, PCSK9 inhibitors, and bempedoic acid. However, other agents that do not target LDL cholesterol show promise, but need additional study, such as fibrates and omega-3 fatty acids. The chapter concludes with what they thinks is a neglected area of diabetic dyslipidemia management, which is the role of diabetes-specific pharmacotherapy. Several drug classes, including metformin, GLP-1 receptor agonists, and thiazolidinediones, target lipoprotein abnormalities and have shown to reduce cardiovascular risk. Thus, cardiovascular risk reduction can be achieved through judicious use of these medications in conjunction with lipid-specific agents.

Michael Roden, Oana Patricia Zaharia, and Vera B. Schrauwen–Hinderling write Chap. 4, "Imaging in Precision Medicine for Diabetes," covering the various imaging tools that can assist in identifying specific abnormal factors in physiological structures that can delineate subgroups of patients for better treatment options. These tools can show specific structural, functional, or molecular abnormalities in groups otherwise classified under the broad umbrella of type 1 diabetes or type 2 diabetes, and provide the basis for optimal preventive or therapeutic measures. For example, different techniques including bioimpedance, hydrostatic weighing, air displacement plethysmography, densitometry (DXA), computed tomography (CT), and magnetic resonance imaging (MRI) can perform an assessment of whole body adiposity, but MRI usually shows the best results.

Ronald C.W. Ma and Juliana C.N. Chan author Chap. 5, "Implementation of Precision Medicine Approaches for Type 1 and 2 Diabetes." The authors cover recent advances in genetics of type 1 diabetes, type 2 diabetes and its associated complications, which have greatly facilitated the potential implementation of precision medicine in diabetes. Personalized approaches to diagnose, prevent, treat, and predict diabetes complications are potential areas to incorporate genomic or other information. However, the implementation of these approaches requires a multipronged approach in biomarker discovery, validation, clinician education and patient empowerment, as well as regulatory support and reimbursement. Development of precision medicine in diabetes represents an important opportunity to improve outcomes and "modernize" diabetes management despite some initial challenges.

Chapter 6, "Precision Medicine for Monogenic Diabetes," by Andrea On Yan Luk and Lee-Ling Lim, covers the methods to diagnose monogenic diabetes, challenges faced, and possible solution to improve case finding. The chapter also addresses common forms of monogenic diabetes including maturity onset diabetes of the young and neonatal diabetes. With monogenic diabetes contributing to 1–3% of diabetes in young people, molecular diagnosis of this condition fully demonstrates the feasibility of precision medicine because it will influence the choice of pharmacotherapy, direct relevant investigation, and prompt screening of at-risk family members. Because of similar clinical symptoms, monogenic diabetes can frequently be misdiagnosed as type 1 diabetes or type 2 diabetes, and over 80% of cases remain unrecognized in clinical practice. Misdiagnosis is mainly due to the lack of initiating genetic testing, the high cost of testing, and a lack of awareness among general physicians.

M. Luiza Caramori and Peter Rossing write Chap. 7, "Diabetic Kidney Disease: Precision Medicine for Identification, Prevention and Treatment." About 10% of the world's population has diabetes, so as a result, diabetes and its complications are a very extensive public health problem. Increased mortality and morbidity are associated with diabetes in large part due to end-stage kidney disease (ESKD) in the USA (47% of new cases) and other developed countries. Type 2 diabetes (T2D) is the major cause of ESKD rather than type 1 diabetes (T1D). However, worldwide, the proportion of individuals starting kidney replacement therapy due to diabetes varies significantly, ranging from 13% in China to 66% in Singapore. Chronic kidney disease (CKD) risk is about 50% for patients with T1D and 30% for those with T2D, and those with T2D and CKD are at higher risk for cardiovascular morbidity and mortality than those without CKD.

Chapter 8, entitled "Precision Medicine for Diabetic Neuropathy," is the work of Eva Feldman, Long Davalos, Amro M. Stino, Dinesh Selvarajah, Stacey A. Sakowski, and Solomon Tesfaye. They note that the most prevalent diabetic and prediabetic complication is diabetic peripheral neuropathy (DPN), which leads to substantial morbidity. Distal symmetric polyneuropathy is the most common manifestation, which can present with tingling, pain, and loss of sensory function. A multi-faceted understanding of evolving concepts in the underlying pathophysiology of DPN is required because DPN due to type 1 (T1D) and type 2 (T2D) diabetes represents largely different disease processes. Particularly in T2D, there is growing evidence suggesting that metabolic syndrome, obesity, and dyslipidemia contribute to the development of DPN. In addition, functional MRI, quantitative sensory testing, and even genomic data assist to more precisely phenotype and classify DPN neuropathic pain. Ultimately, the goal is for treatments to be individualized based on better understanding of underlying pathogenesis and pain processes.

Guillermo E. Umpierrez, Georgia Davis, and Francisco J. Pasquel are the authors of Chap. 9, "Inpatient or Hospital Precision Medicine for Diabetes." In the past few decades, the tools for monitoring and treating patients living with diabetes have expanded exponentially, with opportunities to manage the disease through targeted approaches according to needs and clinical characteristics of individuals. Current advances in genetics and systems biology can identify diabetes phenotypes through data from multiple sources to better determine an individual's needs. However, in the hospital setting, there is still limited application of these concepts. To develop inpatient precision diabetes medicine, they review advances and opportunities in *precision diagnostics* (characterization of unique individual-level data for more accurate disease-state classification and inpatient risk stratification), *precision monitoring* (real-time continuous glucose data with remote monitoring capabilities and patient-specific glycemic control targets), and *precision therapeutics* (addition of non-insulin agents with associated benefits beyond glycemic control, computer-based decision algorithms, and automated insulin delivery).

In Chap. 10, "Precision Medical Management Strategies for Diabetes Remission," Sangeeta R. Kashyap and Saif Borgan write about remission of type 2 diabetes mellitus. Remission is a period of at least 6–12 months to normalization of blood glucose levels to levels below the threshold at which diabetes is diagnosed, in the absence of active pharmacological agents. An area of controversy has been the duration of normalization, which has caused some degree of heterogeneity across studies. Because the genetic and environmental factors that led to the development of this chronic disease still exist in many patients who achieve this state, "remission" is usually the term used, not "cure."

Maria Collazo-Clavell and Maria Daniela Hurtado write Chap. 11, "Precision Surgical Management Strategies for Diabetes Remission." The term "diabesity" is derived from the most important risk factors of overweight and obesity for type 2 diabetes (DM2). Because type 2 is a chronic and progressive disease, "diabesity" is increasing rapidly and is now a public health crisis. Although modest weight loss can improve patients' glucose control, sustained weight loss through lifestyle changes is difficult. Therefore, bariatric surgery has become the most effective and efficient therapy for sustained weight loss and an alternative for patients with "diabesity." Although much evidence has shown that bariatric surgery is associated with 30–95% remission rates of DM2, reasons for remission are not understood fully. Many pre- and post-operative variables are involved, including caloric restriction resulting in massive weight loss, gastrointestinal peptides, bile acids, and microbiomes. Additionally, remission is not always long-term, depending on the individual and these variables.

Chapter 12, "Precision Nutrition for Type 2 Diabetes," by Orly Ben-Yacov and Michal Rein, teaches that precision nutrition aims to affect health outcomes by tailoring dietary recommendations to individuals or population subgroups based on their unique characteristics to effectively promote dietary health. Many recent advances in technologies, such as genomics, metabolomics, and microbiome, and the development of mobile applications and wearable devices offer opportunities for prevention and management of type 2 diabetes mellitus (T2DM). Genetic variants have been identified by nutrigenomics studies related to intake and metabolism of specific nutrients. Potentially modified by diet, individualized fingerprints of food and nutrient consumption and newly uncovered metabolic pathways have been identified by metabolomics. Interpersonal variability of host metabolism and glycemic status and personal postprandial responses are affected by gut microbiome composition and function. Plus, real-time assessment of dietary intake and metabolic state can be detected by mobile applications and wearable devices, which can improve glycemic control and diabetes management. Although the field is rapidly evolving, there are still several challenges impeding the clinical translation of scientific evidence. So, more research is definitely needed before precision nutrition approaches become widely used for prevention and management of T2DM in clinical and public health settings.

Jane Yardley and Normand G Boulé give us Chap. 13, "Precision Exercise and Physical Activity for Diabetes." We know exercise and physical activity improve overall health, but in the management of both type 1 and type 2 diabetes, they are important, in part, due to their ability to decrease risk factors associated with diabetes-related complications. But, just as with any other treatment, a great deal of inter- and intra-individual variation exists in responses to different activity doses (type, timing, intensity, frequency, and duration). This chapter shares the factors that may influence both short- and long-term adaptation to exercise and physical activity in individuals with both type 1 and type 2 diabetes so that the right treatment for the right person at the right time can be designed as an appropriate exercise/physical activity prescription.

Chapter 14, entitled "Diabetes Technology for Precision Therapy in Children, Adults and Pregnancy," is written by Roger S.Mazze, Alice Pik Shan Kong, Goran Petrovski, and Rita Basu. Using case study materials, this chapter reviews the functionality of continuous glucose monitoring (CGM) and continuous insulin infusion (pump) technologies. It addresses their current usage in clinical practice and shows how they contribute to precision medicine, discussing their future applications in the diagnosis and treatment of diabetes. The terms type 1 and type 2 diabetes as well as diabetes in pregnancy are major classifications of a condition and suggest "one term fits all." However, genomics has identified numerous subtypes, suggesting that not all conditions within the same classification are the same. Little emphasis has been on glucose sensing, insulin delivery technologies, and their roles in metabolic profiling to identify the distinguishing features within these subgroups that contribute to greater diagnostic specificity and improved treatment. As a result, the precision medicine paradigm needs to shift to allow for the technologies of continuous glucose monitoring (CGM) and continuous insulin infusion (pump) towards improving metabolic profiling and consequently glycemic control.

Chapter 15, "Adaptive and Individualized Artificial Pancreas for Precision Management of Type 1 Diabetes," is written by Claudio Cobelli, Chiara Toffanin, and Lalo Magni. They describe how automated insulin delivery systems (artificial pancreas, AP) are revolutionizing type 1 diabetes management. Incredible progress in subcutaneous (sc) glucose sensing, sc insulin pumps, and control algorithms make these systems possible. Several control strategies are being explored, for example, proportional derivative integral control and model predictive control, by using the sc insulin delivery route. Also under investigation is AP employing intraperitoneal (ip) insulin delivery. Important issues are control algorithm individualization and adaptivity, that is, capability to adapt to the changing in-time metabolic status of a person. These issues are both very relevant for precision medicine because they would allow the fine-tuning of glucose control to a specific person or a subgroup of people.

Jay S. Skyler authors Chap. 16, "Evolving Precision Medicine Approaches to Type 1 Diabetes Management." There is much progress in therapeutic approaches for type 1 diabetes (T1D). These include automated insulin delivery (AID); prevention of immune destruction, to preserve beta cell mass or function; and replacement or regeneration of insulin-secreting beta cells.

Chapter 1
Precision Medicine Approaches for Management of Type 2 Diabetes

David Chen, Jordan Fulcher, Emma S. Scott, and Alicia J. Jenkins

Introduction

Personalized medicine, sometimes referred to as precision medicine, is defined as "the capacity to predict disease development and influence decisions about lifestyle choices or to tailor medical practice to an individual," and it underpins best practice medicine [1]. Oncologists do this well, often treating patients not just on tumor location(s) but also on their tumor markers and underlying molecular abnormalities, any comorbidities, and patient preferences [2]. Advances in basic and clinical science, molecular medicine, "omics" (e.g., genomics), "big data," electronic health records, and decision support tools increase feasibility of increasingly individualized care for many medical conditions, including diabetes.

D. Chen
Monash School of Medicine, Monash University, Melbourne, VIC, Australia

NHMRC Clinical Trials Centre, University of Sydney, Sydney, NSW, Australia

J. Fulcher
NHMRC Clinical Trials Centre, University of Sydney, Sydney, NSW, Australia

Austin and Repatriation General Hospital, Melbourne, VIC, Australia

E. S. Scott
NHMRC Clinical Trials Centre, University of Sydney, Sydney, NSW, Australia

Royal North Shore Hospital, Sydney, NSW, Australia

A. J. Jenkins (✉)
NHMRC Clinical Trials Centre, University of Sydney, Sydney, NSW, Australia

Department of Medicine, University of Melbourne, Melbourne, VIC, Australia

Department of Endocrinology, St. Vincent's Hospital, Melbourne, VIC, Australia
e-mail: alicia.jenkins@sydney.edu.au

R. Basu (ed.), *Precision Medicine in Diabetes*,
https://doi.org/10.1007/978-3-030-98927-9_1

Diabetes is pandemic, currently affecting 9.3% of the global population aged 20–79 years [3]. Of people with diabetes, an estimated 85–95% have Type 2 diabetes, and about 79% of people with diabetes globally live in disadvantaged regions where access to optimal diabetes care may be limited [3]. Even people with diabetes in advantaged regions may not be able to access or afford all recommended evidence-based therapies. Associated with serious acute and chronic complications, diabetes places significant personal and socioeconomic burdens on the individual, their family and friends, community, healthcare system, and country. Compared to the background population, people with diabetes are more than twofold likely to develop cardiovascular disease (CVD) [4], 15 times more likely to have a non-traumatic lower limb amputation [5], and 25 times more likely to become blind [6]. In addition, diabetes is the leading cause of end-stage renal disease (ESRD) [7], and pregnant women with diabetes have a two- to fourfold greater risk of pre-eclampsia [8], which is also associated with increased risk of Type 2 diabetes, hypertension, CVD, and heart failure [9], both for the mother and her offspring [10–12].

The Metabolic Milieu of Diabetes

The hallmark of diabetes is elevated blood glucose levels, which are used to diagnose diabetes, usually by fasting or random blood glucose levels, an oral glucose tolerance test (OGTT), and/or HbA1c, and to monitor its treatment, usually by serial HbA1c levels and sometimes by self-monitoring of capillary blood or interstitial fluid glucose levels [13, 14]. Yet, the metabolic derangement prior to and during the course of Type 2 diabetes is far more widespread, as summarized in Fig. 1.1.

Diabetes is associated with abnormalities in glucose, lipid, and protein metabolism, changes in insulin secretion and sensitivity, and alterations in the immune system, microbiome, genetics, and epigenetics. It is also associated with increased inflammation, oxidative stress, and advanced glycation end-products (AGEs), as well as abnormalities in β-cell function, hemostasis, fibrinolysis, cell signaling, tissue repair, fibrosis, calcification, angiogenesis, and vascular tone [10, 15–17]. These factors and processes contribute to the pathogenesis of diabetes and its acute and chronic complications. Some of these processes are at least partly modulated by glycemia and insulin and may also be therapeutic targets. Diet and drugs may modulate these processes directly or as pleiotropic effects. It must also be recognized that the metabolic milieu of a person with diabetes may vary substantially over time, with aging; changes in glycemia; weight; diet; kidney, liver, or cardiac function; chronic complication status; intercurrent illnesses; changes in lifestyle; and treatments.

Precision Medicine: Now and Later

There are many genetic and environmental factors that modulate diabetes onset, progression or regression, and response to therapeutics. The person with diabetes can now use an array of devices to collect information, such as their heart rate and

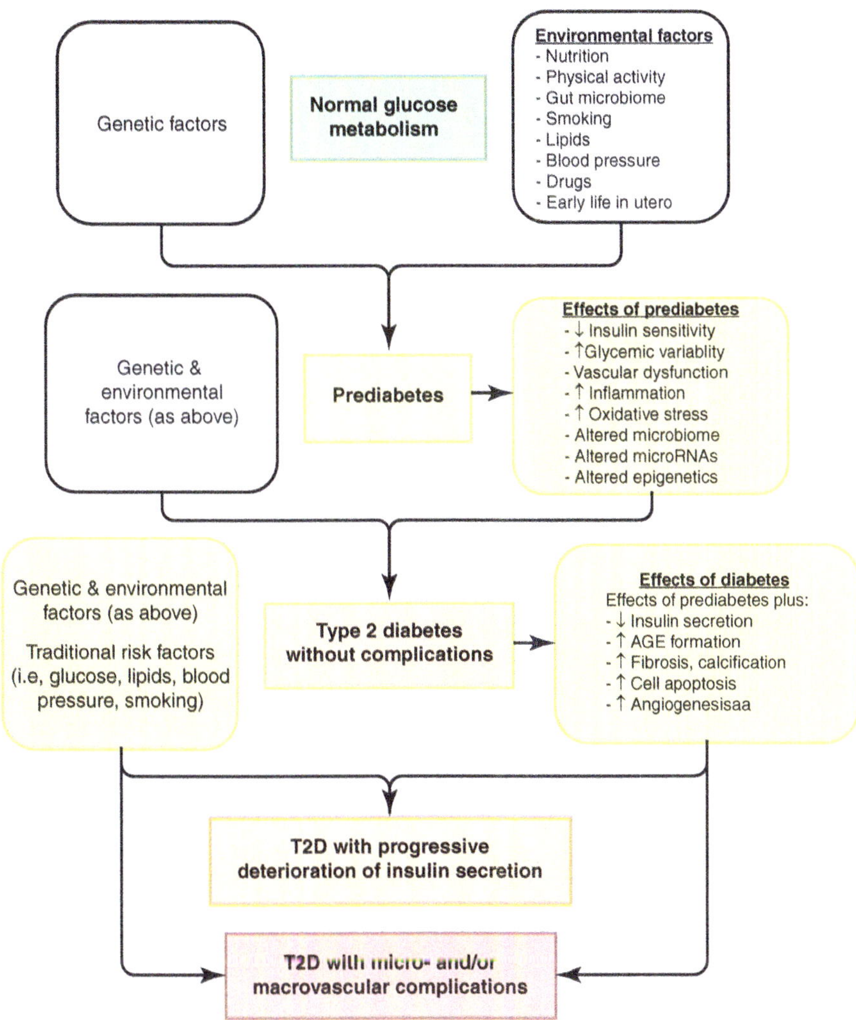

Fig. 1.1 The metabolic milieu of Type 2 diabetes

rhythm, blood pressure, physical activity, food intake, sleep quality, oxygenation, and blood and interstitial fluid glucose levels. It is likely that these data will be increasingly integrated into medical records, complementing other clinical and laboratory data. In this era of molecular biology and advanced biochemistry, such as lipidomics, proteomics, metabolomics, and the capacity to collect and analyze large and complex data sets, new knowledge is emerging, including related to diabetes, that can inform precision medicine. To realize its full potential, there must be more clinical research, advanced accurate and affordable laboratory and computational facilities, and informed participants, including patients, their multidisciplinary healthcare providers, the healthcare system, payers (government or private health insurance), and society.

Many genetic factors have been associated with the risk of Type 2 diabetes, the level of glycemic control, its chronic complications [18–25], and responsiveness to therapies, including nutrition [26–34] and drugs [35, 36]. Some gene chip assays are already available for clinical use, such as for common gene variants that predispose to drug intolerances [37, 38], but having a gene that predisposes one to drug intolerance does not mean that one will be drug intolerant nor that one will be drug tolerant if one does not have the gene. As diabetes and its complications are complex disorders, there are likely multiple genetic factors at play, which may also differ by ethnicity; hence, the use of genetics in diabetes is currently a clinical research tool. In the UK Biobank [39], a GWAS analyses, identified 208 independent SNPs mapping to 69 loci to be associated with Type 2 diabetes. There were age subgroup-specific genetics and causal determinants, supporting the hypothesis that the pathogenesis of Type 2 diabetes changes with age. This increases the challenge for personalized medicine and to the prediction of Type 2 diabetes at different life stages. In less common cases, about 1–5% of people with Type 1 or Type 2 diabetes, a single gene defect is responsible for diabetes—called monogenic diabetes; hence, the clinical use of genetic tests, where available, is useful and enables the practice of precision medicine in diabetes [40]. Some polygenic risk scores have shown utility in predicting diabetes complication risk [41–45]. Other chapters in this book discuss in more detail the genetics of diabetes, including monogenic diabetes.

Acquired factors may alter if and how genes are expressed; this is the field of epigenetics, the study of changes in modification of gene expression rather than of the genetic code itself. Biomarkers in epigenetics include DNA methylation, mRNAs, and microRNAs. MicroRNAs are small non-coding RNAs that modulate gene and mRNA expression and are involved in cell-to-cell communication [46, 47]. Their altered expression has been associated with diabetes and its chronic complications [48–58]. Another molecular factor at the interface of genetics and acquired factors is telomeres, protective caps at chromosome ends, which usually shorten with each cell division. As we recently reviewed in diabetes [59], shorter telomeres in circulating white blood cells have been associated with increased risk of diabetes and its chronic complications, and telomere length is often inversely correlated with traditional cardiometabolic risk factors, such as obesity, hypertension, smoking, and dyslipidemia. In adults with Type 2 diabetes from the Hong Kong Diabetes Register, we showed that shorter relative leukocyte telomere length independently predicted cardiovascular disease and all-cause mortality [60, 61]. Both genetics and environmental factors, including diet, exercise, and medications, impact telomere length and their shortening rate, with drugs commonly used in diabetes, such as metformin, HMG-CoA reductase inhibitors, fenofibrate, and angiotensin converting enzyme (ACE) inhibitors being telomere protective [59, 62, 63]. While there are an increasing number of basic science and clinical studies with positive associations between diabetes and its complications and genetic and epigenetic markers, no such tests are used clinically, apart from monogenic diabetes tests. In addition to a strong evidence base and the dissemination and acceptance of knowledge, an affordable, user-friendly, and practical means of generating and implementing optimal treatments is essential. Advanced computer programs will be required. For simpler data, usually based on traditional risk factors, complication status, and sometimes imaging, such as retinal images or coronary artery calcification, useful risk equations/calculators are already available, such as for Type 2 diabetes itself [64, 65], sight-threatening diabetic retinopathy [66, 67], diabetic kidney disease [68, 69], and cardiovascular disease (CVD) [70], often presented as websites or apps. Artificial intelligence (AI) for the diagnosis of diabetic retinopathy is already being implemented, but further refinements are desirable [71, 72].

While we await further knowledge and translational tools to enhance our ability to tailor lifestyle and therapies to the individual with diabetes, we can already practice some precision medicine for people with diabetes with current resources based on traditional risk factors. Patient preferences, medico-legal considerations, and local resources, such as the ability and preparedness to self-administer injectable drugs and out-of-pocket drug costs, should be considered.

As there are numerous abnormalities in the metabolic milieu of diabetes (Fig. 1.1) and many risk factors for complications, multiple treatments are needed to achieve metabolic control and reduce adverse outcomes. Once Type 2 diabetes is present, there are recommended targets for HbA1c, blood pressure, lipids, albuminuria, BMI, and smoking, and also for vaccinations and complication screening. Table 1.1 summarizes some national/international guidelines. In spite of such guidelines and

Table 1.1 Risk factor targets for diabetes patients from major bodies

	ADA [155]	ESC/EASD [266]	IDF [267]	RACGP/Diabetes Australia [14]
HbA1c	<7% (53 mmol/mol)	<7.0% (53 mmol/mol)	<7% (53 mmol/mol)	≤7% (53 mmol/mol)
SBP	<140 mmHg[a]	<130 mmHg	≤130–140 mmHg	≤140 mmHg
DBP	<90 mmHg[a]	<80 mmHg	≤80 mmHg	≤90 mmHg
LDL-C	–[b]	Moderate CV risk: <2.6 mmol/L High CV risk: <1.8 mmol/L and ≥50% reduction Very high CV risk: <1.4 mmol/L and ≥50% reduction	<2.6 mmol/L Established CVD or high CV risk: <1.8 mmol/L	<2.0 mmol/L <1.8 mmol/L if established CVD
BMI	<25 kg/m^2[c] [78]	–	–	<25 kg/m^2
WHR	–	–	–	–
Waist circumference	–	–	–	♂ < 94 cm ♀ < 80 cm

[a]Target lower by 10 mmHg may be appropriate in individuals at higher CV risk (existing CVD or 10-year ASCVD risk ≥15%)
[b]Prescription of lipid-lowering medications dependent on patient's age and CV risk (as detailed in Fig. 1.2)
[c]<23 kg/m^2 for Asian American individuals

Pre-diabetes
- Lifestyle modifications including the use of technology-assisted tools[82] - Refer to self-management education and support programs[216, 249] - Consider metformin 500mg–2g daily in high-risk individuals[79] - Consider bariatric surgery in morbidly obese, high-risk patients[250] - Annual screening for diabetes - fasting blood glucose, OGTT or HbA1c - Screen for and treat vascular risk factors[251] (GLOBES STRIVED)

Diabetes (no complications) **GLOBES STRIVED** – glucose, lipid control, obesity, BP, emotions, smoking, screening, treatment to target, inflammation/infections, vaccination, education, devices	
Glucose	- Aim for HbA1c ≤7% in most patients[110] o Consider less stringent targets (e.g., 7.5–8%) in certain patients e.g., long duration diabetes, frail, existing CVD, history of severe hypoglycemia o Consider more aggressive target (e.g.,≤6.5%) at diagnosis/early in the course of disease - ADA Standards of Medical Care in Diabetes for guidelines on pharmacologic glycemic treatment[135]
Lipid control‡[154]	- Aim for LDL-C < 2.0mmol/L in most patients o Consider a more aggressive target (e.g., 1.8mmol/L) in those at very high vascular risk (10y ASCVD risk > 20%) o Consider a less aggressive target (e.g., <2.6mmol/L) in those without other vascular risk factors (or 10y ASCVD risk <10%) - Age 40–75y o Moderate intensity statin (e.g., atorvastatin 10–20mg nocte, rosuvastatin 5–10mg daily) – no other CVD risk factors o High intensity statin (e.g., atorvastatin 40–80mg nocte, rosuvastatin 20–40mg daily) – with CVD risk factors, especially if 10y ASCVD risk >10% - Age <40y o Moderate intensity statin in patients with CVD risk factors or long duration diabetes (≥10 years) - Age >75y o Consider initiating statin therapy according to patient discussion weighing vascular risk and other comorbidities - Consider adding ezetimibe in patients at very high vascular risk (10y ASCVD risk >20%) who are not at target LDL-C on maximally tolerated statin therapy - Do not stop statins because of an increase in blood glucose levels or HbA1c
Obesity	- Initial weight loss of 5–10% through lifestyle changes (such as VLCD†) in overweight/obese patients[252] - Consider pharmacological therapies such as orlistat[253] - Consider metabolic/bariatric surgery in morbidly obese (BMI >35) patients with multiple comorbidities[254]
BP	- Aim for BP <140/85mmHg in most patients[255] o Lower targets (e.g.,<130/80mmHg) in high CVD risk patients if achievable - RAAS blocker (ACEI or ARB, not both) recommended as part of treatment[196] - CCB and/or thiazide diuretic – especially in older patients[256, 257] - Consider twodrugs for initial therapy if BP ≥20/10mm Hg above target goal[258] - ≥1BP drug at bedtime[199] - BP self-monitoring at home in hypertensive patients[259]
Emotions	- Formal screening tools for diabetes distress[260] (e.g., PAID, DDS-2) - Ask "How is your diabetes being a pain for you at the moment?" - Consider input from diabetes educators, psychologists and psychiatrists
Smoking	- Counsel for smoking cessation[204] - Refer to support program[204] - Pharmacotherapy (e.g., nicotine, varenicline or bupropion)[204]

Fig. 1.2 Evidence-based clinical practice points for adults with pre-diabetes and diabetes

Screening[14]	- HbA1c 4 times a year - Annual lipids, ocular health and foot care - BP and weight at each clinic visit - Comprehensive eye examination by an ophthalmologist or optometrist at diagnosis and every 2 years thereafter[261] - Annual renal function including a spot urine albumin creatinine ratio or 24h urinary albumin excretion rate and eGFR and serum creatinine levels[78] - Annual screening for neuropathy using simple clinical tests[78, 262]
Treatment to target	- Aim to treat to recommended risk factor targets (Table 1) - Electronic decision support tools can assist with identifying patients not at target
Inflammation / Infections	- People with diabetes are at increased risk of infection (e.g., UTI, fungal infections, periodontal disease)
Vaccination	- Recommend all age-appropriate vaccinations
Education	- Refer for structured diabetes patient education[216, 249] - Refer to dietician for assessment and education[263] - ≥150 minutes of moderate-vigorous exercise over ≥3 days/week & 2–3 sessions of resistance training on non-consecutive days[264]
Devices	- Consider devices such as physical activity trackers, smart phone apps, home BP monitor - Consider glucometers/CGM, particularly for patients requiring insulin therapy
Aspirin	- Not empirically recommended for all patients - Consider on an individual basis in high vascular risk patients (10y ASCVD risk >10%) only after consideration of bleeding risks

Diabetes with CVD complications

See Table 1.6

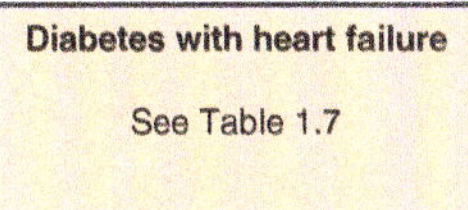

Diabetes with microvascular complications

See Table 1.8

†Prescribe with caution, especially in patients on insulin or sulfonylureas
‡Recommended to use a contemporary risk calculator that is applicable to the population being treated

Lifestyle modifications are first-line therapy for the control of glucose, lipids, obesity, BP and CVD risk
OGTT: oral glucose tolerance test, BP: blood pressure, CVD: cardiovascular disease, VLCD: very low-calorie diet, ACEI: ACE inhibitor, ARB: angiotensin receptor blocker, CCB: calcium channel blocker, PAID: problem areas in diabetes questionnaire, DDS-2: diabetes distress screening scale, p.a.: per annum

Fig. 1.2 (continued)

the proven benefit of optimizing multiple risk factors in diabetes [73], the majority of people with diabetes do not meet recommended treatment targets [74, 75]. Multiple risk factors, even at low severity levels, can place people with diabetes at moderate-to-high risk of complications.

While precision medicine for diabetes will improve, the current evidence base already enables clinicians to personalize diabetes care based on their patients' age, diabetes type, duration, and complication status. In this chapter, we summarize evidence for proven therapies in Type 2 diabetes and its chronic complications. We provide flowcharts, tables, mnemonics, and relevant websites to outline major management points. Other book chapters herein expand some areas.

Targeted Screening for Type 2 Diabetes and Diabetes Prevention

Progression from normal glucose tolerance to Type 2 diabetes is relatively slow, and even when diabetes is present, it can be asymptomatic or symptoms misattributed [76, 77]. National diabetes associations generally recommend testing for Type 2 diabetes in all asymptomatic adults aged ≥45 years (or younger for high-risk ethnic groups) and overweight adults with one or more diabetes risk factors [78]. The American Diabetes Association (ADA)-endorsed guidelines "Standards of Medical Care in Diabetes," which are updated at least annually [13, 78], provide detailed guidance regarding screening and diagnosis (including in the pediatric population).

A range of lifestyle modifications, with an emphasis on weight loss through diet and exercise, medications, and bariatric surgery (discussed in another chapter) can reduce risk of Type 2 diabetes. As shown by the Diabetes Prevention Program (DPP) over 3 years and its ongoing follow-up study (DPPOS), both lifestyle interventions and metformin can reduce progression from pre-diabetes to Type 2 diabetes [79, 80]. The T4DM trial showed that in high BMI middle-aged or elderly men with pre-diabetes or recent-onset Type 2 diabetes and low testosterone levels, testosterone replacement therapy reduced Type 2 diabetes [81]. Technology-mediated interventions, such as Internet-based programs, phone calls, and mobile applications, can deliver lifestyle intervention programs on a much larger scale, and a systematic review found that such interventions improved weight loss and glycemia [82]. A systematic review and meta-analysis of over 49,000 subjects in 43 studies [83] evaluated the sustainability of lifestyle modifications or drugs for Type 2 diabetes prevention. At the end of the intervention phase, the relative risk (RR) reduction for Type 2 diabetes was 39% for lifestyle and 36% for drugs. Following washout or follow-up (mean 7.2 years), the RR reduction was 28% for lifestyle modification, while there was no sustained RR reduction after drug cessation. Bariatric surgery, of various types, discussed in another chapter, is an effective option to prevent and reverse Type 2 diabetes, with both weight-dependent and weight-independent effects [84–86].

Mnemonic to Guide Diabetes Care

In pre-diabetes or Type 2 diabetes, it is important to address more than just glucose (Table 1.1). We previously published a mnemonic checklist for healthcare professional trainees and for clinicians regarding diabetes care: GLOBE^{2}S^2, which stands for *G*lucose, *L*ipids and lipid drugs, *O*besity, *B*lood pressure and blood pressure drugs, *E*ducation and *E*motion, and *S*moking and *S*creening [87]. We now extend this mnemonic to *GLOBES STRIVED*, which stands for *G*lucose, *L*ipids and lipid drugs, *O*besity, *B*lood pressure and blood pressure drugs, *E*motion, and *S*moking (GLOBES) and *S*creening, *TR*eating to target, *I*nfection, *V*accination, *E*ducation, and *D*evices (STRIVED). This is summarized in Table 1.2 and discussed further in this chapter, with various elements being expanded upon in other chapters. There are additional treatments to be considered in people with diabetes complications, and we discuss this later in this chapter, including some mnemonics.

Table 1.2 Mnemonic for clinical factors to address in diabetes care: GLOBES STRIVED

G	Glucose	**S**	Screening
L	Lipids and lipid drugs	**TR**	Treatment to target
O	Obesity	**I**	Inflammation/infections
B	BP and BP drugs	**V**	Vaccination
E	Emotions	**E**	Education
S	Smoking	**D**	Devices

Benefits of Multiple Risk Factor Control

Most people with Type 2 diabetes have multiple vascular risk factors [75]. Substantial reductions of CVD events, sight-threatening retinopathy, end-stage kidney disease, and all-cause mortality of 46–59% have been demonstrated with intensified multifactorial intervention [73]. We now overview recommendations for all people with diabetes (summarized in Fig. 1.2), including those free of clinically evident complications, and then highlight additional recommendations for those with chronic complications. The evidence for various therapeutics for the primary and secondary prevention of CVD and microvascular complications are summarized in Tables 1.3, 1.4, 1.5, 1.6, 1.7, and 1.8.

Lifestyle

Many aspects of daily life are key to diabetes care: physical activity and sedentary time, nutrition, adiposity, smoking status, mental well-being, and self-monitoring of risk factors such as glucose and blood pressure. Exercise and reduced sedentary time benefits, appetite, weight, blood pressure (BP), lipids, (mainly increasing HDL), glycemia, insulin resistance, mental well-being, cardiorespiratory fitness, cardiovascular risk, bone density, and balance.

Exercise Adults with Type 2 diabetes are recommended to undertake ≥150 minutes of moderate-vigorous exercise and 2–3 sessions of resistance training (on nonconsecutive days) every week [78]. While the Look AHEAD trial did not show cardiovascular event or mortality benefits with intensive lifestyle intervention in Type 2 diabetes, there were minimal group differences in weight, waist circumference, physical fitness, and HbA1c after the first year [88]. Longer-term studies may be more informative.

Nutrition A number of diets have shown benefits in Type 2 diabetes. The Dietary Approaches to Stop Hypertension (DASH) diet, comprising foods low in sodium and rich in potassium, magnesium, and calcium, significantly reduced fasting blood glucose, HbA1c, LDL-cholesterol, and BP in people with Type 2 diabetes [89]. In a

Table 1.3 Cardiac and renal effects of novel glucose-lowering drugs

SGLT2 inhibitors
Cardiac effects
Meta-analysis of three RCTs (n = 34,322): Modest secondary prevention of atherosclerotic events Significant reductions in CV mortality or hospitalizations for heart failure (hHF), regardless of prior history of CVD or heart failure [129] Empagliflozin reduced MACE (composite of CV mortality, myocardial infarction, and stroke) by 14%, hHF by 35%, CV mortality by 38%, and all-cause mortality by 32% [268] Canagliflozin reduced MACE by 14% and hHF by 33%, with borderline non-significant all-cause mortality reduction by 13%, but increased amputations by nearly twofold and fractures [269] Dapagliflozin was non-inferior compared to placebo for MACE, with a significant reduction in the composite endpoint (hHF or CV death) [270]
Renal effects
Meta-analysis of four RCTs of empagliflozin, canagliflozin, and dapagliflozin [127]: Reduced composite primary endpoint (dialysis, transplantation, CKD death) by 33% Protected from acute kidney injury and end-stage renal disease (ESRD) Consistent benefits across all baseline eGFR subgroups, and irrespective of albuminuria or use of RAS blockade Canagliflozin significantly reduced the composite endpoint (ESRD, doubling of creatinine level and renal death) by 34%, with no increased risk of amputations or fractures [271] SGLT2 inhibitors were renoprotective irrespective of heart failure status, age, and baseline kidney function [272–277] A combination of an SGLT2 inhibitor with exenatide twice a day may have a synergistic benefit on kidney function in obese Type 2 diabetes patients [278]
Incretin drugs: glucagon-like peptide 1 receptor (GLP-1) agonists
Cardiac effects
Meta-analysis of seven trials (n = 56,004) showed significant reductions in MACE by 12%, cardiovascular mortality by 12%, stroke by 16%, myocardial infarction by 9%, all-cause mortality by 12%, and hHF by 9% [279] Daily liraglutide significantly reduced MACE by 13% and reduced CVD and all-cause mortality by 22% and 15%, respectively [280] Once-weekly semaglutide, albiglutide, and dulagutide all significantly reduced MACE, but semaglutide increased retinopathy complications by 76% [281–283]
Renal effects
GLP-1 agonists reduce albuminuria in Type 2 diabetes [284] Meta-analysis showed reduced composite outcome of new-onset microalbuminuria, eGFR loss, progression to ESRD, or renal death by 17%, mainly due to macroalbuminuria benefit [279]
Incretin drugs: — dipetdiyl-peptidase 4 (DPP-4) inhibitors
Cardiac effects
RCTs showed neutral effects in high-risk T2D patients [285–288] Meta-analysis showed DPP-4 inhibitors may increase risk of heart failure in patients with existing CVD or multiple vascular risk factors [289]
Renal effects
Meta-analysis of 23 RCTs showed reduced albuminuria development or progression in Type 2 diabetes The CARMELINA study, first well-powered RCT of DPP-4 inhibitors for kidney outcomes, showed linagliptin did not reduce the composite kidney outcome (death due to kidney failure, ESRD, or sustained eGFR decrease ≥40%) in high CVD or CKD risk Type 2 diabetes subjects over a median of 2.2 years [286]

Table 1.4 Prevention of CVD complications in patients with Type 2 diabetes

		Primary prevention		Secondary prevention	
Risk factor	Main agents	Reduces CV events	Reduces CV mortality	Reduces CV events	Reduces CV mortality
Thrombosis	Aspirin, clopidogrel (only in patients who cannot tolerate aspirin)	Yes[a] [237] (I)	No [237] (I)	Yes [237] (I)	Yes [237] (I)
Lipids	Statins	Yes [150] (I)	Yes [150] (I)	Yes [150] (I)	Yes [150] (I)
	Ezetimibe	Insufficient evidence[b] [290]	No [290] (I)	Yes [290] (I)	No [290] (I)
	Fibrates	Yes[c] (I)	No [291, 292] (II)	Yes [293][d] (I)	No [293] (I)
	PCKS9 inhibitors (e.g., evolocumab)	Insufficient evidence	Insufficient evidence	Yes [294] (II)	No [295] (II)
Hypertension	ACEi/ARBs, diuretics, calcium channel blockers, beta-blockers, spironolactone	Yes [193, 256] (I)	Yes [193, 256] (I)	Yes [193, 256] (I)	Yes [193, 256] (I)
Hyperglycemia	Biguanides, sulphonylureas, DPP-4 inhibitors[e], thiazolidinediones[e], insulin	Yes, although intense glycemic control has been shown to have greater CV benefits in patients with short-duration diabetes and no known CVD [296] (I)			
	SGLT2-inhibitors	No [129] (I)	Yes [129] (I)	Yes [129] (I)	Yes [129] (I)
	GLP-1 receptor agonists	Insufficient evidence	Insufficient evidence	Yes [280] (I)	Yes [280] (I)
Smoking	Nicotine replacement therapy, varenicline, bupropion	Yes [297] (II)	Yes [297] (II)	Yes [298] (I)	Yes [298] (I)

(continued)

Table 1.4 (continued)

Risk factor	Main agents	Primary prevention		Secondary prevention	
		Reduces CV events	Reduces CV mortality	Reduces CV events	Reduces CV mortality
Obesity	Orlistat	Insufficient evidence	Insufficient evidence	Insufficient evidence	Insufficient evidence
	Bariatric surgery (morbidly obese)	Yes [189] (II)	Yes [189] (II)	Yes, but less effect than in primary prevention [189] (II)	Yes, but less effect than in primary prevention [189] (II)

The levels of evidence (placed in brackets) have been determined using the National Health and Medical Research Council levels of evidence
"No" suggests negative results in ≥1 large RCTs
Lifestyle modifications are recommended first line for all of these risk factors
[a]Only consider in high vascular risk patients (10y ASCVD risk >10%) after consideration of bleeding risks
[b]While a Cochrane review showed limited evidence regarding ezetimibe in the primary prevention of CVD, several major societies recommend ezetimibe in patients at very high vascular risk (10y ASCVD risk >20%) due to the cholesterol hypothesis that vascular risk decreases as LDL-C is reduced
[c]A Cochrane review showed a modest benefit with fibrates in the primary prevention of CVD (absolute risk reductions <1%), while the FIELD and ACCORD trials showed CV benefits with fenofibrate only in diabetes subjects with dyslipidemia
[d]A Cochrane review showed fibrates reduced the primary composite outcome (non-fatal stroke, non-fatal MI, and vascular death) only when including clofibrate data (clofibrate was discontinued in 2012 due to safety concerns), though reduced MI even without clofibrate data
[e]Can cause adverse CVD outcomes in certain settings

Table 1.5 Prevention of microvascular complications in patients with Type 2 diabetes

Risk factors	Main agents	Reduces retinopathy		Reduces nephropathy		Reduces neuropathy	
		Primary prevention	Secondary prevention	Primary prevention	Secondary prevention	Primary prevention	Secondary prevention
Lipids	Statins	Yes, in a meta-analysis of cohort studies [299] (III)	Yes, in a meta-analysis of cohort studies [299] (III)	Reduces albuminuria but not eGFR/BUN[a] [300] (I)	Reduces albuminuria but not eGFR/BUN[a] [300] (I)	Insufficient evidence	Insufficient evidence
	Fibrates	Yes, in a cohort study [301] (III)	Yes [180, 181] (II)	Protective for eGFR and albuminuria. However, rise in serum Cr[a] [182, 183] (II)	Protective for eGFR and albuminuria. However, rise in serum Cr[a] [182, 183] (II)	Yes, in FIELD trial (abstract only) [302]	Yes, in FIELD trial (abstract only) [302]
Hypertension	ACEi/ARBs	Yes [303] (I)	Yes[b] [303, 304]	Yes [305] (II)	Yes [306] (II)	No [307] (II)	Insufficient evidence
	Diuretics, calcium channel blockers, beta-blockers	Yes [303] (I)	No [303]	Yes [308] (II)	Yes [308] (II)	No [307] (II)	Insufficient evidence
Hyperglycemia	Biguanides, sulphonylureas, SGLT-2 inhibitors, DPP-4 inhibitors, GLP-1 agonist, thiazolidinediones, insulin	Yes [99] (I)	Yes, in recently diagnosed diabetes [131–133] (II)	Yes [99] (II)	Yes [309] (II)	Yes [132, 310] (I)	Yes [311] (II)

The levels of evidence (placed in brackets) have been determined using the National Health and Medical Research Council levels of evidence

"No" suggests negative results in ≥1 large RCTs

Lifestyle modifications are recommended first line for all of these risk factors

[a]Currently no renal indication for statins or fenofibrates

[b]A RCT showed candesartan non-significantly reduced risk of retinopathy progression and significantly increased regression on active treatment, though a Cochrane review found that lowering BP did not slow retinopathy progression

[c]Currently no indication for antihypertensive agents in the primary prevention of diabetic nephropathy

Table 1.6 Clinical practice points for management of diabetes with cardiovascular disease

Diabetes with CVD complications Refer to cardiologist Fairly fast SA²A²B: fish oil, fibrate, statin, antiplatelets (dual), ACEi/ARB, aldosterone antagonist, beta-blocker	
Glucose	Consider relaxing HbA1c target to mitigate risk of hypoglycemia (e.g., patients on insulin or sulfonylureas, patients with history of hypoglycemia) [110, 312] Consider cardioprotective glucose-lowering agents (e.g., SGLT2 inhibitors, GLP-1 analogues) [268, 280]
Fish oil	Current evidence does not support use nor cessation of fish oils. Systematic review showed nil reduction in CV events, but reduced CVD mortality [313] Consider highly purified fish oils (on statin background) if high triglycerides [314]
Fibrate	Fenofibrate if patient has dyslipidemia (elevated triglycerides, low HDL-C) [291, 292]
Statin	High-dose statin therapy (e.g., atorvastatin 40–80 mg nocte, rosuvastatin 20–40 mg daily) [150] Consider combination therapy with ezetimibe [315] 10 mg daily if LDL-C >1.6 mmol/L or PCSK9 inhibitor [295] if not reaching targets
Antiplatelets (dual)	Aspirin 75–162 mg daily (reduces major vascular events by 25%) [237] Use clopidogrel if patient is allergic to aspirin ACS: aspirin + ticagrelor 90 mg bd [316] (or clopidogrel 75 mg daily [317]) for up to a year ACS treated with coronary stent: aspirin + ticagrelor 90 mg bd [316]/ prasugrel 10 mg daily [318] (or clopidogrel 75 mg daily) for 12 months (minimum duration of DAPT depends on stent type – consult cardiologist for early cessation) 2016 ACC/AHA guidelines recommend prasugrel for ACS patients not at high risk of bleeding and with no history of cerebrovascular events and ticagrelor in other ACS patients [319] Seek input from cardiology team
ACEi/ARB	Long-term therapy is recommended, including in normotensive individuals [320, 321] Aim for BP <130/80 mmHg if achievable If BP not achieved with monotherapy, add CBB or thiazide [259] Monitor potassium, especially with CKD, or on ACEi/ARB or aldosterone antagonist
Aldosterone antagonist	Recommended in post-MI patients with LVEF ≤40% [322] Equal CV benefits of spironolactone (lower cost) and eplerenone (fewer side effects) [323]
Beta blocker	Long-term therapy is recommended, unless contraindicated [324]

ACS acute coronary syndrome, *DAPT* dual antiplatelet therapy, *HFrEF* heart failure with reduced ejection fraction

RCT of which 50% of subjects had Type 2 diabetes, the Mediterranean diet, characterized by abundant olive oil, fruits, vegetables, nuts, and cereals, significantly lowered the risk of a major cardiovascular event by 31% [90].

Table 1.7 Clinical practice points for management of diabetes with symptomatic HFrEF

Diabetes with symptomatic HFrEF Refer to cardiologist *BANDAID*[2]: beta-blocker, ACEi/ARB, nitrate-hydralazine, diuretic, aldosterone antagonist, ivabradine, device (AICD, CRT), and digoxin Most patients will also benefit from fish oils, statins, and antiplatelet medications (e.g., aspirin)	
Glucose	Consider relaxing HbA1c target to mitigate risk of hypoglycemia (e.g., in patients on insulin or sulfonylureas, patients with history of hypoglycemia) [110] Consider SGLT2 inhibitors (i.e., empagliflozin, canagliflozin), or GLP-1 analogues with proven CVD benefits if SGLT2 inhibitors are contraindicated or not tolerated [268, 280, 325]
Beta-blocker	Recommended for all patients [326] Ensure that the patient is clinically stable and euvolemic before commencing
ACEi/ARB	Recommended for all patients [327, 328] ARNI recommended as replacement for ACEi/ARB (with at least 36-hour washout window) in patients with LVEF ≤40% despite maximal ACEi/ARB and beta-blocker dosage [249]
Nitrate-hydralazine	Recommended if an ACEi/ARB is contraindicated or if there are no other therapeutic options [329, 330]
Diuretic	Recommended to achieve euvolemia in fluid-overloaded patients [331]
Aldosterone antagonist	Recommended for all patients [332] Avoid/use cautiously in patients with stage 4–5 CKD or *K* >5 mmol/K
Ivabradine	Consider in patients with LVEF ≤35% who are receiving appropriate therapy with sinus rhythm and HR ≥70 bpm despite maximum beta-blocker dosage [333]
AICD	Recommended in NYHA II-III HFrEF patients at least 1 month post-MI with LVEF ≤35% and a prognosis of ≥12 months [334]
CRT	Recommended in patients with LVEF ≤35%, sinus rhythm, and QRS duration ≥150 ms Consider in patients with LVEF ≤35%, sinus rhythm, and QRS duration 130–149 ms [335]
Digoxin	Consider in patients with sinus rhythm and moderate-severe symptoms (NYHA class III-IV) despite maximum ACEi/ARB dosage (reduces hospitalizations for recurrent heart failure but has not been shown to clearly reduce all-cause mortality) [336]

ARNI angiotensin receptor-neprilysin inhibitor, *AICD* automatic implantable cardioverter-defibrillator, *CRT* cardiac resynchronization therapy, *NYHA* New York Heart Association, *LVEF* left ventricular ejection fraction, *LBBB* left bundle branch block

Calorie restriction diets In motivated patients with short-duration Type 2 diabetes, a medically supervised very-low-calorie diet (VLCD) can have significant benefits, as shown in the DiRECT trial where nearly half (46%) of the intervention group (825–853 kcal/day for 3–5 months and withdrawal of antihypertensive and antidiabetic medications) achieved diabetes remission at 12 months versus only 6% in the control group [91, 92].

Table 1.8 Clinical practice points for management of diabetes with microvascular complications

Diabetic retinopathy
Screening
Annual comprehensive dilated exam by an ophthalmologist or optometrist
More frequent for progressive or sight-threatening retinopathy
Treatment
Optimizing glycemia slows retinopathy progression in short-duration diabetes, but there is little benefit in older patients [102, 132, 133]
Consider avoiding semaglutide in patients with retinopathy due to association with early retinopathy worsening related to rapid and substantial HbA1c reduction [337]
A Cochrane review found that better BP control did not slow retinopathy progression, despite some trial evidence of ACEi/ARB therapy benefit [303, 304]
While not the primary trial endpoint, fenofibrate may slow retinopathy progression in Type 2 diabetes with some retinopathy, independent of traditional lipid levels [180, 181, 338]
Several RCTs of fenofibrate with a diabetic retinopathy endpoint are underway, e.g., LENS trial (https://clinicaltrials.gov/ct2/show/NCT03439345)
In late-stage retinopathy, anti-VEGF injections, intraocular steroids, laser therapy, or vitrectomy can reduce risk of vision loss [339]
An ophthalmologist can advise regarding treatment choice and delivery
Referral
Refer to ophthalmologist if:
Sudden onset or slowly progressive vision loss, or increased "floaters"
Any level of diabetic macular edema, severe non-proliferative or proliferative diabetic retinopathy
Diabetic nephropathy
Screening
Monitor renal function, electrolytes, Ca, PO4, and Hb every 6 months at eGFR of 45–60 and every 3 months at eGFR <45
Annual bone density scan, parathyroid hormone, and vitamin D levels at eGFR <60
Treatment
Smoking cessation, a healthy weight and diet (protein intake of <0.8 g/kg/day in non-dialysis patients) [177], better glycemia [99, 131], and ACEi/ARB therapy [306, 340] can slow nephropathy progression
Consider a SGLT2 inhibitor in albuminuric CKD [341]
Effects are unclear in patients with eGFR <30 mL/min/1.73 m^2
If SGLT2 inhibitors are not tolerated or contraindicated, consider GLP-1 analogues with CVD benefit [135]
No lipid-lowering drugs have regulatory approval for nephropathy, although fenofibrate was renoprotective in FIELD and ACCORD Lipid trials in spite of an apparent rise (≈12–20%) in serum creatinine [182, 183, 342, 343]
Statins can reduce albuminuria, but not eGFR, serum creatinine, and blood urea nitrogen [300]
For late-stage renal disease, a nephrologist can guide use (or non-use) of renal replacement therapy (dialysis or transplant)
Referral
Refer to nephrologist if:
Doubt about cause of nephropathy
Rapid decline in renal function
GFR <30 ml/min/1.73m^2

Table 1.8 (continued)

Diabetic neuropathy
Screening
Large nerve: loss of vibration, ankle reflexes, and 10 g monofilament sensation
Small nerve: loss of sensation to pinprick and temperature
Consider investigations to exclude other causes of neuropathy
Treatment
Optimizing glycemia reduces onset and progression [311]
Minimize alcohol consumption
Vitamin B12 supplements if levels are low
In the FIELD trial, long-term fenofibrate reduced new neuropathy and increased reversal of known neuropathy (abstract only) [302]
For painful neuropathy, pregabalin and duloxetine are usually effective [344–346]
Tricyclic depressants alpha lipoic acid and topical treatments (e.g., capsaicin creams, lignocaine sprays/patches) may be tried in individual patients, but have a less robust evidence base [347–350]
Referral
Refer to neurologist (or relevant specialist) if:
Doubt about cause of neuropathy
Issues with clinical management (e.g., difficulty controlling neuropathic pain)

A 12-week pilot study found similar glycemic and weight improvements with a 5:2 diet (2 days of severe energy restriction (1670–2500 kJ/day) and 5 days of habitual eating) and moderate continuous energy restriction (5000–6500 kJ/day) [93]. While no long-term studies have been reported, this study provides promising evidence that a 5:2 diet may be a suitable alternative for those who prefer intermittent fasting.

We will now discuss in order the elements of our GLOBES STRIVED mnemonic. We then briefly comment on aspirin usage in people with diabetes.

Glycemia

There are several aspects of glucose control that should be addressed in diabetes care, including the mean glucose level, usually assessed by HbA1c levels, time in the recommended target glucose range and above and below it (if continuous glucose monitoring (CGM) is used), hypoglycemia, and glucose variability. A standardized Average Glucose Profile (AGP) report summarizing the CGM profile has been developed, and CGM-related targets for people with Type 2 diabetes recommended [94]. Glucose variability (discussed more below) may be assessed by variability in interstitial fluid glucose levels (by CGM) or serial blood glucose or HbA1c levels. All aspects of glucose control, including hyperglycemia, hypoglycemia, and higher glucose variability, have been linked with increased risk of micro- and macrovascular complications and with mortality [95–98]. Given the slow development of the chronic complications of diabetes, years will need to pass until robust prospective evidence linking CGM-related glucose metrics to future complications is available.

Personalizing Glucose Targets

Meta-analyses have shown substantially reduced risk of microvascular complications with better glycemia, usually measured by HbA1c, and some CVD benefit, albeit less than for microvascular complications [99, 100].

A HbA1c <7% (53 mmol/mol) is recommended for most people with diabetes (Table 1.1), although recently, the American College of Physicians suggested a general HbA1c target of 7–8% (53–64 mmol/mol) [101]. Glucose targets can be personalized to optimize clinical outcomes. While lowering glycemia usually reduces the risk of complications, overtreatment may increase the risk of hypoglycemia, subsequent CVD events, and mortality [13–15], which subsequently increase care costs for the patient and for the healthcare system. Hypoglycemia is associated with increased CVD and mortality risk [102–104]. Potential mechanisms by which hypoglycemia may increase adverse vascular events include prolongation of the cardiac QT interval, which combined with hypoglycemia-related catecholamine surges and the relative excess of insulin-induced hypokalemia may induce a cardiac arrhythmia and sudden death. This is sometimes referred to as the "dead-in-bed" syndrome, which was first recognized in young people with Type 1 diabetes [105, 106]. Severe hypoglycemia may also lead to a seizure. Other adverse effects of hypoglycemia include vascular endothelial dysfunction (with vasoconstriction), increased inflammation, oxidative stress, and a prothrombotic tendency, which can last for several days after the hypoglycemic event [107]. Another indirect association between hypoglycemia and cardiovascular events may be that frailty and reduced ability for self-care may increase risk of both cardiovascular events, death, and of hypoglycemia [108].

Subset analyses of major trials suggest that more intensive glucose control may have cardiovascular benefits in patients with short-duration Type 2 diabetes; hence, a more stringent target (e.g., HbA1c ≤6 or 6.5%, 42 or 48 mmol/mol) should be considered in patients with (a) Type 2 diabetes for less than 5 years, (b) Type 2 diabetes treated with lifestyle and oral hypoglycemic agents (OHAs) with minimal side effects, and (c) women with Type 2 diabetes who are pregnant or anticipating pregnancy (HbA1c target ≤6%) [109, 110]. To mitigate risk of *hypoglycemia*, a less stringent HbA1c target (e.g., ≤8%, 64 mmol/mol) is reasonable in patients with (a) a history of severe hypoglycemia or impaired hypoglycemia awareness or (b) multiple comorbidities with limited life expectancy (6). Diabetes care guidelines now often recommend personalization of HbA1c targets, taking into consideration such factors as patient age, diabetes duration, pregnancy, comorbidities including CVD and kidney disease, risk of and problems from hypoglycemia, level of independence, and types of medications. Less stringent HbA1c targets should be considered in frail people living alone or in care facilities [109].

Particular care must be taken to the prescription of medications for people with impaired kidney function, which is common in diabetes and may be secondary to aging, diabetic kidney disease, hypertension, or other comorbidities. Kidney dysfunction-related pharmacokinetic changes may increase the risk of hypoglycemia and other side effects, which are likely to be higher for people with chronic kidney disease (CKD) stages 4 and 5 (estimated glomerular filtration rates (eGFR) <30 and <15 ml/min/1.73 m^2, respectively) [109]. Several large studies have demonstrated that even for metformin, which is often the first-line drug for pre-diabetes and for Type 2 diabetes, errors in its prescription, usually to people with more severe CKD than recommended, are common [111–113]. Over the past three decades, there has been progressive relaxation of the lower limit of renal function deemed safe for metformin use and also a shift from using serum creatinine levels to eGFR, with metformin usually being regarded as safe to commence in those with an eGFR over 45 ml/min/1.73 m^2 [114, 115] and can be continued in those with eGFR over 30 ml ml/min/1.73 m^2 [116]. A major concern related to metformin use in moderate-to-severe CKD, liver disease, or heart failure is that of metformin-associated lactic acidosis (MALA). While MALA is of low incidence (<10 cases per 100,000 patient-years), it has a mortality rate of approximately 50% [117]. Further research into this widely used, low-cost, and generally well-tolerated OHA may provide more detail regarding its safety and efficacy in people with more severe CKD. Another glucose-related complication of OHA drugs, in particular with sodium glucose transporter 2 (SGLT2) inhibitors, is that of diabetic ketoacidosis, which may be associated with normal or relatively mildly elevated glucose levels, so-called euglycemic DKA [118–120]. As many drugs used in diabetes care may require dosage adjustment or cessation with kidney or liver disease, regular monitoring of kidney and liver function and review of medications are required.

Higher *glucose variability* (*GV*), usually assessed by CGM or blood glucose levels in the short term (over days to 2 weeks) and by HbA1c standard deviation (SD) or coefficient of variation (CV) in the long term (months–years), has been independently associated with higher risk of micro- and macrovascular complications and mortality [121–123]. In a post hoc analysis of the Fenofibrate Intervention and Event Lowering in Diabetes (FIELD) study, GV was calculated as the SD and CV of HbA1c and of fasting plasma glucose in 9795 adults with Type 2 diabetes. Baseline factors associated with higher on-study GV included younger age, longer-known diabetes duration, male sex, and higher use of drug therapies. HbA1c and/or fasting glucose CV in the first 2 years were significantly associated with increased risk of on-trial complications for the remaining trial time (a total of a median of 5 years) including microvascular complications, CVD, stroke, and increased total, coronary, and non-coronary mortality [97]. Impaired vasodilation, increased oxidative stress and inflammation, prothrombotic effects, and epigenetic changes may be mediators [124]. Means to lower GV include diet, exercise, some glucose control drugs such as SGLT2 inhibitors [125] and GLP 1 analogues [125], and insulin, optimal insulin dosing times, and medication adherence [126]. The use of CGM can assist with patient education and guide clinicians regarding GV. Electronic medical records and pathology reports could automate the calculation of HbA1c variability.

Rationale for Glucose Targets

Personalization of the intensity of glucose control is supported by some clinical trials. Some glucose drugs have pleiotropic effects that may reduce complication risk above and beyond their glucose benefits. The favorable effects of SGLT2 inhibitors on cardiovascular, heart failure, and diabetic kidney disease are key examples [127–129].

Macrovascular disease benefit Type 2 diabetes trials contrast in their findings. Supportive trials of benefit include The United Kingdom Prospective Diabetes Study (UKPDS) and the Veterans Affairs Diabetes Trial (VADT). Their 10-year observational follow-up studies showed long-term reductions in CVD events with intensive glucose control (median achieved HbA1c ≈7% in both trials) [130, 131]. In contrast, the Action to Control Cardiovascular Risk in Diabetes (ACCORD) and Action in Diabetes and Vascular Disease: Preterax and Diamicron MR Controlled Evaluation (ADVANCE) trials, which studied high cardiovascular risk adults with Type 2 diabetes and achieved lower median HbA1c levels of ≈6.4% in their intensively treated group, were not favorable. ADVANCE demonstrated no differences in macrovascular events or cardiovascular mortality between the intensive and standard treatment groups [104], while ACCORD was stopped early due to a 22% increased mortality with intensive glucose treatment [102]. The ACCORD trial participants had long-duration diabetes with greater prevalence of complications. More antidiabetic drugs (including insulin and thiazolidinediones) were required to achieve tight glycemic control, and there were issues relating to weight gain and increased severe hypoglycemia in the intensively treated group [110]. This is in contrast to the UKPDS study, which evaluated newly diagnosed T2D patients where tight glucose control was easier to achieve. It is now mandated that before glucose control agents are approved by regulatory bodies such as the USA's Therapeutic Goods Association (TGA) for clinical use, trials must demonstrate their cardiovascular safety. Very large and moderately long-duration clinical trials are required.

Microvascular disease benefit Multiple trials have demonstrated benefits of better glycemia. In the UKPDS, intensive glucose treatment reduced cumulative microvascular endpoints by 25% [131], while a recent meta-analysis found significant reductions in kidney and eye events (20% and 13% respectively), but not in nerve events [99]. Retinal benefits may be greater in younger patients with shorter-duration diabetes. The ACCORD and ADVANCE trials in older subjects showed no or marginal retinal benefits with intensive glucose control [102, 132], while the

VADT found benefits in younger patients but harm in older patients [133]. Trial differences may relate to differences in participant ages, diabetes duration, HbA1c starting points and targets, their rate of achievement, and in drugs used and their pleiotropic effects.

Novel Glucose Control Agents

Recently, several large RCTs have demonstrated exciting major clinical benefits with SGLT-2 inhibitors and GLP-1 analogues, reducing CVD events, heart failure, diabetic kidney disease, and mortality, with much benefit independent of their HbA1c reductions (summarized in Table 1.3). These trials are already changing guidelines and clinical practice, often becoming first- or second-line glucose control drugs in advantaged regions [13, 134].

Individualizing Glucose-Lowering Medications

There are now regularly (at least annually) updated guidelines on how to personalize glucose-lowering medications [134, 135]. Given the dynamic nature of available drugs, for example, with the increasing longer-acting injectable GLP-1 agonists [136–140], and results of newly completed clinical trials, we recommend readers review the regularly updated guidelines on websites such as by the ADA [141] and the Australian Diabetes Society [134, 135, 142] for guidance. Along with the patient's age, diabetes duration, complications, kidney function, pregnancy status, and other medications, treatment options will also be influenced by national drug approval, local drug availability, affordability, and patient preference (e.g., injectable or non-injectable drugs). Formulations combining drug classes to reduce pill burden and subsidies to minimize drug costs may promote patient adherence.

Lipids and Lipid Drugs

Associations Between Lipids, Diabetes, and Chronic Diabetes Complications

Adverse traditional lipid profiles, including elevated triglycerides, LDL-cholesterol (LDL-C), and low HDL-cholesterol (HDL-C) levels, have been both associated with and predictive of Type 2 diabetes *per se* and of its chronic complications [143–146]. This dyslipidemia may be exacerbated by poor glycemic control, obesity, kidney or liver dysfunction, suboptimal lifestyle, genetics, and some drugs (e.g., thiazides) [147]. Links between abnormal lipids and CVD are stronger and more consistent than for microvascular complications. Associations between lipids and complications may be direct and/or indirect such as via obesity and lifestyle-related factors [148].

Statins and Diabetes Complications

Cardiovascular disease The initial low-dose statin lowers LDL-C levels by about 50%, and each doubling of the dose usually lowers LDL-C by an additional 6% [149]. The primary and secondary cardioprotective effects of statins in people with Type 2 diabetes are well established. In the Cholesterol Treatment Trialists' Collaboration (CTTC) meta-analysis of 14 trials (18,686 subjects), statins reduced cardiovascular events by 25%, all-cause mortality by 9%, and CV death by 13% for every 1 mmol/L reduction in LDL-C levels [150], comparable to results of the CTTC's meta-analysis of statin trials in the general population [151]. Unless contraindicated or not tolerated, statins are the recommended first-line lipid-lowering therapy for the secondary prevention of CVD. For primary prevention in people with diabetes, a CVD risk calculator [152–154] can be used to derive risk levels and guide statin therapy. Some national diabetes care guidelines, such as the those by the ADA, do not recommend the routine assessment of subclinical coronary artery disease in asymptomatic people, such as by coronary artery calcification (CAC) or CT coronary angiography as it will not change management or outcomes, providing there is judicious attention to risk factor management as per guidelines [155]. In some cases, a non-evidence-based specialist consensus exists for consideration of screening for people who have "atypical" symptoms which might be angina variants, other markers of atherosclerosis, ischemic ECG changes, or in people wishing to start strenuous physical activity in the absence of regular exercise. Such testing may include exercise testing, CAC or CT angiography, nuclear imaging, or pharmacologic stress echocardiography. It is recognized that some patients and some clinicians are more likely to initiate and to adhere to proven effective therapies, such as statins if they are aware of a clinically silent atheroma burden [147]. Referral to a cardiologist for advice regarding the most appropriate and cost-effective investigation and management may be appropriate.

Microvascular disease Statins' effects on microvascular complications are less well studied, with there being a lack of robust randomized controlled trials with a microvascular complication primary endpoint. Most results are from databases or meta-analyses, briefly summarized below.

Early statin studies did not report any diabetic microvascular benefit. More recent evidence, predominantly from very large databases and meta-analyses of statin trials, suggest some retinopathy benefit, including for sight-threatening retinopathy [156–161]. The literature is mixed regarding renoprotection. In a meta-analysis (11 statin RCTs, 543 CKD diabetes subjects), statins reduced albuminuria but not proteinuria nor eGFR [162]. In a 28 trial meta-analysis (n = 183,419) of cardioprotection by eGFR categories, statins significantly reduced the risk of a first major vascular event by 21% per mmol/L reduction in LDL-C, with less benefit as eGFR declined [163]. Diabetic neuropathy studies are lacking. Statin studies mainly in the general population [164] and a meta-analysis did not find any links between statins and neuropathy [165].

Statins and new-onset diabetes (NOD) Statins can increase the risk of Type 2 diabetes by 9–12% [141, 166–168]. As this usually occurs in people with pre-diabetes or other risk factors for diabetes and/or CVD, the risk benefit ratio is seen as favorable. Underlying mechanisms may relate to impaired insulin secretion and increased peripheral insulin resistance [169]. Some risk may be mediated by the lower LDL levels [170].

Other LDL-Lowering Drugs

A subset of people with diabetes may be statin intolerant. We have reviewed its diagnosis and provided a management algorithm [171]. Other LDL-C-lowering drugs which can be used for statin-intolerant subjects or added to a statin in those not meeting their LDL-C target are a once daily tablet of ezetimibe; less well-tolerated bile acid binding resins, usually taken 2–3 times a day with food, which reduce lipid absorption from the gut; bempedoic acid; and injectable PCSK9 inhibitors [172]. Combinations such as of a statin, ezetrol, and bempedoic acid may be used to lower LDL-C adequately [173, 174].

Ezetimibe acts by inhibiting the cholesterol transport protein Nieman Pick C1-like 1 protein in small intestine enterocytes, lowering LDL-C by about 20% if used alone and when added to a statin [174]. In the IMPROVE-IT trial, including 5000 adults with diabetes and acute coronary syndrome, the addition of ezetimibe to a statin reduced the composite cardiovascular primary endpoint by 14% versus 2% in subjects without diabetes [175].

Resins lower LDL-C levels by 10–30% by binding cholesterol-rich bile acids in the gut and removing them via the fecal route, which necessitates synthesis of more bile acids. They also improve glucose control in diabetes. Tolerability is often low due to gastrointestinal side effects, the inconvenience of multiple daily doses, and the potential need to separate its dosing from other oral medications due to its impairment of absorption of some drugs [174].

Bempedoic acid is the first drug in a new class of lipid-lowering agents, the adenosine triphosphate-citrate lyase (ACL) inhibitors, which act two steps upstream of HMG-CoA reductase to inhibit cholesterol production. In a meta-analysis (11 trials, $n = 4391$ general population subjects), bempedoic acid significantly reduced LDL-C (median −22.9, 95% CI −27.3 to −18.5%), CRP (median −24.7, 95% CI −32.1 to −17.3%), composite cardiovascular events (RR 0.75, 95% CI 0.56–0.99), and rates of new-onset or worsening diabetes (RR 0.65, 95% CI 0.44–0.96). Hence, this drug is not associated with higher rates of NOD or worsening metabolic control [176]. As yet, there are no Type 2 diabetes-specific drug trial results.

PCSK9 inhibitors Proprotein Convertase Subtilisin-kexin type 9 (PCSK9) is a proprotein convertase involved in the degradation of hepatic LDL receptors; hence, PCSK9 inhibitors inhibit LDL-receptor recycling, which increases LDL clearance. There are currently two fully human monoclonal antibodies (evolocumab and alirocumab) that inhibit PCSK9 approved for clinical use. These drugs are usually given by subcutaneous injection every 2 weeks and can lower LDL-C levels by 60% and be used in conjunction with a statin [177]. In the Further Cardiovascular Outcomes Research with PCSK9 Inhibition in Subjects with Elevated Risk (FOURIER) trial in the general population, evolocumab added to a statin significantly lowered LDL-C by 59% and reduced the risk of a composite cardiovascular endpoint (HR 0.86, 95% CI 0.79–0.92, $p < 0.001$), with similar benefits in people with versus without diabetes (of which 97.2% had Type 2 diabetes). A meta-analysis of PCSK9 inhibitors suggested that more potent PCSK9 inhibitors and longer-term use may be associated with increased risk of NOD and worsening glycemia [178]. Detailed analyses of glycemia, long-term follow-up, and further PCSK9 trials in diabetes are merited. Local injection site reactions and drug cost may limit drug use.

Triglyceride-Lowering Drugs

Most predominantly LDL-C-lowering drugs also have some triglyceride-lowering effects [172].

Fibrates The major triglyceride-lowering drug, fenofibrate, did not reduce CVD in the (T2D) FIELD or ACCORD trials, except in those with dyslipidemia (elevated triglycerides and low HDL-C) [179, 180], which is common in Type 2 diabetes. In both studies, fenofibrate significantly reduced retinopathy [180, 181] independent of lipid levels and was renoprotective [182, 183]. In the FIELD trial, fenofibrate also reduced microvascular-related amputations [184]. Trials of fenofibrate with diabetic retinopathy as the primary endpoint are in progress. The active form of fenofibrate, fenofibric acid, is now available for clinical use; however, its efficacy in reducing diabetic retinopathy progression has not been evaluated in clinical trials.

Unlike the fibrate gemfibrozil, where there is an increased risk of statin intolerance and rhabdomyolysis, fenofibrate can be taken with a statin [185].

Fish oils can also lower triglycerides, but there is no evidence of protection against the microvascular or macrovascular complications of Type 2 diabetes. In a RCT of 15,480 diabetes patients without CVD, there was no difference in the risk of serious vascular events for $n-3$ fatty acid supplements vs. placebo [186].

Suggested Lipid Drug Use in People with Type 2 Diabetes

In addition to lifestyle measures, statin therapy is indicated for people with a prior CVD event (secondary prevention) and high CVD risk adults (primary prevention), usually assessed by a cardiovascular risk calculator, with treatment to evidence-based lipid targets. If moderate-to-high-dose statin therapy does not achieve adequate LDL-C levels, the usual next step would be to add ezetimibe. If additional LDL-C lowering is desirable (or nil or only low-dose statin therapy can be tolerated), then other lowering drugs such as bempedoic acid or PCSK9 inhibitors can be used. While not FDA approved for use in the USA, fenofibrate has been approved for use in Australia and some other (mainly low- and middle-income) countries for protection against progression of diabetic retinopathy in people with Type 2 diabetes and existent retinopathy, independent of lipid levels. For people with Type 2 diabetes with high triglycerides and low HDL-cholesterol levels, fenofibrate (either alone or on statin background) can reduce cardiovascular events. For people with diabetes and severe hypertriglyceridemia (fasting triglycerides over 6.5 mmol/l), fibrate therapy is appropriate to reduce the risk of acute pancreatitis. If a statin is being prescribed, fenofibrate is the only fibrate approved for statin-fibrate combination therapy due to the lower risk of rhabdomyolysis [185]. As for glucose and BP control, people with diabetes may require and benefit from combination therapy of lipid-lowering agents.

Obesity

Being overweight or obese is commonly associated with Type 2 diabetes, and its coexistence usually increases risk factors such as dyslipidemia and hypertension. An initial weight loss of 5–10% of body weight for overweight or obese patients is recommended [187]. In obese patients with Type 2 diabetes, a very-low-carbohydrate, high-unsaturated fat, low-saturated fat diet produced greater improvements in lipids, glycemia, and diabetes medication reductions compared to a high-carbohydrate, low-fat diet [188]. In addition to lifestyle changes, doctors should aim to prescribe glucose-lowering drugs that promote weight loss (e.g., metformin, SGLT-2 inhibitors, GLP-1 analogues) or are weight neutral (e.g., DPP-4 inhibitors), as well as pharmacological therapies (e.g., orlistat) if the benefits of weight loss outweigh medication risks. In morbidly obese diabetic patients with multiple comorbidities, bariatric/metabolic surgery improves glucose control and may even reverse Type 2 diabetes [189]. Benefits on diabetes prevention and regression have been shown with bariatric surgery at less severe levels of obesity (BMI 30–35 kg/m^2) and even in those with a BMI <30 kg/m^2 [190, 191], but more studies with longer follow-up, standardized definitions of diabetes remission and consideration of the type of bariatric surgery, duration of dysglycemia, and ethnicity are desirable. There are various types of bariatric surgery, which are discussed in detail in another book chapter herein.

Blood Pressure

Hypertension is common in many non-diabetic populations, and its incidence is usually increased in people with Type 2 diabetes. Due to BP lability and "white-coat hypertension," 24-hour BP monitoring and at-home measurements are more reliable than in-clinic measures [192]. In addition to individual trials (including UKPDS), a meta-analysis of 40 trials found that that among Type 2 diabetes patients, each

10 mmHg reduction in systolic BP lowered all-cause mortality by 13%, CVD events by 11%, albuminuria by 17%, and diabetic retinopathy by 13% [193].

Individualizing BP Targets

Recommended BP targets vary depending on the Type 2 diabetic patient's cardiovascular and renal risk. While a BP target of <140/90 mmHg is reasonable in patients at lower CVD risk (ASCVD risk <15%), a lower BP target of 130/80 mmHg is advised in those at higher CVD risk (ASCVD risk >15%) if achievable [78]. Targeting lower systolic BPs (e.g., <120 mmHg) has not been shown to reduce major CVD in diabetic patients but increases serious adverse events of hypotension and renal dysfunction [194]. A combination of lifestyle (low salt, minimum alcohol, DASH diet, weight loss, exercise, non-smoking) and pharmacological treatments is recommended to optimize BP.

Selecting BP-Lowering Drugs

In patients with existing CVD or renal or retinal disease, angiotensin-converting enzyme inhibitors (ACEi) or angiotensin receptor blockers (ARB) are recommended as first-line therapy [78]. In Black patients, a calcium channel blocker (CCB) or a thiazide diuretic is preferred as the first-line agent [195] as hypertension is more often salt responsive in Black populations than in Caucasian groups. Thiazide diuretics are recommended first line in the elderly population [196] but can be associated with worsening of glucose, lipid, and uric acid levels. This is not a feature of the once-daily indapamide (Natrilix) member of the thiazide class, which is also available as a slow-release preparation. Otherwise, ACEis, ARBs, CCBs, and thiazide diuretics are all reasonable therapies for primary prevention. A meta-analysis including both primary and secondary prevention trials, but excluding patients with heart failure, revealed that RAAS drugs were not superior to other classes of BP agents (e.g., CCBs, thiazides, beta-blockers) at reducing hard CVD and renal endpoints in diabetic patients [197]. In patients with a systolic BP 20 mmHg above goal, dual antihypertensive therapy is advised [198], but a combination of ACEis and ARBs should not be used due to adverse effects on renal function [199]. In addition, taking antihypertensive medications at bedtime is recommended. In a Type 2 diabetes RCT, taking antihypertensive treatment at bedtime compared to upon wakening improved ambulatory control BP and significantly reduced cardiovascular risk by 67% [200]. Often multiple BP-lowering drugs may be needed to meet recommended BP targets and to avoid side effects associated with high drug dosages. Combination tablets can help with patient adherence. In general, drug doses can be titrated after 4 weeks of a regimen.

A suggested flow-chart covering hypertension therapy is shown in Fig. 1.3. Other excellent guidelines are available such as from the ADA [13].

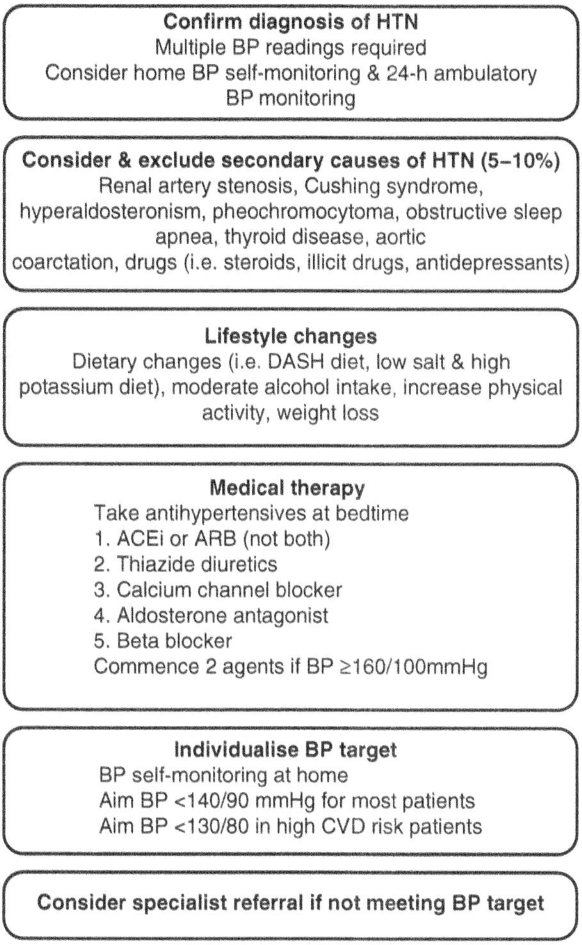

Confirm diagnosis of HTN
Multiple BP readings required
Consider home BP self-monitoring & 24-h ambulatory BP monitoring

Consider & exclude secondary causes of HTN (5–10%)
Renal artery stenosis, Cushing syndrome, hyperaldosteronism, pheochromocytoma, obstructive sleep apnea, thyroid disease, aortic coarctation, drugs (i.e. steroids, illicit drugs, antidepressants)

Lifestyle changes
Dietary changes (i.e. DASH diet, low salt & high potassium diet), moderate alcohol intake, increase physical activity, weight loss

Medical therapy
Take antihypertensives at bedtime
1. ACEi or ARB (not both)
2. Thiazide diuretics
3. Calcium channel blocker
4. Aldosterone antagonist
5. Beta blocker
Commence 2 agents if BP ≥160/100mmHg

Individualise BP target
BP self-monitoring at home
Aim BP <140/90 mmHg for most patients
Aim BP <130/80 in high CVD risk patients

Consider specialist referral if not meeting BP target

Fig. 1.3 Management of hypertension in adults with Type 2 diabetes

Emotion

Approximately 25% of people with Type 2 diabetes will experience depression, and 40–45% will experience diabetes distress [201]. Suboptimal mental health is associated with poorer self-care and higher HbA1c levels [202]. Short survey tools (e.g., PAID and DDS-2) are recommended to screen for diabetes distress. For patients experiencing psychological problems, a diabetes educator, psychologist, or psychiatrist can be helpful.

Smoking

Smoking cessation reduces mortality risk by one third over only a few years [203]. Smokers are more likely to develop Type 2 diabetes, and people with Type 2 diabetes are likely to stop smoking if they receive the appropriate counseling and support [204]. In the motivated patient, combining pharmacological therapy (e.g., nicotine patches) with counseling is more effective than either therapy alone [205]. E-cigarette or "vaping" is not recommended as an aid to smoking cessation, although a 2016 meta-analysis of 18 observational studies showed that e-cigarette users had a 28% lower odds ratio of stopping smoking compared to non-users [206].

Screening

All people with Type 2 diabetes should undergo regular screening, usually annually, for complications and risk factors (Fig. 1.2). Identified risk factors should be reassessed after several months of therapy. This screening also applies to youth with Type 2 diabetes, as they are at a particularly high risk of complications (even higher than those with comparable duration of Type 1 diabetes) [207], likely related to risk factors such as obesity, hypertension, and dyslipidemia.

People with Type 2 diabetes should also undergo appropriate screening for cancers as they are at the same or increased risk of cancers, except for prostate cancer, than their non-diabetic peers [208, 209]. Some anticancer immunotherapies or chemotherapy regimens can also induce diabetes or worsen glucose control [210].

TReating to Target

Many people with diabetes do not meet recommended risk factor targets, with multiple factors likely being contributory, including clinical inertia by the care team [211] and patient non-adherence. Clinical inertia may be mitigated by educational or learning interventions and by empowered patients. Clinician diligence, a regular review of targets met, and audits may be helpful. Electronic decision support tools can assist with identifying subjects not at target and suggesting therapeutic steps [211]. Patient non-adherence may arise due to complexity of treatment regimens, perceived or real drug side effects or risks, inability to afford medications, and mental health issues.

Inflammation/Infections

People with diabetes, particularly with suboptimal glucose control, are at increased risk of infection. Common infections include urinary tract infections, which can be asymptomatic, fungal infections of the skin and genitourinary tract, and periodontal disease. Periodontal disease has been associated with increased risk of CVD, microvascular complications, and death [212, 213].

As recently observed in the COVID-19 pandemic, people with diabetes are also at increased risk of adverse outcomes such as requiring hospitalization, ventilation, and death [214–216].

Vaccinations

Due to their increased risk of infection, people with Type 2 diabetes should have all age-appropriate vaccinations such as against influenza, pneumococcal pneumonia, tetanus, and COVID-19, and others as appropriate to age, sex, occupation, environment, and travel.

Education

In an American Association of Diabetes Educators systematic review, diabetes self-management education was associated with a 0.74% HbA1c reduction [217]. People should be educated at diabetes diagnosis with further education over their lifetime. Diabetes is a complex condition, and personalized treatment goals and available medications will change over time. Ideally, patients should be referred for structured diabetes education and to a dietician, and care team members should avoid providing conflicting advice. Clinicians may assist patient education by referral to reliable websites, such as those by the ADA (www.diabetes.org) and Diabetes Australia (www.diabetesaustralia.com.au). Accurate information may still be misunderstood by the patient, and some social media sites or lay people may provide unreliable information, including the use of unproven therapies. Clinicians should be open to discussing such topics.

Devices

An increasing array of devices may assist diabetes care. Some people with diabetes may choose to use food, weight, and physical activity trackers or smartphone apps. Body weight, body composition scales, and a BP cuff for at-home use may be helpful. Clinician-prescribed 24-hour BP monitoring can help diagnose hypertension and monitor therapy. Loss of nocturnal BP dipping is often the first sign of hypertension and has been associated with increased risk of chronic diabetes complications [218, 219].

Glucose Monitoring

Devices Glucose levels can be assessed by self-monitoring of capillary blood, which is usually reserved for people requiring insulin therapy. Some blood glucose meters have in-built bolus calculators which can guide insulin dosing for meals or high glucose corrections [220]. In a study of Type 1 and insulin-using Type 2 diabetes subjects, the use of a blood glucose meter to estimate insulin doses was associated with significantly less insulin dosing errors than manual calculations and was preferred by patients [221].

More recently, CGM or flash glucose monitoring (FGM) can provide interstitial fluid glucose measures at 5–15-minute intervals over 6–14 days, depending on which system is used. Current systems are based on glucose oxidase chemistry, as are blood glucose test strips. Both masked and real-time systems are available, some of which are factory calibrated and do not require blood glucose calibration by the user. Data from masked systems are uploaded for review by a clinician, and unlike real-time CGM or FGM systems, the glucose data are not immediately available to the wearer. Real-time systems provide glucose data to the wearer via a glucose meter device or a smartphone app. Most have alarms to alert the wearer (and sometimes a remote carer) to low, high, and rapidly changing glucose levels. Data downloads (via the Cloud) enable more detailed data analyses and sharing [222–226]. CGM and FGM data can be particularly helpful in revealing otherwise unrecognized nocturnal hypoglycemia and rebound hyperglycemia, preventing the potential harmful increase in basal insulin doses and in drawing attention to the need for the addition of bolus insulin to basal insulin. For example, in the primacy-care based INITATION trial of adults with suboptimal glucose control of their Type 2 diabetes, episodic masked CGM use (3 monthly for 12 months) did not improve HbA1c levels differentially between the intervention and standard care group, but three times more of the CGM group were commenced on bolus insulin than in the control group [227].

Advantages and disadvantages of interstitial fluid glucose monitoring Advantages of interstitial fluid glucose monitoring include reduced finger-prick burden, an abundance of glucose data, alarms for glucose levels which may require intervention, and the ability to measure GV. Unlike HbA1c, interstitial fluid glucose monitors are not adversely impacted by anemia or hemoglobinopathies, but can be impacted by substances such as paracetamol (aminocetaphen), salicyclic acid, and high-dose vitamin C [228, 229]. While simultaneous interstitial fluid and blood glucose levels may be well aligned, particularly when the person is not in the post-prandial state or has exercised, the mean average difference between interstitial fluid and blood glucose levels is about 10% and can be much higher [223]. Interstitial fluid glucose levels usually lag about 10 minutes behind changes in blood glucose levels, with about 6 minutes being physiological and the rest device-related. All sensors tend to perform better on and after Day 2 of use, due to initial tissue reactions around the inserted sensor [224].

Disadvantages include the need to be "attached" to a device continuously, and the abundance of glucose data, which some may find distressing, particularly if they spend substantial time out of their desired glucose range. Some people are upset and lack trust in the system due to differences between interstitial fluid and blood glucose levels. Common problems include skin irritation, which may be reduced by barrier creams, sensor failures and dislodgement, and high financial costs if subsidies are not available [230].

Publications and experience report feasibility, safety, acceptable accuracy, and informative use of CGM or FGM in special circumstances such as fasting (for weight loss or religious reasons), pregnancy, extreme sports, hemodialysis, and within inpatients and intensive care unit settings.

Interstitial fluid glucose monitoring can facilitate patient education, motivation, monitoring, decisions regarding glucose control regimens, and also clinical research.

Treatment targets based on interstitial fluid glucose monitoring There are international consensus recommendations for standardized reporting of CGM and FGM data, including mean glucose, SD and CV of glucose levels, GV, an estimated HbA1c and time (%) in target range (3.9–10 mmol/l), time above 10 and above 13.9 mmol/l, and time below 3.9 and below 3.0 mmol/l. This is usually presented as a color-coded bar graph. A daily graph of each glucose trace from midnight to midnight is recommended as an overlay plot with a line for median glucose levels and shaded areas for 25–75th and 10–90th percentiles. Recommended times in each glucose range are suggested. For non-high-risk adults with Type 2 diabetes, the recommended time in target range (TIR) is over 70%. Recommended time above 10 and above 13.9 mmol/l is less than 25% and 5%, respectively, and time below 3.9 and below 3.0 mmol/l is less than 4% and 1%, respectively. Recommended glucose CV is less than 36%. For high-risk adults with Type 2 diabetes, avoidance of low glucose levels and less TIR are suggested. High-risk adults may include people with CVD, multiple comorbidities, limited life expectancy, impaired cognition, frailty, or those living in assisted care facilities. For this group, general recommendations are above 50% for TIR; time above 10 mmol/l and above 13.9 mmol/l are less than 50% and 10%, respectively; and time below 3.9 mmol/l less than 1%, with no time below 3.0 mmol/l. As yet, there are no recommendations for pregnant women with Type 2 diabetes due to limited evidence, but such data will likely become available [94].Of course, the treating clinician should always personalize targets. TIR has been shown to correlate with HbA1c levels, in spite of the different time frames. It has been calculated that an increase in TIR by 10% correlates with a HbA1c reduction by 0.9% [231]. It is recommended that decisions regarding clinical care be based on at least 2 weeks of CGM (or FGM) data with data available for at least 70% of the time [94].

Glucose benefits Relative to Type 1 diabetes, the benefits of CGM and FGM use on HbA1c levels and TIR are more modest in Type 2 diabetes. Meta-analyses suggest modest (0.35% or less) or no statistically significant impact on HbA1c in Type 2 diabetes [232–234].TIR is usually improved with CGM or FGM use, and in some studies, low glucose time and hypoglycemia are reduced [232–234]. Wearer acceptability is generally good, but there is potential for selection bias in trials and user bias in clinical practice. Further research is merited to guide user choice and optimal frequency of use.

Future directions Interstitial fluid glucose-monitoring devices are continuing to evolve and will likely have improved accuracy, factory calibration, duration of use, capacity for long-term implantation, and ability to measure analytes other than glucose such as ketones, lactate, and physical movement [235, 236].

Antiplatelet Agents

While recommended for secondary CVD protection, aspirin is not routinely recommended for primary prevention in diabetes, but there may be a role in those at high risk. An Antithrombotic Treatment Trialists' meta-analysis concluded that aspirin was reasonable in high-CVD-risk (5-year risk >5%) patients who are not at increased bleeding risk. There was a clear recommendation against aspirin in those at low CVD risk (5-year risk <2.5%) [237]. However, the ASCENDRCT (5480 people ≥40 years old with Type 2 diabetes and no clinically evident CVD) showed daily 100 mg enteric-coated aspirin reduced vascular events by 12% but increased major (mostly GI) bleeding by 29%, with no effect on all-cause mortality or cancer [238]. Results were broadly consistent across CVD risk levels [238]. It is important to consider that the impact of an MI or stroke may be very different to that of a GI bleed.

Management of Type 2 Diabetes Patients with Known CVD

While there are many features in common for the care of people with Type 2 diabetes with and without complications, there are also differences, such as more aggressive treatment targets for secondary prevention and benefits of additional therapies. Some drugs used in complication-free people with diabetes may require dosage adjustment or cessation in the presence of complications, such as CKD.

With 60% of deaths in people with diabetes being due to CVD, clinicians should implement proven secondary prevention therapies. *Fairly fast* SA^2A^2B (fish oil, fibrate, statin, dual-antiplatelet therapy, ACEi, aldosterone antagonist, beta-blocker) is an evidence-based mnemonic for the secondary prevention of CVD in the general population [239]. As there are other related chapters in this book, we list some key practice points for the management of CVD and heart failure (Tables 1.6 and 1.7).

Management of Arterial Disease and Heart Failure

A cardiologist, neurologist, or vascular surgeon and vascular imaging can guide decisions regarding medical therapy alone or surgery. Current evidence suggests that diabetic patients have a better prognosis with bypass grafts (preferably arterial vs. venous [240]) compared to angioplasty or stent procedures [241]. Drug-eluting stents are more effective than non-drug-eluting stents [242], with both requiring temporary antiplatelet cover.

We and others have reviewed heart failure in diabetes [243–247], and it is covered in detail in another chapter. Heart failure, which may be due to ischemia, hypertension, or diabetic cardiomyopathy, or a combination thereof, is more common and has a poorer prognosis in people with Type 2 diabetes than in non-diabetic subjects. Heart failure can be divided into that with reduced or preserved ejection fraction (heart failure with reduced ejection fraction (HFrEF) or HFpEF), with the latter accounting for about 50% of heart failure. Table 1.7 provides key points for HFrEF care. A long subclinical phase is recognized, but no routine cardiac imaging for its diagnosis, such as echocardiography or cardiac MRI, is recommended. Treatment of HFpEF is particularly difficult as there are no specific treatments yet and no therapies shown to reduce mortality.

An evidence-based mnemonic for treatment of HFrEF [248], devised by co-authors (JF) and colleagues, is **BANDAID^2** (beta-blocker, ACEi/ARB/angiotensin receptor-neprilysin inhibitor (ARNI), nitrate-hydralazine, diuretics, aldosterone antagonist, ivabradine, devices, and digoxin). Further detail is provided in Table 1.7 and in the original paper [248]. In addition, SGLT-2 inhibitors or GLP-1 analogues should be considered in Type 2 diabetic patients with heart failure [78]. In class II or III HFrEF patients without prior angioedema, current guidelines recommend switching ACEi/ARB therapy to an ARNI (e.g., Entresto). In a large RCT, ARNI reduced the composite outcome of cardiovascular mortality or HF by 20% [249].

Management of Microvascular Complications in Type 2 Diabetes

As there are other relevant chapters in this book, we summarize proven prevention treatments in Table 1.5 and list some key practice points for the management of existent microvascular complications in Table 1.8.

Conclusions

We already have the evidence base to practice personalized medicine in people with Type 2 diabetes, and we hope that the mnemonics, tables, and figures in this book chapter are useful guides for the busy clinician. A holistic multidisciplinary team approach to patient-centered care is ideal, but this can be challenging given the large number of people with diabetes and increasing complexity of care. Given the rapid evolution of new clinical evidence, drugs, and devices, ongoing education of the diabetes care team and of the person with diabetes is key. More electronic decision support tools and AI, ideally integrated with electronic medical records, will likely become available to assist in optimizing the choice of therapies for the person with diabetes. The approach will need to be modified as new proven therapies become available and the person's health status changes. While care should always be personalized to the person living with Type 2 diabetes, there will be constraints related to the resources of the patient and the local healthcare system. Clinical inertia must be prevented and overcome when it occurs. Advocacy at individual, local, and global levels is also important to ensure more equitable access to quality diabetes care for all people with or at risk of Type 2 diabetes.

Acknowledgments DC was supported by a University of Sydney and Australian National Health and Medical Research Council (NHMRC) Clinical Trials Centre (CTC) Summer Research Scholarship. AJJ is supported by an NHMRC Practitioner Fellowship. This work is dedicated to DC's parents, Mary Liu and Phillip Chen, who have been DC's greatest supports throughout his medical training.

References

1. National Health and Medical Research Council. Clinical utility of personalised medicine: Information for health professionals 2011. Available from: https://www.nhmrc.gov.au/_files_nhmrc/publications/attachments/ps0001_clinical_utility_personalised_medicine_feb_2011.pdf.
2. Li X, Oprea-Ilies GM, Krishnamurti U. New developments in breast cancer and their impact on daily practice in pathology. Arch Pathol Lab Med. 2017;141(4):490–8.
3. International Diabetes Federation. IDF diabetes atlas. 9th ed. Brussels: International Diabetes Federation; 2019.
4. Chowdhury TA, Shaho S, Moolla A. Complications of diabetes: progress, but significant challenges ahead. Ann Transl Med. 2014;2(12):120.
5. Most RS, Sinnock P. The epidemiology of lower extremity amputations in diabetic individuals. Diabetes Care. 1983;6(1):87–91.
6. National Eye Institute. Health education leads to more eye exams in group at risk for vision loss 1999. Available from: https://nei.nih.gov/news/pressreleases/morexam.
7. Ghaderian SB, Hayati F, Shayanpour S, Beladi Mousavi SS. Diabetes and end-stage renal disease; a review article on new concepts. J Renal Inj Prev. 2015;4(2):28–33.
8. Weissgerber TL, Mudd LM. Preeclampsia and diabetes. Curr Diab Rep. 2015;15(3):9.
9. Leslie MS, Briggs LA. Preeclampsia and the risk of future vascular disease and mortality: a review. J Midwifery Womens Health. 2016;61(3):315–24.
10. Golden TN, Simmons RA. Immune dysfunction in developmental programming of type 2 diabetes mellitus. Nat Rev Endocrinol. 2021;17(4):235–45.

11. Kurbasic A, Fraser A, Mogren I, Hallmans G, Franks PW, Rich-Edwards JW, et al. Maternal hypertensive disorders of pregnancy and offspring risk of hypertension: a population-based cohort and sibling study. Am J Hypertens. 2019;32(4):331–4.
12. Rughani A, Friedman JE, Tryggestad JB. Type 2 diabetes in youth: the role of early life exposures. Curr Diab Rep. 2020;20(9):45.
13. American Diabetes Association. Classification and diagnosis of diabetes: standards of medical care in diabetes2021. Diabetes Care. 2021;44(Suppl 1):S15–33.
14. The Royal Australian College of General Practitioners. Management of type 2 diabetes: A handbook for general practice. East Melbourne, Vic: RACGP, 2020. ISBN: 978-0-86906-577-8 (web).
15. Jenkins AJ, Best JD, Klein RL, Lyons TJ. Lipoproteins, glycoxidation and diabetic angiopathy. Diabetes Metab Res Rev. 2004;20(5):349–68.
16. Salamone D, Rivellese AA, Vetrani C. The relationship between gut microbiota, short-chain fatty acids and type 2 diabetes mellitus: the possible role of dietary fibre. Acta Diabetol. 2021;58(9):1131–8.
17. Yehualashet AS, Yikna BB. Microbial ecosystem in diabetes mellitus: consideration of the gastrointestinal system. Diabetes Metab Syndr Obes. 2021;14:1841–54.
18. Abuhendi N, Qush A, Naji F, Abunada H, Al Buainain R, Shi Z, et al. Genetic polymorphisms associated with type 2 diabetes in the Arab world: a systematic review and meta-analysis. Diabetes Res Clin Pract. 2019;151:198–208.
19. Doumatey AP, Ekoru K, Adeyemo A, Rotimi CN. Genetic basis of obesity and type 2 diabetes in Africans: impact on precision medicine. Curr Diab Rep. 2019;19(10):105.
20. Guan M, Keaton JM, Dimitrov L, Hicks PJ, Xu J, Palmer ND, et al. Genome-wide association study identifies novel loci for type 2 diabetes-attributed end-stage kidney disease in African Americans. Hum Genomics. 2019;13(1):21.
21. Jia X, Yang Y, Chen Y, Xia Z, Zhang W, Feng Y, et al. Multivariate analysis of genome-wide data to identify potential pleiotropic genes for type 2 diabetes, obesity and coronary artery disease using metacca. Int J Cardiol. 2019;283:144–50.
22. Jonas W, Schurmann A. Genetic and epigenetic factors determining NAFLD risk. Mol Metab. 2020;50:101111.
23. Sayed S, Nabi A. Diabetes and genetics: a relationship between genetic risk alleles, clinical phenotypes and therapeutic approaches. Adv Exp Med Biol. 2021;1307:457–98.
24. Witka BZ, Oktaviani DJ, Marcellino M, Barliana MI, Abdulah R. Type 2 diabetes-associated genetic polymorphisms as potential disease predictors. Diabetes Metab Syndr Obes. 2019;12:2689–706.
25. Zhang Y, Li S, Cao Z, Cheng Y, Xu C, Yang H, et al. A network analysis framework of genetic and nongenetic risks for type 2 diabetes. Rev Endocr Metab Disord. 2021;22(2):461–9.
26. Aronica L, Volek J, Poff A, D'Agostino DP. Genetic variants for personalised management of very low carbohydrate ketogenic diets. BMJ Nutr Prev Health. 2020;3(2):363–73.
27. Berry SE, Valdes AM, Drew DA, Asnicar F, Mazidi M, Wolf J, et al. Human postprandial responses to food and potential for precision nutrition. Nat Med. 2020;26(6):964–73.
28. Chen Y, Zhou T, Sun D, Li X, Ma H, Liang Z, et al. Distinct genetic subtypes of adiposity and glycemic changes in response to weight-loss diet intervention: the POUNDS LOST trial. Eur J Nutr. 2021;60(1):249–58.
29. Correa TAF, Quintanilha BJ, Norde MM, Pinhel MAS, Nonino CB, Rogero MM. Nutritional genomics, inflammation and obesity. Arch Endocrinol Metab. 2020;64(3):205–22.
30. Franzago M, Santurbano D, Vitacolonna E, Stuppia L. Genes and diet in the prevention of chronic diseases in future generations. Int J Mol Sci. 2020;21(7):2633.
31. Li X, Zhou T, Ma H, Heianza Y, Champagne CM, Williamson DA, et al. Genetic variation in lean body mass, changes of appetite and weight loss in response to diet interventions: the POUNDS LOST trial. Diabetes Obes Metab. 2020;22(12):2305–15.
32. Malekizadeh A, Rahbaran M, Afshari M, Abbasi D, Aghaei Meybodi HR, Hasanzad M. Association of common genetic variants of KCNJ11 gene with the risk of type 2 diabetes mellitus. Nucleosides Nucleotides Nucleic Acids. 2021;40(5):530–41.

33. Shahcheraghi SH, Aljabali AAA, Al Zoubi MS, Mishra V, Charbe NB, Haggag YA, et al. Overview of key molecular and pharmacological targets for diabetes and associated diseases. Life Sci. 2021;278:119632.
34. Spracklen CN, Sim X. Progress in defining the genetic contribution to type 2 diabetes in individuals of East Asian ancestry. Curr Diab Rep. 2021;21(6):17.
35. Frazier-Wood AC, Ordovas JM, Straka RJ, Hixson JE, Borecki IB, Tiwari HK, et al. The PPAR-alpha gene is associated with triglyceride, low-density cholesterol and inflammation marker response to fenofibrate intervention: the GOLDN study. Pharmacogenomics J. 2013;13(4):312–7.
36. Morieri ML, Shah HS, Sjaarda J, Lenzini PA, Campbell H, Motsinger-Reif AA, et al. PPARa polymorphism influences the cardiovascular benefit of fenofibrate in type 2 diabetes: findings from ACCORD-LIPID. Diabetes. 2020;69(4):771–83.
37. Sivashanmugarajah A, Fulcher J, Sullivan D, Elam M, Jenkins A, Keech A. Author reply. Intern Med J. 2020;50(4):507–8.
38. Suthers G, Somogyi AA. Pharmacogenetics of statin intolerance. Intern Med J. 2020;50(4):506–7.
39. Noordam R, Lall K, Smit RA, Laisk T, Estonian Biobank Research, Loos RJ, et al. Stratification of type 2 diabetes mellitus by age of diagnosis in the UK biobank reveals subgroup-specific genetic associations and causal risk profiles. Diabetes. 2021;70(8):1816–25.
40. Zhang H, Colclough K, Gloyn AL, Pollin TI. Monogenic diabetes: a gateway to precision medicine in diabetes. J Clin Invest. 2021;131(3):e142244.
41. Bebu I, Schade D, Braffett B, Kosiborod M, Lopes-Virella M, Soliman EZ, et al. Risk factors for first and subsequent CVD events in type 1 diabetes: the DCCT/EDIC study. Diabetes Care. 2020;43(4):867–74.
42. Forrest IS, Chaudhary K, Paranjpe I, Vy HMT, Marquez-Luna C, Rocheleau G, et al. Genome-wide polygenic risk score for retinopathy of type 2 diabetes. Hum Mol Genet. 2021;30(10):952–60.
43. Jiang G, Luk AO, Tam CHT, Lau ES, Ozaki R, Chow EYK, et al. Obesity, clinical, and genetic predictors for glycemic progression in Chinese patients with type 2 diabetes: a cohort study using the Hong Kong Diabetes Register and Hong Kong Diabetes Biobank. PLoS Med. 2020;17(7):e1003209.
44. Tam CHT, Lim CKP, Luk AOY, Ng ACW, Lee HM, Jiang G, et al. Development of genome-wide polygenic risk scores for lipid traits and clinical applications for dyslipidemia, subclinical atherosclerosis, and diabetes cardiovascular complications among East Asians. Genome Med. 2021;13(1):29.
45. Vujkovic M, Keaton JM, Lynch JA, Miller DR, Zhou J, Tcheandjieu C, et al. Discovery of 318 new risk loci for type 2 diabetes and related vascular outcomes among 1.4 million participants in a multi-ancestry meta-analysis. Nat Genet. 2020;52(7):680–91.
46. O'Brien J, Hayder H, Zayed Y, Peng C. Overview of microRNA biogenesis, mechanisms of actions, and circulation. Front Endocrinol (Lausanne). 2018;9:402.
47. Su X, Nie M, Zhang G, Wang B. MicroRNA in cardio-metabolic disorders. Clin Chim Acta. 2021;518:134–41.
48. Akbari Kordkheyli V, Amir Mishan M, Khonakdar Tarsi A, Mahrooz A, Rezaei Kanavi M, Hafezi-Moghadam A, et al. MicroRNAs may provide new strategies in the treatment and diagnosis of diabetic retinopathy: importance of VEGF. Iran J Basic Med Sci. 2021;24(3):267–79.
49. Bielska A, Niemira M, Kretowski A. Recent highlights of research on miRNAs as early potential biomarkers for cardiovascular complications of type 2 diabetes mellitus. Int J Mol Sci. 2021;22(6):3153.
50. Fujita Y, Murakami T, Nakamura A. Recent advances in biomarkers and regenerative medicine for diabetic neuropathy. Int J Mol Sci. 2021;22(5):2301.

51. Jakubik D, Fitas A, Eyileten C, Jarosz-Popek J, Nowak A, Czajka P, et al. MicroRNAs and long non-coding RNAs in the pathophysiological processes of diabetic cardiomyopathy: emerging biomarkers and potential therapeutics. Cardiovasc Diabetol. 2021;20(1):55.
52. Joglekar MV, Januszewski AS, Jenkins AJ, Hardikar AA. Circulating microRNA biomarkers of diabetic retinopathy. Diabetes. 2016;65(1):22–4.
53. Kaidonis G, Gillies MC, Abhary S, Liu E, Essex RW, Chang JH, et al. A single-nucleotide polymorphism in the microRNA-146a gene is associated with diabetic nephropathy and sight-threatening diabetic retinopathy in Caucasian patients. Acta Diabetol. 2016;53(4):643–50.
54. Mathur P, Rani V. Micrornas: a critical regulator and a promising therapeutic and diagnostic molecule for diabetic cardiomyopathy. Curr Gene Ther. 2021;21(4):313–26.
55. Rai AK, Lee B, Gomez R, Rajendran D, Khan M, Garikipati VNS. Current status and potential therapeutic strategies for using non-coding RNA to treat diabetic cardiomyopathy. Front Physiol. 2020;11:612722.
56. Ren H, Wang Q. Non-coding RNA and diabetic kidney disease. DNA Cell Biol. 2021;40(4):553–67.
57. Verduci L, Tarcitano E, Strano S, Yarden Y, Blandino G. CircRNAs: role in human diseases and potential use as biomarkers. Cell Death Dis. 2021;12(5):468.
58. Zhou H, Ni WJ, Meng XM, Tang LQ. MicroRNAs as regulators of immune and inflammatory responses: potential therapeutic targets in diabetic nephropathy. Front Cell Dev Biol. 2020;8:618536.
59. Cheng F, Carroll L, Joglekar MV, Januszewski AS, Wong KK, Hardikar AA, et al. Diabetes, metabolic disease, and telomere length. Lancet Diabetes Endocrinol. 2021;9(2):117–26.
60. Cheng F, Luk AO, Wu H, Lim CKP, Carroll L, Tam CHT, et al. Shortened relative leukocyte telomere length is associated with all-cause mortality in type 2 diabetes- analysis from the Hong Kong Diabetes Register. Diabetes Res Clin Pract. 2021;173:108649.
61. Cheng F, Luk AO, Tam CHT, Fan B, Wu H, Yang A, et al. Shortened relative leukocyte telomere length is associated with prevalent and incident cardiovascular complications in type 2 diabetes: analysis from the Hong Kong Diabetes Register. Diabetes Care. 2020;43(9):2257–65.
62. Libertini G, Corbi G, Cellurale M, Ferrara N. Age-related dysfunctions: evidence and relationship with some risk factors and protective drugs. Biochemistry (Mosc). 2019;84(12):1442–50.
63. Sutanto SSI, McLennan SV, Keech AC, Twigg SM. Shortening of telomere length by metabolic factors in diabetes: protective effects of fenofibrate. J Cell Commun Signal. 2019;13(4):523–30.
64. American Diabetes Association. Type 2 diabetes risk test. Available from: https://www.diabetes.org/risk-test.
65. Diabetes Australia. Are you at risk? Available from: https://www.diabetesaustralia.com.au/about-diabetes/are-you-at-risk-type-2/.
66. Aspelund T, Thornorisdottir O, Olafsdottir E, Gudmundsdottir A, Einarsdottir AB, Mehlsen J, et al. Individual risk assessment and information technology to optimise screening frequency for diabetic retinopathy. Diabetologia. 2011;54(10):2525–32.
67. Lund SH, Aspelund T, Kirby P, Russell G, Einarsson S, Palsson O, et al. Individualised risk assessment for diabetic retinopathy and optimisation of screening intervals: a scientific approach to reducing healthcare costs. Br J Ophthalmol. 2016;100(5):683–7.
68. Ali I, Donne RL, Kalra PA. A validation study of the kidney failure risk equation in advanced chronic kidney disease according to disease aetiology with evaluation of discrimination, calibration and clinical utility. BMC Nephrol. 2021;22(1):194.
69. Australian Chronic Disease Prevention Alliance. Australian absolute cardiovascular disease risk calculator. Available from: https://www.cvdcheck.org.au/.
70. Choi Y, Yang Y, Hwang BH, Lee EY, Yoon KH, Chang K, et al. Practical cardiovascular risk calculator for asymptomatic patients with type 2 diabetes mellitus: precise-DM risk score. Clin Cardiol. 2020;43(9):1040–7.
71. Grzybowski A, Brona P, Lim G, Ruamviboonsuk P, Tan GSW, Abramoff M, et al. Artificial intelligence for diabetic retinopathy screening: a review. Eye (Lond). 2020;34(3):451–60.

72. Quinn N, Brazionis L, Zhu B, Ryan C, D'Aloisio R, Lilian Tang H, et al. Facilitating diabetic retinopathy screening using automated retinal image analysis in underresourced settings. Diabet Med. 2021;38(9):e14582.
73. Gaede P, Lund-Andersen H, Parving HH, Pedersen O. Effect of a multifactorial intervention on mortality in type 2 diabetes. N Engl J Med. 2008;358(6):580–91.
74. Atkinson-Briggs S, Jenkins A, Keech A, Ryan C, Brazionis L, on behalf of the Centre of Research Excellence in Diabetic Retinopathy Study Group. Nurse-led vascular risk assessment in a regional Victorian Indigenous primary care diabetes clinic: An integrated Diabetes Education and Eye disease Screening [iDEES] study. Journal of Advanced Nursing in press. Accepted Dec 2021.
75. Australian Institute of Health and Welfare. Cardiovascular disease, diabetes and chronic kidney disease: Australian facts mortality 2014 [cited 2018 25 January]. Available from: https://www.aihw.gov.au/reports/heart-stroke-vasculardisease/cardiovascular-diabetes-chronic-kidney-mortality/contents/table-of-contents.
76. Royal Australian College of General Practitioners. Guidelines for preventive activities in general practice. 9th ed. East Melbourne: Royal Australian College of General Practitioners; 2016.
77. Beagley J, Guariguata L, Weil C, Motala AA. Global estimates of undiagnosed diabetes in adults. Diabetes Res Clin Pract. 2014;103(2):150–60.
78. American Diabetes Association. 2. Classification and diagnosis of diabetes: standards of medical care in diabetes-2019. Diabetes Care. 2019;42(Suppl 1):S13–S28. https://doi.org/10.2337/dc19-S002. PMID: 30559228.
79. Knowler WC, Barrett-Connor E, Fowler SE, Hamman RF, Lachin JM, Walker EA, et al. Reduction in the incidence of type 2 diabetes with lifestyle intervention or metformin. N Engl J Med. 2002;346(6):393–403.
80. Diabetes Prevention Program Research Group. Long-term effects of lifestyle intervention or metformin on diabetes development and microvascular complications over 15-year follow-up: the Diabetes Prevention Program Outcomes Study. Lancet Diabetes Endocrinol. 2015;3(11):866–75.
81. Wittert G, Bracken K, Robledo KP, Grossmann M, Yeap BB, Handelsman DJ, et al. Testosterone treatment to prevent or revert type 2 diabetes in men enrolled in a lifestyle programme (T4DM): a randomised, double-blind, placebo-controlled, 2-year, phase 3b trial. Lancet Diabetes Endocrinol. 2021;9(1):32–45.
82. Bian RR, Piatt GA, Sen A, Plegue MA, De Michele ML, Hafez D, et al. The effect of technology-mediated diabetes prevention interventions on weight: a meta-analysis. J Med Internet Res. 2017;19(3):e76.
83. Haw JS, Galaviz KI, Straus AN, Kowalski AJ, Magee MJ, Weber MB, et al. Long-term sustainability of diabetes prevention approaches: a systematic review and meta-analysis of randomized clinical trials. JAMA Intern Med. 2017;177(12):1808–17.
84. Affinati AH, Esfandiari NH, Oral EA, Kraftson AT. Bariatric surgery in the treatment of type 2 diabetes. Curr Diab Rep. 2019;19(12):156.
85. Cummings DE, Cohen RV. Bariatric/metabolic surgery to treat type 2 diabetes in patients with a BMI<35 kg/m2. Diabetes Care. 2016;39(6):924–33.
86. Koliaki C, Liatis S, le Roux CW, Kokkinos A. The role of bariatric surgery to treat diabetes: current challenges and perspectives. BMC Endocr Disord. 2017;17(1):50.
87. Jenkins A, Januszewski AS, O'Neal D. Addressing vascular risk factors in diabetes. Endocrinol Today. 2015;4(4):35–8.
88. Look ARG, Wing RR, Bolin P, Brancati FL, Bray GA, Clark JM, et al. Cardiovascular effects of intensive lifestyle intervention in type 2 diabetes. N Engl J Med. 2013;369(2):145–54.
89. Azadbakht L, Fard NR, Karimi M, Baghaei MH, Surkan PJ, Rahimi M, et al. Effects of the dietary approaches to stop hypertension (DASH) eating plan on cardiovascular risks among type 2 diabetic patients: a randomized crossover clinical trial. Diabetes Care. 2011;34(1):55–7.
90. Estruch R, Ros E, Salas-Salvado J, Covas MI, Corella D, Aros F, et al. Primary prevention of cardiovascular disease with a Mediterranean diet supplemented with extra-virgin olive oil or nuts. N Engl J Med. 2018;378(25):e34.

91. Lean ME, Leslie WS, Barnes AC, Brosnahan N, Thom G, McCombie L, et al. Primary care-led weight management for remission of type 2 diabetes (DIRECT): an open-label, cluster-randomised trial. Lancet. 2018;391(10120):541–51.
92. Newcastle University. Reversing type 2 diabetes. Available from: https://www.ncl.ac.uk/magres/research/diabetes/reversal/#publicinformation.
93. Carter S, Clifton PM, Keogh JB. The effects of intermittent compared to continuous energy restriction on glycaemic control in type 2 diabetes; a pragmatic pilot trial. Diabetes Res Clin Pract. 2016;122:106–12.
94. Battelino T, Danne T, Bergenstal RM, Amiel SA, Beck R, Biester T, et al. Clinical targets for continuous glucose monitoring data interpretation: recommendations from the International Consensus on Time in Range. Diabetes Care. 2019;42(8):1593–603.
95. Foreman YD, van Doorn W, Schaper NC, van Greevenbroek MMJ, van der Kallen CJH, Henry RMA, et al. Greater daily glucose variability and lower time in range assessed with continuous glucose monitoring are associated with greater aortic stiffness: the Maastricht study. Diabetologia. 2021;64(8):1880–92.
96. Handa T, Nakamura A, Miya A, Nomoto H, Kameda H, Cho KY, et al. The association between hypoglycemia and glycemic variability in elderly patients with type 2 diabetes: a prospective observational study. Diabetol Metab Syndr. 2021;13(1):37.
97. Scott ES, Januszewski AS, O'Connell R, Fulcher G, Scott R, Kesaniemi A, et al. Long-term glycemic variability and vascular complications in type 2 diabetes: post hoc analysis of the FIELD study. J Clin Endocrinol Metab. 2020;105(10):dgaa361.
98. Zhang J, Yang J, Liu L, Li L, Cui J, Wu S, et al. Significant abnormal glycemic variability increased the risk for arrhythmias in elderly type 2 diabetic patients. BMC Endocr Disord. 2021;21(1):83.
99. Zoungas S, Arima H, Gerstein HC, Holman RR, Woodward M, Reaven P, et al. Effects of intensive glucose control on microvascular outcomes in patients with type 2 diabetes: a meta-analysis of individual participant data from randomised controlled trials. Lancet Diabetes Endocrinol. 2017;5(6):431–7.
100. Ray KK, Seshasai SR, Wijesuriya S, Sivakumaran R, Nethercott S, Preiss D, et al. Effect of intensive control of glucose on cardiovascular outcomes and death in patients with diabetes mellitus: a meta-analysis of randomised controlled trials. Lancet. 2009;373(9677):1765–72.
101. Qaseem A, Wilt TJ, Kansagara D, Horwitch C, Barry MJ, Forciea MA, et al. Hemoglobin A1c targets for glycemic control with pharmacologic therapy for nonpregnant adults with type 2 diabetes mellitus: a guidance statement update from the American college of physicians. Ann Intern Med. 2018;168(8):569–76.
102. Action to Control Cardiovascular Risk in Diabetes Study Group, Gerstein HC, Miller ME, Byington RP, Goff DC Jr, Bigger JT, et al. Effects of intensive glucose lowering in type 2 diabetes. N Engl J Med. 2008;358(24):2545–59.
103. Duckworth W, Abraira C, Moritz T, Reda D, Emanuele N, Reaven PD, et al. Glucose control and vascular complications in veterans with type 2 diabetes. N Engl J Med. 2009;360(2):129–39.
104. Group AC, Patel A, MacMahon S, Chalmers J, Neal B, Billot L, et al. Intensive blood glucose control and vascular outcomes in patients with type 2 diabetes. N Engl J Med. 2008;358(24):2560–72.
105. Andersen A, Jorgensen PG, Knop FK, Vilsboll T. Hypoglycemia and cardiac arrhythmias in diabetes. Ther Adv Endocrinol Metab. 2020;11:2042018820911803.
106. Heller SR. Abnormalities of the electrocardiogram during hypoglycemia: the cause of the dead in bed syndrome? Int J Clin Pract Suppl. 2002;129:27–32.
107. Gogitidze Joy N, Hedrington MS, Briscoe VJ, Tate DB, Ertl AC, Davis SN. Effects of acute hypoglycemia on inflammatory and pro-atherothrombotic biomarkers in individuals with type 1 diabetes and healthy individuals. Diabetes Care. 2010;33(7):1529–35.
108. Yun JS, Park YM, Han K, Cha SA, Ahn YB, Ko SH. Association between BMI and risk of severe hypoglycemia in type 2 diabetes. Diabetes Metab. 2019;45(1):19–25.

109. Cheung NW, Conn JJ, d'Emden MC, Gunton JE, Jenkins AJ, Ross GP, et al. Position statement of the Australian Diabetes Society: individualisation of glycated haemoglobin targets for adults with diabetes mellitus. Med J Aust. 2009;191(6):339–44.
110. Skyler JS, Bergenstal R, Bonow RO, Buse J, Deedwania P, Gale EA, et al. Intensive glycemic control and the prevention of cardiovascular events: implications of the ACCORD, ADVANCE, and VA diabetes trials: a position statement of the American Diabetes Association and a scientific statement of the American College of Cardiology Foundation and the American Heart Association. Diabetes Care. 2009;32(1):187–92.
111. Huang DL, Abrass IB, Young BA. Medication safety and chronic kidney disease in older adults prescribed metformin: a cross-sectional analysis. BMC Nephrol. 2014;15:86.
112. Manski-Nankervis JA, Thuraisingam S, Sluggett JK, Kilov G, Furler J, O'Neal D, et al. Prescribing of diabetes medications to people with type 2 diabetes and chronic kidney disease: a national cross-sectional study. BMC Fam Pract. 2019;20(1):29.
113. Tuot DS, Lin F, Shlipak MG, Grubbs V, Hsu CY, Yee J, et al. Potential impact of prescribing metformin according to EGFR rather than serum creatinine. Diabetes Care. 2015;38(11):2059–67.
114. Crowley MJ, Diamantidis CJ, McDuffie JR, Cameron B, Stanifer J, Mock CK, et al. Metformin use in patients with historical contraindications or precautions. VA evidence-based synthesis program reports. Washington, DC: Department of Veterans Affairs; 2016.
115. Crowley MJ, Diamantidis CJ, McDuffie JR, Cameron CB, Stanifer JW, Mock CK, et al. Clinical outcomes of metformin use in populations with chronic kidney disease, congestive heart failure, or chronic liver disease: a systematic review. Ann Intern Med. 2017;166(3):191–200.
116. Gosmanov AR, Gemoets DE, Kaminsky LS, Kovesdy CP, Gosmanova EO. Efficacy of metformin monotherapy in US veterans with type 2 diabetes and preexisting chronic kidney disease stage 3. Diabetes Obes Metab. 2021;23(8):1879–85.
117. DeFronzo R, Fleming GA, Chen K, Bicsak TA. Metformin-associated lactic acidosis: current perspectives on causes and risk. Metabolism. 2016;65(2):20–9.
118. Bonora BM, Avogaro A, Fadini GP. Euglycemic ketoacidosis. Curr Diab Rep. 2020;20(7):25.
119. Goldenberg RM, Berard LD, Cheng AYY, Gilbert JD, Verma S, Woo VC, et al. SGLT2 inhibitor-associated diabetic ketoacidosis: clinical review and recommendations for prevention and diagnosis. Clin Ther. 2016;38(12):2654–64. e2651.
120. Modi A, Agrawal A, Morgan F. Euglycemic diabetic ketoacidosis: a review. Curr Diabetes Rev. 2017;13(3):315–21.
121. Hirakawa Y, Arima H, Zoungas S, Ninomiya T, Cooper M, Hamet P, et al. Impact of visit-to-visit glycemic variability on the risks of macrovascular and microvascular events and all-cause mortality in type 2 diabetes: the ADVANCE trial. Diabetes Care. 2014;37(8):2359–65.
122. Su G, Mi SH, Li Z, Tao H, Yang HX, Zheng H. Prognostic value of early in-hospital glycemic excursion in elderly patients with acute myocardial infarction. Cardiovasc Diabetol. 2013;12:33.
123. Nalysnyk L, Hernandez-Medina M, Krishnarajah G. Glycaemic variability and complications in patients with diabetes mellitus: evidence from a systematic review of the literature. Diabetes Obes Metab. 2010;12(4):288–98.
124. Costantino S, Paneni F, Battista R, Castello L, Capretti G, Chiandotto S, et al. Impact of glycemic variability on chromatin remodeling, oxidative stress, and endothelial dysfunction in patients with type 2 diabetes and with target HbA1c levels. Diabetes. 2017;66(9):2472–82.
125. Henry RR, Rosenstock J, Edelman S, Mudaliar S, Chalamandaris AG, Kasichayanula S, et al. Exploring the potential of the SGLT2 inhibitor dapagliflozin in type 1 diabetes: a randomized, double-blind, placebo-controlled pilot study. Diabetes Care. 2015;38(3):412–9.
126. Suh S, Kim JH. Glycemic variability: how do we measure it and why is it important? Diabetes Metab J. 2015;39(4):273–82.

127. Neuen BL, Young T, Heerspink HJL, Neal B, Perkovic V, Billot L, et al. SGLT2 inhibitors for the prevention of kidney failure in patients with type 2 diabetes: a systematic review and meta-analysis. Lancet Diabetes Endocrinol. 2019;7(11):845–54.
128. Toyama T, Neuen BL, Jun M, Ohkuma T, Neal B, Jardine MJ, et al. Effect of SGLT2 inhibitors on cardiovascular, renal and safety outcomes in patients with type 2 diabetes mellitus and chronic kidney disease: a systematic review and meta-analysis. Diabetes Obes Metab. 2019;21(5):1237–50.
129. Zelniker TA, Wiviott SD, Raz I, Im K, Goodrich EL, Bonaca MP, et al. SGLT2 inhibitors for primary and secondary prevention of cardiovascular and renal outcomes in type 2 diabetes: a systematic review and meta-analysis of cardiovascular outcome trials. Lancet. 2019;393(10166):31–9.
130. Hayward RA, Reaven PD, Wiitala WL, Bahn GD, Reda DJ, Ge L, et al. Follow-up of glycemic control and cardiovascular outcomes in type 2 diabetes. N Engl J Med. 2015;372(23):2197–206.
131. UK Prospective Diabetes Study (UKPDS) Group. Intensive blood-glucose control with sulphonylureas or insulin compared with conventional treatment and risk of complications in patients with type 2 diabetes (UKPDS 33). Lancet. 1998;352(9131):837–53.
132. Ismail-Beigi F, Craven T, Banerji MA, Basile J, Calles J, Cohen RM, et al. Effect of intensive treatment of hyperglycemia on microvascular outcomes in type 2 diabetes: an analysis of the accord randomised trial. Lancet. 2010;376(9739):419–30.
133. Azad N, Agrawal L, Emanuele NV, Klein R, Bahn GD, Reaven P, et al. Association of blood glucose control and pancreatic reserve with diabetic retinopathy in the Veterans Affairs Diabetes Trial (VADT). Diabetologia. 2014;57(6):1124–31.
134. Australian Diabetes Society. A new blood glucose management algorithm for type 2 diabetes: a position statement of the Australian Diabetes Society 2016. Available from: https://t2d.diabetessociety.com.au/documents/92f4CL73.pdf.
135. American Diabetes Association. Pharmacologic approaches to glycemic treatment: standards of medical care in diabetes-2021. Diabetes Care. 2021;44(Suppl 1):S111–24.
136. Chun JH, Butts A. Long-acting GLP-1ras: an overview of efficacy, safety, and their role in type 2 diabetes management. JAAPA. 2020;33(S8 Suppl 1):3–18.
137. Cornell S. A review of GLP-1 receptor agonists in type 2 diabetes: a focus on the mechanism of action of once-weekly agents. J Clin Pharm Ther. 2020;45(Suppl 1):17–27.
138. Jain AB, Ali A, Gorgojo Martinez JJ, Hramiak I, Kavia K, Madsbad S, et al. Switching between GLP-1 receptor agonists in clinical practice: expert consensus and practical guidance. Int J Clin Pract. 2021;75(2):e13731.
139. Ma J, Zhang B, Hou J, Peng Y. Efficacy and safety of once weekly dulaglutide in East Asian patients with type 2 diabetes: subgroup analysis by potential influential factors. Diabetes Ther. 2021;12(1):211–22.
140. Mirabelli M, Chiefari E, Tocci V, Caroleo P, Giuliano S, Greco E, et al. Clinical effectiveness and safety of once-weekly glp-1 receptor agonist dulaglutide as add-on to metformin or metformin plus insulin secretagogues in obesity and type 2 diabetes. J Clin Med. 2021;10(5):985.
141. Guber K, Pemmasani G, Malik A, Aronow WS, Yandrapalli S, Frishman WH. Statins and higher diabetes mellitus risk: incidence, proposed mechanisms and clinical implications. Cardiol Rev. 2021;29(6):314–22.
142. American Diabetes Association. American Diabetes Association. Available from: https://www.diabetes.org/.
143. Atchison E, Barkmeier A. The role of systemic risk factors in diabetic retinopathy. Curr Ophthalmol Rep. 2016;4(2):84–9.
144. Cai Z, Yang Y, Zhang J. A systematic review and meta-analysis of the serum lipid profile in prediction of diabetic neuropathy. Sci Rep. 2021;11(1):499.
145. Eid S, Sas KM, Abcouwer SF, Feldman EL, Gardner TW, Pennathur S, et al. New insights into the mechanisms of diabetic complications: role of lipids and lipid metabolism. Diabetologia. 2019;62(9):1539–49.

146. Howard BV, Robbins DC, Sievers ML, Lee ET, Rhoades D, Devereux RB, et al. LDL cholesterol as a strong predictor of coronary heart disease in diabetic individuals with insulin resistance and low LDL: the Strong Heart Study. Arterioscler Thromb Vasc Biol. 2000;20(3):830–5.
147. Jenkins AJ, Scott ES, Fulcher J, Kilov G, Januszewski AS. Management of diabetes mellitus. In: Toth PP, Cannon CP, editors. Comprehensive cardiovascular medicine in the primary care setting. 2nd ed. Totowa: Humana Press; 2018.
148. Sobrin L, Chong YH, Fan Q, Gan A, Stanwyck LK, Kaidonis G, et al. Genetically determined plasma lipid levels and risk of diabetic retinopathy: a Mendelian randomization study. Diabetes. 2017;66(12):3130–41.
149. Leitersdorf E. Cholesterol absorption inhibition: filling an unmet need in lipid-lowering management. Eur Heart J Suppl. 2001;3(suppl E):E17–23.
150. Cholesterol Treatment Trialists Collaboration, Kearney PM, Blackwell L, Collins R, Keech A, Simes J, et al. Efficacy of cholesterol-lowering therapy in 18,686 people with diabetes in 14 randomised trials of statins: a meta-analysis. Lancet. 2008;371(9607):117–25.
151. Cholesterol Treatment Trialists Collaboration, Fulcher J, O'Connell R, Voysey M, Emberson J, Blackwell L, et al. Efficacy and safety of LDL-lowering therapy among men and women: meta-analysis of individual data from 174,000 participants in 27 randomised trials. Lancet. 2015;385(9976):1397–405.
152. University of Oxford. UKPDS risk engine. Available from: https://www.dtu.ox.ac.uk/riskengine/download.php.
153. ClinRisk. Qrisk®3-2017 risk calculator 2017. Available from: https://qrisk.org/three/index.php.
154. American College of Cardiology. ASCVD risk estimator plus. Available from: http://tools.acc.org/ASCVD-Risk-Estimator-Plus/#!/calculate/estimate/.
155. American Diabetes Association. Cardiovascular disease and risk management: standards of medical care in diabetes-2021. Diabetes Care. 2021;44(Suppl 1):S125–50.
156. Kang EY, Chen TH, Garg SJ, Sun CC, Kang JH, Wu WC, et al. Association of statin therapy with prevention of vision-threatening diabetic retinopathy. JAMA Ophthalmol. 2019;137(4):363–71.
157. Kawasaki R, Konta T, Nishida K. Lipid-lowering medication is associated with decreased risk of diabetic retinopathy and the need for treatment in patients with type 2 diabetes: a real-world observational analysis of a health claims database. Diabetes Obes Metab. 2018;20(10):2351–60.
158. Mozetic V, Pacheco RL, Latorraca COC, Riera R. Statins and/or fibrates for diabetic retinopathy: a systematic review and meta-analysis. Diabetol Metab Syndr. 2019;11:92.
159. Murakami T, Kato S, Shigeeda T, Itoh H, Komuro I, Takeuchi M, et al. Intensive treat-to-target statin therapy and severity of diabetic retinopathy complicated by hypercholesterolaemia. Eye (Lond). 2021;35(8):2221–8.
160. Pranata R, Vania R, Victor AA. Statin reduces the incidence of diabetic retinopathy and its need for intervention: a systematic review and meta-analysis. Eur J Ophthalmol. 2020;31(3):1216–24. https://doi.org/10.1177/1120672120922444.
161. Vail D, Callaway NF, Ludwig CA, Saroj N, Moshfeghi DM. Lipid-lowering medications are associated with lower risk of retinopathy and ophthalmic interventions among United States patients with diabetes. Am J Ophthalmol. 2019;207:378–84.
162. Qin X, Dong H, Fang K, Lu F. The effect of statins on renal outcomes in patients with diabetic kidney disease: a systematic review and meta-analysis. Diabetes Metab Res Rev. 2017;33(6) https://doi.org/10.1002/dmrr.2901.
163. Cholesterol Treatment Trialists' (CTT) Collaboration, Herrington WG, Emberson J, Mihaylova B, Blackwell L, Reith C, et al. Impact of renal function on the effects of LDL cholesterol lowering with statin-based regimens: a meta-analysis of individual participant data from 28 randomised trials. Lancet Diabetes Endocrinol. 2016;4(10):829–39.
164. Pergolizzi JV Jr, Magnusson P, LeQuang JA, Razmi R, Zampogna G, Taylor R Jr. Statins and neuropathic pain: a narrative review. Pain Ther. 2020;9(1):97–111.

165. Wang M, Li M, Xie Y. The association between statins exposure and peripheral neuropathy risk: a meta-analysis. J Clin Pharm Ther. 2021;46(4):1046–54.
166. Keni R, Sekhar A, Gourishetti K, Nayak PG, Kinra M, Kumar N, et al. Role of statins in new-onset diabetes mellitus: the underlying cause, mechanisms involved, and strategies to combat. Curr Drug Targets. 2021;22(10):1121–8.
167. Masson W, Lobo M, Lavalle-Cobo A, Masson G, Molinero G. Effect of bempedoic acid on new onset or worsening diabetes: a meta-analysis. Diabetes Res Clin Pract. 2020;168:108369.
168. Szili-Torok T, Bakker SJL, Tietge UJF. Statin use is prospectively associated with new-onset diabetes after transplantation in renal transplant recipients. Diabetes Care. 2020;43(8):1945–7.
169. Anyanwagu U, Idris I, Donnelly R. Drug-induced diabetes mellitus: evidence for statins and other drugs affecting glucose metabolism. Clin Pharmacol Ther. 2016;99(4):390–400.
170. Schmidt AF, Swerdlow DI, Holmes MV, Patel RS, Fairhurst-Hunter Z, Lyall DM, et al. PCSK9 genetic variants and risk of type 2 diabetes: a Mendelian randomisation study. Lancet Diabetes Endocrinol. 2017;5(2):97–105.
171. Sivashanmugarajah A, Fulcher J, Sullivan D, Elam M, Jenkins A, Keech A. Suggested clinical approach for the diagnosis and management of 'statin intolerance' with an emphasis on muscle-related side-effects. Intern Med J. 2019;49(9):1081–91.
172. Beshir SA, Hussain N, Elnor AA, Said ASA. Umbrella review on non-statin lipid-lowering therapy. J Cardiovasc Pharmacol Ther. 2021;26(5):437–52. https://doi.org/10.1177/10742484211002943.
173. Ballantyne CM, Laufs U, Ray KK, Leiter LA, Bays HE, Goldberg AC, et al. Bempedoic acid plus ezetimibe fixed-dose combination in patients with hypercholesterolemia and high CVD risk treated with maximally tolerated statin therapy. Eur J Prev Cardiol. 2020;27(6):593–603.
174. Feingold KR. Cholesterol lowering drugs. In: Feingold KR, Anawalt B, Boyce A, Chrousos G, de Herder WW, Dhatariya K, et al., editors. Endotext. South Dartmouth: MDText.com; 2021.
175. Giugliano RP, Cannon CP, Blazing MA, Nicolau JC, Corbalan R, Spinar J, et al. Benefit of adding ezetimibe to statin therapy on cardiovascular outcomes and safety in patients with versus without diabetes mellitus: results from IMPROVE-IT (improved reduction of outcomes: Vytorin efficacy international trial). Circulation. 2018;137(15):1571–82.
176. Wang X, Zhang Y, Tan H, Wang P, Zha X, Chong W, et al. Efficacy and safety of bempedoic acid for prevention of cardiovascular events and diabetes: a systematic review and meta-analysis. Cardiovasc Diabetol. 2020;19(1):128.
177. Robinson JG et al. ODYSSEY LONG TERM Investigators. Efficacy and safety of alirocumab in reducing lipids and cardiovasuclar events. New Engl J Med. 2015;372(16):1489–99. PMID 25773378.
178. de Carvalho LSF, Campos AM, Sposito AC. Proprotein convertase subtilisin/kexin type 9 (PCSK9) inhibitors and incident type 2 diabetes: a systematic review and meta-analysis with over 96,000 patient-years. Diabetes Care. 2018;41(2):364–7.
179. Keech A, Simes RJ, Barter P, Best J, Scott R, Taskinen MR, et al. Effects of long-term fenofibrate therapy on cardiovascular events in 9795 people with type 2 diabetes mellitus (the FIELD study): randomised controlled trial. Lancet. 2005;366(9500):1849–61.
180. ACCORD Study Group, ACCORD-Eye Study Group, Chew EY, Ambrosius WT, Davis MD, Danis RP, et al. Effects of medical therapies on retinopathy progression in type 2 diabetes. N Engl J Med. 2010;363(3):233–44.
181. Keech AC, Mitchell P, Summanen PA, O'Day J, Davis TM, Moffitt MS, et al. Effect of fenofibrate on the need for laser treatment for diabetic retinopathy (FIELD study): a randomised controlled trial. Lancet. 2007;370(9600):1687–97.
182. Davis TM, Ting R, Best JD, Donoghoe MW, Drury PL, Sullivan DR, et al. Effects of fenofibrate on renal function in patients with type 2 diabetes mellitus: the Fenofibrate Intervention and Event Lowering in Diabetes (FIELD) study. Diabetologia. 2011;54(2):280–90.
183. Bonds DE, Craven TE, Buse J, Crouse JR, Cuddihy R, Elam M, et al. Fenofibrate-associated changes in renal function and relationship to clinical outcomes among individuals with type

2 diabetes: the Action to Control Cardiovascular Risk in Diabetes (ACCORD) experience. Diabetologia. 2012;55(6):1641–50.
184. Rajamani K, Colman PG, Li LP, Best JD, Voysey M, D'Emden MC, et al. Effect of fenofibrate on amputation events in people with type 2 diabetes mellitus (FIELD study): a prespecified analysis of a randomised controlled trial. Lancet. 2009;373(9677):1780–8.
185. Medscape. Combining statins and fibrates. Available from: https://www.medscape.org/viewarticle/563490.
186. Group ASC, Bowman L, Mafham M, Wallendszus K, Stevens W, Buck G, et al. Effects of n-3 fatty acid supplements in diabetes mellitus. N Engl J Med. 2018;379(16):1540–50.
187. The Royal Australian College of General Practitioners and Diabetes Australia. General practice management of type 2 diabetes. 2016–18.
188. Tay J, Luscombe-Marsh ND, Thompson CH, Noakes M, Buckley JD, Wittert GA, et al. Comparison of low- and high-carbohydrate diets for type 2 diabetes management: a randomized trial. Am J Clin Nutr. 2015;102(4):780–90.
189. Mingrone G, Panunzi S, De Gaetano A, Guidone C, Iaconelli A, Nanni G, et al. Bariatric-metabolic surgery versus conventional medical treatment in obese patients with type 2 diabetes: 5 year follow-up of an open-label, single-centre, randomised controlled trial. Lancet. 2015;386(9997):964–73.
190. Kim JH, Pyo JS, Cho WJ, Kim SY. The effects of bariatric surgery on type 2 diabetes in Asian populations: a meta-analysis of randomized controlled trials. Obes Surg. 2020;30(3):910–23.
191. Rubio-Almanza M, Hervas-Marin D, Camara-Gomez R, Caudet-Esteban J, Merino-Torres JF. Does metabolic surgery lead to diabetes remission in patients with BMI <30 kg/m(2)?: a meta-analysis. Obes Surg. 2019;29(4):1105–16.
192. Pickering TG, White WB, Giles TD, Black HR, Izzo JL, Materson BJ, et al. When and how to use self (home) and ambulatory blood pressure monitoring. J Am Soc Hypertens. 2010;4(2):56–61.
193. Emdin CA, Rahimi K, Neal B, Callender T, Perkovic V, Patel A. Blood pressure lowering in type 2 diabetes: a systematic review and meta-analysis. JAMA. 2015;313(6):603–15.
194. ACCORD Study Group, Cushman WC, Evans GW, Byington RP, Goff DC Jr, Grimm RH Jr, et al. Effects of intensive blood-pressure control in type 2 diabetes mellitus. N Engl J Med. 2010;362(17):1575–85.
195. Flack JM, Sica DA, Bakris G, Brown AL, Ferdinand KC, Grimm RH Jr, et al. Management of high blood pressure in blacks: an update of the International Society on Hypertension in Blacks Consensus Statement. Hypertension. 2010;56(5):780–800.
196. Nguyen QT, Anderson SR, Sanders L, Nguyen LD. Managing hypertension in the elderly: a common chronic disease with increasing age. Am Health Drug Benefits. 2012;5(3):146–53.
197. Bangalore S, Fakheri R, Toklu B, Messerli FH. Diabetes mellitus as a compelling indication for use of renin angiotensin system blockers: systematic review and meta-analysis of randomized trials. BMJ. 2016;352:i438.
198. Guerrero-Garcia C, Rubio-Guerra AF. Combination therapy in the treatment of hypertension. Drugs Context. 2018;7:212531.
199. Yusuf S, Teo KK, Pogue J, Dyal L, Copland I, Schumacher H, et al. Telmisartan, ramipril, or both in patients at high risk for vascular events. N Engl J Med. 2008;358(15):1547–59.
200. Hermida RC, Ayala DE, Mojon A, Fernandez JR. Influence of time of day of blood pressure-lowering treatment on cardiovascular risk in hypertensive patients with type 2 diabetes. Diabetes Care. 2011;34(6):1270–6.
201. Nicolucci A, Kovacs Burns K, Holt RI, Comaschi M, Hermanns N, Ishii H, et al. Diabetes attitudes, wishes and needs second study (DAWN2): cross-national benchmarking of diabetes-related psychosocial outcomes for people with diabetes. Diabet Med. 2013;30(7):767–77.
202. Nanayakkara N, Pease A, Ranasinha S, Wischer N, Andrikopoulos S, Speight J, et al. Depression and diabetes distress in adults with type 2 diabetes: results from the Australian National Diabetes Audit (ANDA) 2016. Sci Rep. 2018;8(1):7846.

203. Critchley JA, Capewell S. Mortality risk reduction associated with smoking cessation in patients with coronary heart disease: a systematic review. JAMA. 2003;290(1):86–97.
204. Wilkes S, Evans A. A cross-sectional study comparing the motivation for smoking cessation in apparently healthy patients who smoke to those who smoke and have ischaemic heart disease, hypertension or diabetes. Fam Pract. 1999;16(6):608–10.
205. West R. Tobacco smoking: health impact, prevalence, correlates and interventions. Psychol Health. 2017;32(8):1018–36.
206. Kalkhoran S, Glantz SA. E-cigarettes and smoking cessation in real-world and clinical settings: a systematic review and meta-analysis. Lancet Respir Med. 2016;4(2):116–28.
207. Dabelea D, Stafford JM, Mayer-Davis EJ, D'Agostino R Jr, Dolan L, Imperatore G, et al. Association of type 1 diabetes vs type 2 diabetes diagnosed during childhood and adolescence with complications during teenage years and young adulthood. JAMA. 2017;317(8):825–35.
208. Feng X, Song M, Preston MA, Ma W, Hu Y, Pernar CH, et al. The association of diabetes with risk of prostate cancer defined by clinical and molecular features. Br J Cancer. 2020;123(4):657–65.
209. Suh S, Kim KW. Diabetes and cancer: cancer should be screened in routine diabetes assessment. Diabetes Metab J. 2019;43(6):733–43.
210. Marchand L, Disse E, Dalle S, Reffet S, Vouillarmet J, Fabien N, et al. The multifaceted nature of diabetes mellitus induced by checkpoint inhibitors. Acta Diabetol. 2019;56(12):1239–45.
211. Gabbay RA, Kendall D, Beebe C, Cuddeback J, Hobbs T, Khan ND, et al. Addressing therapeutic inertia in 2020 and beyond: a 3-year initiative of the American Diabetes Association. Clin Diabetes. 2020;38(4):371–81.
212. Nguyen ATM, Akhter R, Garde S, Scott C, Twigg SM, Colagiuri S, et al. The association of periodontal disease with the complications of diabetes mellitus. A systematic review. Diabetes Res Clin Pract. 2020;165:108244.
213. Paul O, Arora P, Mayer M, Chatterjee S. Inflammation in periodontal disease: possible link to vascular disease. Front Physiol. 2020;11:609614.
214. Hwang Y, Khasag A, Jia W, Jenkins A, Huang CN, Yabe D, et al. Diabetes and COVID-19: IDF perspective in the Western Pacific region. Diabetes Res Clin Pract. 2020;166:108278.
215. Scott ES, Jenkins AJ, Fulcher GR. Challenges of diabetes management during the COVID-19 pandemic. Med J Aust. 2020;213(2):56–57 e51.
216. Prattichizzo F, de Candia P, Nicolucci A, Ceriello A. Elevated HbA1c levels in pre-COVID-19 infection increases the risk of mortality: a systematic review and meta-analysis. Diabetes Metab Res Rev. 2021;38:e3476.
217. Chrvala CA, Sherr D, Lipman RD. Diabetes self-management education for adults with type 2 diabetes mellitus: a systematic review of the effect on glycemic control. Patient Educ Couns. 2016;99(6):926–43.
218. Gunawan F, Ng HY, Gilfillan C, Anpalahan M. Ambulatory blood pressure monitoring in type 2 diabetes mellitus: a cross-sectional study. Curr Hypertens Rev. 2019;15(2):135–43.
219. Najafi MT, Khaloo P, Alemi H, Jaafarinia A, Blaha MJ, Mirbolouk M, et al. Ambulatory blood pressure monitoring and diabetes complications: targeting morning blood pressure surge and nocturnal dipping. Medicine (Baltimore). 2018;97(38):e12185.
220. Schwartz FL, Marling CR. Use of automated bolus calculators for diabetes management. Eur Endocrinol. 2013;9(2):92–5.
221. Sussman A, Taylor EJ, Patel M, Ward J, Alva S, Lawrence A, et al. Performance of a glucose meter with a built-in automated bolus calculator versus manual bolus calculation in insulin-using subjects. J Diabetes Sci Technol. 2012;6(2):339–44.
222. Cappon G, Vettoretti M, Sparacino G, Facchinetti A. Continuous glucose monitoring sensors for diabetes management: a review of technologies and applications. Diabetes Metab J. 2019;43(4):383–97.

223. Freckmann G, Pleus S, Grady M, Setford S, Levy B. Measures of accuracy for continuous glucose monitoring and blood glucose monitoring devices. J Diabetes Sci Technol. 2019;13(3):575–83.
224. Mian Z, Hermayer KL, Jenkins A. Continuous glucose monitoring: review of an innovation in diabetes management. Am J Med Sci. 2019;358(5):332–9.
225. Taylor PJ, Thompson CH, Brinkworth GD. Effectiveness and acceptability of continuous glucose monitoring for type 2 diabetes management: a narrative review. J Diabetes Investig. 2018;9(4):713–25.
226. Vigersky R, Shrivastav M. Role of continuous glucose monitoring for type 2 in diabetes management and research. J Diabetes Complicat. 2017;31(1):280–7.
227. Manski-Nankervis J, Yates CJ, Blackberry I, Furler J, Ginnivan L, Cohen N, et al. Impact of insulin initiation on glycaemic variability and glucose profiles in a primary healthcare type 2 diabetes cohort: analysis of continuous glucose monitoring data from the initiation study. Diabet Med. 2016;33(6):803–11.
228. Basu A, Veettil S, Dyer R, Peyser T, Basu R. Direct evidence of acetaminophen interference with subcutaneous glucose sensing in humans: a pilot study. Diabetes Technol Ther. 2016;18(Suppl 2):S243–7.
229. Basu A, Slama MQ, Nicholson WT, Langman L, Peyser T, Carter R, et al. Continuous glucose monitor interference with commonly prescribed medications: a pilot study. J Diabetes Sci Technol. 2017;11(5):936–41.
230. Tanenbaum ML, Hanes SJ, Miller KM, Naranjo D, Bensen R, Hood KK. Diabetes device use in adults with type 1 diabetes: barriers to uptake and potential intervention targets. Diabetes Care. 2017;40(2):181–7.
231. Vigersky RA, McMahon C. The relationship of hemoglobin A1c to time-in-range in patients with diabetes. Diabetes Technol Ther. 2019;21(2):81–5.
232. Ida S, Kaneko R, Murata K. Utility of real-time and retrospective continuous glucose monitoring in patients with type 2 diabetes mellitus: a meta-analysis of randomized controlled trials. J Diabetes Res. 2019;2019:4684815.
233. Janapala RN, Jayaraj JS, Fathima N, Kashif T, Usman N, Dasari A, et al. Continuous glucose monitoring versus self-monitoring of blood glucose in type 2 diabetes mellitus: a systematic review with meta-analysis. Cureus. 2019;11(9):e5634.
234. Park C, Le QA. The effectiveness of continuous glucose monitoring in patients with type 2 diabetes: a systematic review of literature and meta-analysis. Diabetes Technol Ther. 2018;20(9):613–21.
235. Shokrekhodaei M, Quinones S. Review of non-invasive glucose sensing techniques: optical, electrical and breath acetone. Sensors (Basel). 2020;20(5):1251.
236. Teymourian H, Moonla C, Tehrani F, Vargas E, Aghavali R, Barfidokht A, et al. Microneedle-based detection of ketone bodies along with glucose and lactate: toward real-time continuous interstitial fluid monitoring of diabetic ketosis and ketoacidosis. Anal Chem. 2020;92(2):2291–300.
237. Antithrombotic Trialists Collaboration, Baigent C, Blackwell L, Collins R, Emberson J, Godwin J, et al. Aspirin in the primary and secondary prevention of vascular disease: collaborative meta-analysis of individual participant data from randomised trials. Lancet. 2009;373(9678):1849–60.
238. Group ASC, Bowman L, Mafham M, Wallendszus K, Stevens W, Buck G, et al. Effects of aspirin for primary prevention in persons with diabetes mellitus. N Engl J Med. 2018;379(16):1529–39.
239. Chin J, Fulcher J, Jenkins A, Keech A. Is it time to repair a fairly fast SAAB convertible? Testing an evidence-based mnemonic for the secondary prevention of cardiovascular disease. Heart Lung Circ. 2015;24(5):480–7.
240. Raza S, Blackstone EH, Houghtaling PL, Rajeswaran J, Riaz H, Bakaeen FG, et al. Influence of diabetes on long-term coronary artery bypass graft patency. J Am Coll Cardiol. 2017;70(5):515–24.

241. Castelvecchio S, Menicanti L, Garatti A, Tramarin R, Volpe M, Parolari A. Myocardial revascularization for patients with diabetes: coronary artery bypass grafting or percutaneous coronary intervention? Ann Thorac Surg. 2016;102(3):1012–22.
242. Jimenez-Quevedo P, Sabate M, Angiolillo DJ, Alfonso F, Hernandez-Antolin R, SanMartin M, et al. Long-term clinical benefit of sirolimus-eluting stent implantation in diabetic patients with de novo coronary stenoses: long-term results of the diabetes trial. Eur Heart J. 2007;28(16):1946–52.
243. Delbridge L, Mellor K, Ritchie R, Jenkins A. The heart's performance when diabetes is the puppeteer. Diabetes Manag J. 2020;8–12.
244. Dunlay SM, Givertz MM, Aguilar D, Allen LA, Chan M, Desai AS, et al. Type 2 diabetes mellitus and heart failure: a scientific statement from the American Heart Association and the Heart Failure Society of America: this statement does not represent an update of the 2017 ACC/AHA/HFSA heart failure guideline update. Circulation. 2019;140(7):e294–324.
245. Kenny HC, Abel ED. Heart failure in type 2 diabetes mellitus. Circ Res. 2019;124(1):121–41.
246. McHugh K, DeVore AD, Wu J, Matsouaka RA, Fonarow GC, Heidenreich PA, et al. Heart failure with preserved ejection fraction and diabetes: JACC state-of-the-art review. J Am Coll Cardiol. 2019;73(5):602–11.
247. Sohrabi C, Saberwal B, Lim WY, Tousoulis D, Ahsan S, Papageorgiou N. Heart failure in diabetes mellitus: an updated review. Curr Pharm Des. 2020;26(46):5933–52.
248. Chia N, Fulcher J, Keech A. Beta-blocker, angiotensin-converting enzyme inhibitor/angiotensin receptor blocker, nitrate-hydralazine, diuretics, aldosterone antagonist, ivabradine, devices and digoxin (BANDAID(2)): an evidence-based mnemonic for the treatment of systolic heart failure. Intern Med J. 2016;46(6):653–62.
249. McMurray JJ, Packer M, Desai AS, Gong J, Lefkowitz MP, Rizkala AR, et al. Angiotensin-neprilysin inhibition versus enalapril in heart failure. N Engl J Med. 2014;371(11):993–1004.
250. He X, Li J, Wang B, Yao Q, Li L, Song R, et al. Diabetes self-management education reduces risk of all-cause mortality in type 2 diabetes patients: a systematic review and meta-analysis. Endocrine. 2017;55(3):712–31.
251. Carlsson LM, Peltonen M, Ahlin S, Anveden A, Bouchard C, Carlsson B, et al. Bariatric surgery and prevention of type 2 diabetes in Swedish obese subjects. N Engl J Med. 2012;367(8):695–704.
252. Ford ES, Zhao G, Li C. Pre-diabetes and the risk for cardiovascular disease: a systematic review of the evidence. J Am Coll Cardiol. 2010;55(13):1310–7.
253. Look ARG, Pi-Sunyer X, Blackburn G, Brancati FL, Bray GA, Bright R, et al. Reduction in weight and cardiovascular disease risk factors in individuals with type 2 diabetes: one-year results of the LOOK AHEAD trial. Diabetes Care. 2007;30(6):1374–83.
254. Rucker D, Padwal R, Li SK, Curioni C, Lau DC. Long term pharmacotherapy for obesity and overweight: updated meta-analysis. BMJ. 2007;335(7631):1194–9.
255. Panunzi S, Carlsson L, De Gaetano A, Peltonen M, Rice T, Sjostrom L, et al. Determinants of diabetes remission and glycemic control after bariatric surgery. Diabetes Care. 2016;39(1):166–74.
256. Brunström M, Carlberg B. Effect of antihypertensive treatment at different blood pressure levels in patients with diabetes mellitus: systematic review and meta-analyses. BMJ. 2016;352:i717.
257. Officers A, Coordinators for the ACRGTA, Lipid-Lowering Treatment to Prevent Heart Attack Trial. Major outcomes in high-risk hypertensive patients randomized to angiotensin-converting enzyme inhibitor or calcium channel blocker vs diuretic: the Antihypertensive and Lipid-Lowering treatment to prevent Heart Attack Trial (ALLHAT). JAMA. 2002;288(23):2981–97.
258. Staessen JA, Fagard R, Thijs L, Celis H, Arabidze GG, Birkenhager WH, et al. Randomised double-blind comparison of placebo and active treatment for older patients with isolated systolic hypertension. The Systolic Hypertension in Europe (SYST-EUR) Trial Investigators. Lancet. 1997;350(9080):757–64.

259. Bakris GL, Weir MR, Study of Hypertension and the Efficacy of Lotrel in Diabetes (SHIELD) Investigators. Achieving goal blood pressure in patients with type 2 diabetes: conventional versus fixed-dose combination approaches. J Clin Hypertens (Greenwich). 2003;5(3):202–9.
260. Omboni S, Gazzola T, Carabelli G, Parati G. Clinical usefulness and cost effectiveness of home blood pressure telemonitoring: meta-analysis of randomized controlled studies. J Hypertens. 2013;31(3):455–67; discussion 467–458.
261. Snoek FJ, Bremmer MA, Hermanns N. Constructs of depression and distress in diabetes: time for an appraisal. Lancet Diabetes Endocrinol. 2015;3(6):450–60.
262. Hutchinson A, McIntosh A, Peters J, O'Keeffe C, Khunti K, Baker R, et al. Effectiveness of screening and monitoring tests for diabetic retinopathy—a systematic review. Diabet Med. 2000;17(7):495–506.
263. Perkins BA, Olaleye D, Zinman B, Bril V. Simple screening tests for peripheral neuropathy in the diabetes clinic. Diabetes Care. 2001;24(2):250–6.
264. Franz MJ, MacLeod J, Evert A, Brown C, Gradwell E, Handu D, et al. Academy of nutrition and dietetics nutrition practice guideline for type 1 and type 2 diabetes in adults: systematic review of evidence for medical nutrition therapy effectiveness and recommendations for integration into the nutrition care process. J Acad Nutr Diet. 2017;117(10):1659–79.
265. Colberg SR, Sigal RJ, Fernhall B, Regensteiner JG, Blissmer BJ, Rubin RR, et al. Exercise and type 2 diabetes: the American College of Sports Medicine and the American Diabetes Association: joint position statement executive summary. Diabetes Care. 2010;33(12):2692–6.
266. Cosentino F, Grant PJ, Aboyans V, Bailey CJ, Ceriello A, Delgado V, et al. 2019 ESC guidelines on diabetes, pre-diabetes, and cardiovascular diseases developed in collaboration with the EASD. Eur Heart J. 2020;41(2):255–323.
267. Aschner P. New IDF clinical practice recommendations for managing type 2 diabetes in primary care. Diabetes Res Clin Pract. 2017;132:169–70.
268. Zinman B, Wanner C, Lachin JM, Fitchett D, Bluhmki E, Hantel S, et al. Empagliflozin, cardiovascular outcomes, and mortality in type 2 diabetes. N Engl J Med. 2015;373(22):2117–28.
269. Neal B, Perkovic V, Mahaffey KW, de Zeeuw D, Fulcher G, Erondu N, et al. Canagliflozin and cardiovascular and renal events in type 2 diabetes. N Engl J Med. 2017;377(7):644–57.
270. Wiviott SD, Raz I, Bonaca MP, Mosenzon O, Kato ET, Cahn A, et al. Dapagliflozin and cardiovascular outcomes in type 2 diabetes. N Engl J Med. 2019;380(4):347–57.
271. Perkovic V, Jardine MJ, Neal B, Bompoint S, Heerspink HJL, Charytan DM, et al. Canagliflozin and renal outcomes in type 2 diabetes and nephropathy. N Engl J Med. 2019;380(24):2295–306.
272. Butler J, Zannad F, Fitchett D, Zinman B, Koitka-Weber A, von Eynatten M, et al. Empagliflozin improves kidney outcomes in patients with or without heart failure. Circ Heart Fail. 2019;12(6):e005875.
273. Inzucchi SE, Fitchett D, Jurisic-Erzen D, Woo V, Hantel S, Janista C, et al. Are the cardiovascular and kidney benefits of empagliflozin influenced by baseline glucose-lowering therapy? Diabetes Obes Metab. 2020;22(4):631–9.
274. Levin A, Perkovic V, Wheeler DC, Hantel S, George JT, von Eynatten M, et al. Empagliflozin and cardiovascular and kidney outcomes across KDIGO risk categories: post hoc analysis of a randomized, double-blind, placebo-controlled, multinational trial. Clin J Am Soc Nephrol. 2020;15(10):1433–44.
275. Monteiro P, Bergenstal RM, Toural E, Inzucchi SE, Zinman B, Hantel S, et al. Efficacy and safety of empagliflozin in older patients in the EMPA-REG outcome(r) trial. Age Ageing. 2019;48(6):859–66.
276. Roy A, Maiti A, Sinha A, Baidya A, Basu AK, Sarkar D, et al. Kidney disease in type 2 diabetes mellitus and benefits of sodium-glucose cotransporter 2 inhibitors: a consensus statement. Diabetes Ther. 2020;11(12):2791–827.
277. Williams DM, Nawaz A, Evans M. Renal outcomes in type 2 diabetes: a review of cardiovascular and renal outcome trials. Diabetes Ther. 2020;11(2):369–86.

278. van Ruiten CC, van der Aart-van der Beek AB, Ijzerman RG, Nieuwdorp M, Hoogenberg K, van Raalte DH, et al. Effect of exenatide twice daily and dapagliflozin, alone and in combination, on markers of kidney function in obese patients with type 2 diabetes: a prespecified secondary analysis of a randomized controlled clinical trial. Diabetes Obes Metab. 2021;23(8):1851–8.
279. Kristensen SL, Rorth R, Jhund PS, Docherty KF, Sattar N, Preiss D, et al. Cardiovascular, mortality, and kidney outcomes with GLP-1 receptor agonists in patients with type 2 diabetes: a systematic review and meta-analysis of cardiovascular outcome trials. Lancet Diabetes Endocrinol. 2019;7(10):776–85.
280. Marso SP, Daniels GH, Brown-Frandsen K, Kristensen P, Mann JF, Nauck MA, et al. Liraglutide and cardiovascular outcomes in type 2 diabetes. N Engl J Med. 2016;375(4):311–22.
281. Marso SP, Bain SC, Consoli A, Eliaschewitz FG, Jodar E, Leiter LA, et al. Semaglutide and cardiovascular outcomes in patients with type 2 diabetes. N Engl J Med. 2016;375(19):1834–44.
282. Gerstein HC, Colhoun HM, Dagenais GR, Diaz R, Lakshmanan M, Pais P, et al. Dulaglutide and cardiovascular outcomes in type 2 diabetes (REWIND): a double-blind, randomised placebo-controlled trial. Lancet. 2019;394(10193):121–30.
283. Hernandez AF, Green JB, Janmohamed S, D'Agostino RB Sr, Granger CB, Jones NP, et al. Albiglutide and cardiovascular outcomes in patients with type 2 diabetes and cardiovascular disease (HARMONY outcomes): a double-blind, randomised placebo-controlled trial. Lancet. 2018;392(10157):1519–29.
284. Greco EV, Russo G, Giandalia A, Viazzi F, Pontremoli R, De Cosmo S. GLP-1 receptor agonists and kidney protection. Medicina (Kaunas). 2019;55(6):233.
285. Green JB, Bethel MA, Armstrong PW, Buse JB, Engel SS, Garg J, et al. Effect of sitagliptin on cardiovascular outcomes in type 2 diabetes. N Engl J Med. 2015;373(3):232–42.
286. Rosenstock J, Perkovic V, Johansen OE, Cooper ME, Kahn SE, Marx N, et al. Effect of linagliptin vs placebo on major cardiovascular events in adults with type 2 diabetes and high cardiovascular and renal risk: the Carmelina randomized clinical trial. JAMA. 2019;321(1):69–79.
287. Scirica BM, Bhatt DL, Braunwald E, Steg PG, Davidson J, Hirshberg B, et al. Saxagliptin and cardiovascular outcomes in patients with type 2 diabetes mellitus. N Engl J Med. 2013;369(14):1317–26.
288. White WB, Cannon CP, Heller SR, Nissen SE, Bergenstal RM, Bakris GL, et al. Alogliptin after acute coronary syndrome in patients with type 2 diabetes. N Engl J Med. 2013;369(14):1327–35.
289. Li L, Li S, Deng K, Liu J, Vandvik PO, Zhao P, et al. Dipeptidyl peptidase-4 inhibitors and risk of heart failure in type 2 diabetes: systematic review and meta-analysis of randomised and observational studies. BMJ. 2016;352:i610.
290. Zhan S, Tang M, Liu F, Xia P, Shu M, Wu X. Ezetimibe for the prevention of cardiovascular disease and all-cause mortality events. Cochrane Database Syst Rev. 2018;11:CD012502.
291. Scott R, O'Brien R, Fulcher G, Pardy C, D'Emden M, Tse D, et al. Effects of fenofibrate treatment on cardiovascular disease risk in 9,795 individuals with type 2 diabetes and various components of the metabolic syndrome: the Fenofibrate Intervention and Event Lowering in Diabetes (FIELD) study. Diabetes Care. 2009;32(3):493–8.
292. Ginsberg HN. The ACCORD (Action to Control Cardiovascular Risk in Diabetes) lipid trial: what we learn from subgroup analyses. Diabetes Care. 2011;34(Suppl 2):S107–8.
293. Millan J, Pinto X, Brea A, Blasco M, Hernandez-Mijares A, Ascaso J, et al. Fibrates in the secondary prevention of cardiovascular disease (infarction and stroke). Results of a systematic review and meta-analysis of the Cochrane collaboration. Clin Investig Arterioscler. 2018;30(1):30–5.
294. Schmidt AF, Carter JL, Pearce LS, Wilkins JT, Overington JP, Hingorani AD, et al. PCSK9 monoclonal antibodies for the primary and secondary prevention of cardiovascular disease. Cochrane Database Syst Rev. 2020;10:CD011748.

295. Sabatine MS, Giugliano RP, Keech AC, Honarpour N, Wiviott SD, Murphy SA, et al. Evolocumab and clinical outcomes in patients with cardiovascular disease. N Engl J Med. 2017;376(18):1713–22.
296. Prattichizzo F, de Candia P, De Nigris V, Nicolucci A, Ceriello A. Legacy effect of intensive glucose control on major adverse cardiovascular outcome: systematic review and meta-analyses of trials according to different scenarios. Metabolism. 2020;110:154308.
297. Wang X, Qin LQ, Arafa A, Eshak ES, Hu Y, Dong JY. Smoking cessation, weight gain, cardiovascular risk, and all-cause mortality: a meta-analysis. Nicotine Tob Res. 2021;23(12):1987–94.
298. Critchley J, Capewell S. Smoking cessation for the secondary prevention of coronary heart disease. Cochrane Database Syst Rev. 2004;(1):CD003041.
299. Pranata R, Vania R, Victor AA. Statin reduces the incidence of diabetic retinopathy and its need for intervention: a systematic review and meta-analysis. Eur J Ophthalmol. 2021;31(3):1216–24.
300. Shen X, Zhang Z, Zhang X, Zhao J, Zhou X, Xu Q, et al. Efficacy of statins in patients with diabetic nephropathy: a meta-analysis of randomized controlled trials. Lipids Health Dis. 2016;15(1):179.
301. Morgan CL, Owens DR, Aubonnet P, Carr ES, Jenkins-Jones S, Poole CD, et al. Primary prevention of diabetic retinopathy with fibrates: a retrospective, matched cohort study. BMJ Open. 2013;3(12):e004025.
302. Rajamani K, Donoghoe M, Li L, Ting R-D, Colman PG, Drury P, et al. Abstract 18987: Fenofibrate reduces peripheral neuropathy in type 2 diabetes: the Fenofibrate Intervention and Event Lowering in Diabetes (FIELD) study. Circulation. 2010;122(suppl_21):A18987.
303. Do DV, Wang X, Vedula SS, Marrone M, Sleilati G, Hawkins BS, et al. Blood pressure control for diabetic retinopathy. Cochrane Database Syst Rev. 2015;1:CD006127.
304. Sjolie AK, Klein R, Porta M, Orchard T, Fuller J, Parving HH, et al. Effect of candesartan on progression and regression of retinopathy in type 2 diabetes (DIRECT-PROTECT 2): a randomised placebo-controlled trial. Lancet. 2008;372(9647):1385–93.
305. Haller H, Ito S, Izzo JL Jr, Januszewicz A, Katayama S, Menne J, et al. Olmesartan for the delay or prevention of microalbuminuria in type 2 diabetes. N Engl J Med. 2011;364(10):907–17.
306. Heart Outcomes Prevention Evaluation Study Investigators. Effects of ramipril on cardiovascular and microvascular outcomes in people with diabetes mellitus: results of the hope study and micro-hope substudy. Lancet. 2000;355(9200):253–9.
307. Estacio RO, Jeffers BW, Gifford N, Schrier RW. Effect of blood pressure control on diabetic microvascular complications in patients with hypertension and type 2 diabetes. Diabetes Care. 2000;23(Suppl 2):B54–64.
308. Schrier RW, Estacio RO, Esler A, Mehler P. Effects of aggressive blood pressure control in normotensive type 2 diabetic patients on albuminuria, retinopathy and strokes. Kidney Int. 2002;61(3):1086–97.
309. MacIsaac RJ, Jerums G, Ekinci EI. Effects of glycaemic management on diabetic kidney disease. World J Diabetes. 2017;8(5):172–86.
310. Callaghan BC, Little AA, Feldman EL, Hughes RA. Enhanced glucose control for preventing and treating diabetic neuropathy. Cochrane Database Syst Rev. 2012;(6):CD007543.
311. Ang L, Jaiswal M, Martin C, Pop-Busui R. Glucose control and diabetic neuropathy: lessons from recent large clinical trials. Curr Diab Rep. 2014;14(9):528.
312. Zoungas S, Patel A, Chalmers J, de Galan BE, Li Q, Billot L, et al. Severe hypoglycemia and risks of vascular events and death. N Engl J Med. 2010;363(15):1410–8.
313. Kotwal S, Jun M, Sullivan D, Perkovic V, Neal B. Omega 3 fatty acids and cardiovascular outcomes: systematic review and meta-analysis. Circ Cardiovasc Qual Outcomes. 2012;5(6):808–18.
314. Bhatt DL, Steg PG, Miller M, Brinton EA, Jacobson TA, Ketchum SB, et al. Cardiovascular risk reduction with icosapent ethyl for hypertriglyceridemia. N Engl J Med. 2019;380(1):11–22.
315. Cannon CP, Blazing MA, Giugliano RP, McCagg A, White JA, Theroux P, et al. Ezetimibe added to statin therapy after acute coronary syndromes. N Engl J Med. 2015;372(25):2387–97.

316. Wallentin L, Becker RC, Budaj A, Cannon CP, Emanuelsson H, Held C, et al. Ticagrelor versus clopidogrel in patients with acute coronary syndromes. N Engl J Med. 2009;361(11):1045–57.
317. Aradi D, Komocsi A, Vorobcsuk A, Serebruany VL. Impact of clopidogrel and potent P2Y 12 -inhibitors on mortality and stroke in patients with acute coronary syndrome or undergoing percutaneous coronary intervention: a systematic review and meta-analysis. Thromb Haemost. 2013;109(1):93–101.
318. Wiviott SD, Braunwald E, McCabe CH, Montalescot G, Ruzyllo W, Gottlieb S, et al. Prasugrel versus clopidogrel in patients with acute coronary syndromes. N Engl J Med. 2007;357(20):2001–15.
319. Levine GN, Bates ER, Bittl JA, Brindis RG, Fihn SD, Fleisher LA, et al. 2016 ACC/AHA guideline focused update on duration of dual antiplatelet therapy in patients with coronary artery disease: a report of the American College of Cardiology/American Heart Association task force on clinical practice guidelines: an update of the 2011 ACCF/AHA/SCAI guideline for percutaneous coronary intervention, 2011 ACCF/AHA guideline for coronary artery bypass graft surgery, 2012 ACC/AHA/ACP/AATS/PCNA/SCAI/STS guideline for the diagnosis and management of patients with stable ischemic heart disease, 2013 ACCF/AHA guideline for the management of ST-elevation myocardial infarction, 2014 AHA/ACC guideline for the management of patients with non-ST-elevation acute coronary syndromes, and 2014 ACC/AHA guideline on perioperative cardiovascular evaluation and management of patients undergoing noncardiac surgery. Circulation. 2016;134(10):e123–55.
320. Saha SA, Molnar J, Arora RR. Tissue ace inhibitors for secondary prevention of cardiovascular disease in patients with preserved left ventricular function: a pooled meta-analysis of randomized placebo-controlled trials. J Cardiovasc Pharmacol Ther. 2007;12(3):192–204.
321. Saha SA, Molnar J, Arora RR. Tissue angiotensin-converting enzyme inhibitors for the prevention of cardiovascular disease in patients with diabetes mellitus without left ventricular systolic dysfunction or clinical evidence of heart failure: a pooled meta-analysis of randomized placebo-controlled clinical trials. Diabetes Obes Metab. 2008;10(1):41–52.
322. Pitt B, Remme W, Zannad F, Neaton J, Martinez F, Roniker B, et al. Eplerenone, a selective aldosterone blocker, in patients with left ventricular dysfunction after myocardial infarction. N Engl J Med. 2003;348(14):1309–21.
323. Chatterjee S, Moeller C, Shah N, Bolorunduro O, Lichstein E, Moskovits N, et al. Eplerenone is not superior to older and less expensive aldosterone antagonists. Am J Med. 2012;125(8):817–25.
324. Freemantle N, Cleland J, Young P, Mason J, Harrison J. Beta blockade after myocardial infarction: systematic review and meta regression analysis. BMJ. 1999;318(7200):1730–7.
325. Davies MJ, D'Alessio DA, Fradkin J, Kernan WN, Mathieu C, Mingrone G, et al. Management of hyperglycemia in type 2 diabetes, 2018. A consensus report by the American Diabetes Association (ADA) and the European Association for the Study of Diabetes (EASD). Diabetes Care. 2018;41(12):2669–701.
326. Brophy JM, Joseph L, Rouleau JL. Beta-blockers in congestive heart failure. A Bayesian meta-analysis. Ann Intern Med. 2001;134(7):550–60.
327. Garg R, Yusuf S. Overview of randomized trials of angiotensin-converting enzyme inhibitors on mortality and morbidity in patients with heart failure. Collaborative group on ACE inhibitor trials. JAMA. 1995;273(18):1450–6.
328. Heran BS, Musini VM, Bassett K, Taylor RS, Wright JM. Angiotensin receptor blockers for heart failure. Cochrane Database Syst Rev. 2012;(4):CD003040.
329. Cohn JN, Archibald DG, Ziesche S, Franciosa JA, Harston WE, Tristani FE, et al. Effect of vasodilator therapy on mortality in chronic congestive heart failure. Results of a Veterans Administration cooperative study. N Engl J Med. 1986;314(24):1547–52.
330. Cohn JN, Johnson G, Ziesche S, Cobb F, Francis G, Tristani F, et al. A comparison of enalapril with hydralazine-isosorbide dinitrate in the treatment of chronic congestive heart failure. N Engl J Med. 1991;325(5):303–10.

331. Faris RF, Flather M, Purcell H, Poole-Wilson PA, Coats AJ. Diuretics for heart failure. Cochrane Database Syst Rev. 2012;(2):CD003838.
332. Ezekowitz JA, McAlister FA. Aldosterone blockade and left ventricular dysfunction: a systematic review of randomized clinical trials. Eur Heart J. 2009;30(4):469–77.
333. Swedberg K, Komajda M, Bohm M, Borer JS, Ford I, Dubost-Brama A, et al. Ivabradine and outcomes in chronic heart failure (shift): a randomised placebo-controlled study. Lancet. 2010;376(9744):875–85.
334. Nanthakumar K, Epstein AE, Kay GN, Plumb VJ, Lee DS. Prophylactic implantable cardioverter-defibrillator therapy in patients with left ventricular systolic dysfunction: a pooled analysis of 10 primary prevention trials. J Am Coll Cardiol. 2004;44(11):2166–72.
335. Cleland JG, Abraham WT, Linde C, Gold MR, Young JB, Claude Daubert J, et al. An individual patient meta-analysis of five randomized trials assessing the effects of cardiac resynchronization therapy on morbidity and mortality in patients with symptomatic heart failure. Eur Heart J. 2013;34(46):3547–56.
336. Hood WB Jr, Dans AL, Guyatt GH, Jaeschke R, McMurray JJ. Digitalis for treatment of congestive heart failure in patients in sinus rhythm. Cochrane Database Syst Rev. 2004;(2):CD002901.
337. Vilsboll T, Bain SC, Leiter LA, Lingvay I, Matthews D, Simo R, et al. Semaglutide, reduction in glycated haemoglobin and the risk of diabetic retinopathy. Diabetes Obes Metab. 2018;20(4):889–97.
338. Wright AD, Dodson PM. Medical management of diabetic retinopathy: Fenofibrate and accord eye studies. Eye (Lond). 2011;25(7):843–9.
339. Duh EJ, Sun JK, Stitt AW. Diabetic retinopathy: current understanding, mechanisms, and treatment strategies. JCI Insight. 2017;2(14):e93751.
340. Barnett AH, Bain SC, Bouter P, Karlberg B, Madsbad S, Jervell J, et al. Angiotensin-receptor blockade versus converting-enzyme inhibition in type 2 diabetes and nephropathy. N Engl J Med. 2004;351(19):1952–61.
341. Neumiller JJ, Kalyani RR. How does credence inform best use of SGLT2 inhibitors in CKD? Clin J Am Soc Nephrol. 2019;14(11):1667–9.
342. Ting RD, Keech AC, Drury PL, Donoghoe MW, Hedley J, Jenkins AJ, et al. Benefits and safety of long-term fenofibrate therapy in people with type 2 diabetes and renal impairment: the FIELD study. Diabetes Care. 2012;35(2):218–25.
343. Mychaleckyj JC, Craven T, Nayak U, Buse J, Crouse JR, Elam M, et al. Reversibility of fenofibrate therapy-induced renal function impairment in accord type 2 diabetic participants. Diabetes Care. 2012;35(5):1008–14.
344. Freeman R, Durso-Decruz E, Emir B. Efficacy, safety, and tolerability of pregabalin treatment for painful diabetic peripheral neuropathy: findings from seven randomized, controlled trials across a range of doses. Diabetes Care. 2008;31(7):1448–54.
345. Quilici S, Chancellor J, Lothgren M, Simon D, Said G, Le TK, et al. Meta-analysis of duloxetine vs. Pregabalin and gabapentin in the treatment of diabetic peripheral neuropathic pain. BMC Neurol. 2009;9:6.
346. Wernicke JF, Pritchett YL, D'Souza DN, Waninger A, Tran P, Iyengar S, et al. A randomized controlled trial of duloxetine in diabetic peripheral neuropathic pain. Neurology. 2006;67(8):1411–20.
347. Joss JD. Tricyclic antidepressant use in diabetic neuropathy. Ann Pharmacother. 1999;33(9):996–1000.
348. Vallianou N, Evangelopoulos A, Koutalas P. Alpha-lipoic acid and diabetic neuropathy. Rev Diabet Stud. 2009;6(4):230–6.
349. Treatment of painful diabetic neuropathy with topical capsaicin. A multicenter, double-blind, vehicle-controlled study. The capsaicin study group. Arch Intern Med. 1991;151(11):2225–9.
350. Derry S, Wiffen PJ, Moore RA, Quinlan J. Topical lidocaine for neuropathic pain in adults. Cochrane Database Syst Rev. 2014;(7):CD010958.

Chapter 2
Precision Medicine for Diabetes and Cardiovascular Disease

Siu-Hin Wan and Horng H. Chen

Introduction

Cardiovascular disease is one of the leading causes of morbidity and mortality in the world, and diabetes mellitus plays a significant role in the development and progression of the most common types of heart disease. Understanding how these two entities are intricately connected allows for better risk stratification, prevention, prognostication, and management of patients with both diabetes and heart disease.

Cardiovascular and Metabolic Cross-talk

The development of heart failure in diabetes mellitus is complex and involves multiple mechanisms. Diabetes can lead to heart failure development, and heart failure can lead to diabetes development. Diabetes leads to hyperglycemia, insulin resistance, and hyperinsulinemia, resulting in heart failure development. This promotes coronary artery disease due to increased inflammation, hyperlipidemia, microvascular and macrovascular disease, and endothelial dysfunction. Additionally, diabetes results in direct hypertrophy of cardiomyocytes, increased fibrosis due to activation of the renin angiotensin aldosterone system, and formation of advanced glycation end products [1, 2]. These mechanisms comprise diabetic cardiomyopathy and subsequently lead to heart failure.

S.-H. Wan
Minneapolis Heart Institute, United Hospital, Saint Paul, MN, USA

H. H. Chen (✉)
Department of Cardiovascular Diseases, Mayo Clinic, Rochester, MN, USA
e-mail: chen.horng@mayo.edu

R. Basu (ed.), *Precision Medicine in Diabetes*,
https://doi.org/10.1007/978-3-030-98927-9_2

Heart failure also leads to the development of diabetes. In heart failure, increased sympathetic nervous system activation and increased renin angiotensin aldosterone activation lead to cytokine release and vasoconstriction. Increased free fatty acids and effects on the pancreas, muscles, and liver result in hyperglycemia as well as insulin resistance, leading to diabetes [3].

Heart failure is a risk factor for diabetes mellitus development. Whereas the general population incidence of diabetes is approximately 10 per 1000 person years, those with heart failure have an incidence of 20–30 per 1000 person years [4]. Additionally, those with heart failure and the following comorbidities are at even higher risk of incident diabetes development: obesity, tobacco history, elevated HbA1c, higher blood pressure, longer duration of heart failure, diuretic therapy, and worse NYHA functional class.

There is increasingly greater evidence that natriuretic peptides have favorable cardiometabolic effects, including on fat metabolism and glucose handling [5]. Several studies have demonstrated an inverse relationship between plasma natriuretic peptides levels and the risk for development of type 2 diabetes [6–8]. In obesity, as well as exogenous insulin administration, natriuretic peptide levels are low with downregulation of the receptor, and this deficiency of the natriuretic peptide system may be linked to diabetes development [9]. Natriuretic peptide deficiency therefore is associated with an increased risk for diabetes. Genetic variants that result in an elevation of natriuretic peptides are linked to lower risk of metabolic syndrome and diabetes [10]. Infusion of BNP was shown to improve insulin sensitivity and blood glucose control [11, 12].

Given the cardiometabolic and neurohormonal dysfunction in diabetes and heart failure, natriuretic peptides play an important role in rescuing the failing heart. Natriuretic peptides ANP and BNP are released when there is fluid overload. For the cardiovascular system, natriuretic peptides result in natriuresis, vasodilation, inhibition of the renin angiotensin aldosterone system, and anti-fibrosis and relaxation. For metabolic effects, ANP results in increased fatty oxidation in the muscles, increased lipolysis, decreased inflammation, and subsequent increase in insulin sensitivity and improved glycemic control [13]. Therefore, natriuretic peptides have beneficial cardiovascular and endocrine effects, making them potential treatment candidates for diabetic heart disease.

Cardiovascular Complications of Diabetes

Diabetes promotes heart disease, including accelerated atherosclerosis, hypertension, direct damage to the myocardium, and subsequent development of heart failure (Fig. 2.1).

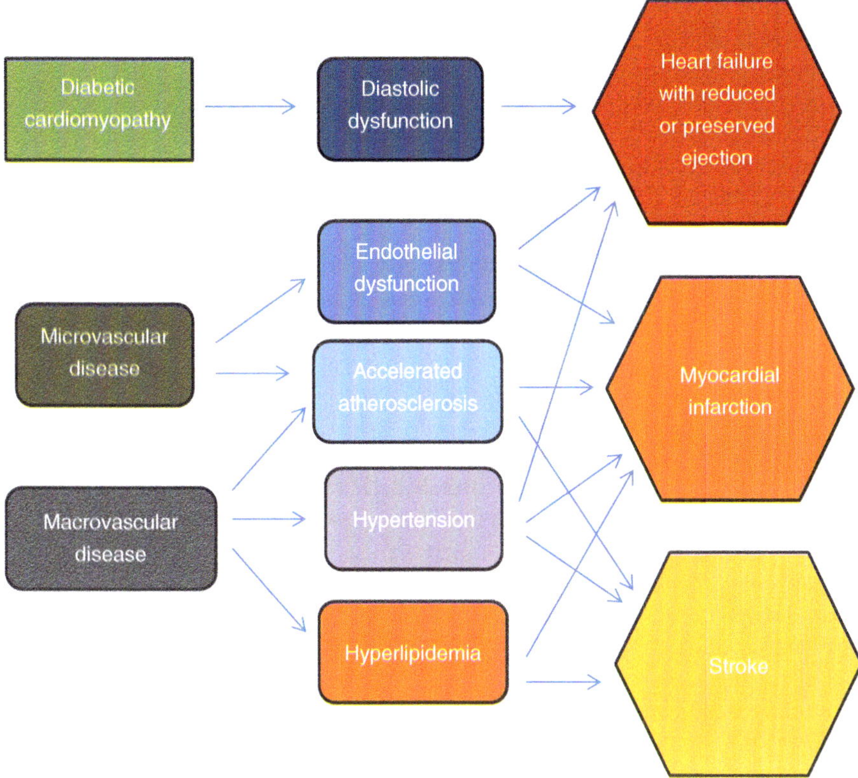

Fig. 2.1 Mechanisms of heart disease in diabetes

Coronary Artery Disease

Hyperglycemia in diabetes mellitus leads to multiple mechanisms that accelerate coronary artery disease, including inflammation and damage of coronary arteries, proliferation of vascular smooth muscle, hyperlipidemia, and endothelial dysfunction. Microvascular and macrovascular disease is a hallmark of diabetes sequalae. Angiographic studies in patients with diabetes demonstrate greater disease burden and greater likelihood of multivessel coronary artery disease [14, 15]. Coronary artery calcification on CT imaging and myocardial flow reserve by PET imaging also demonstrate greater coronary disease among those with diabetes [16, 17]. Furthermore, disease burden is directly associated with blood glucose.

Mechanisms of increased cardiovascular risk include endothelial dysfunction and increased thrombosis risk. Endothelial dysfunction is one of the mechanisms by which diabetes leads to worse coronary outcomes. Insulin resistance is thought to contribute to this pathophysiology, and antiglycemic agents appear to reverse endothelial dysfunction [18, 19].

There is also increased risk of coronary thrombosis and plaque rupture in diabetes. There is platelet dysfunction and increased platelet activation and aggregation in diabetes [20]. Other mechanisms include increase in fibrinogen with reduction in fibrinolysis, increased lipid composition of plaque, and greater risk of rupture [21–23]. These mechanisms result in greater risk of myocardial infarctions and strokes.

One of the challenges of managing patients with coronary artery disease and diabetes is that the variety of mechanisms by which diabetes acts result in atypical patient presentations. Symptoms of coronary artery disease may be atypical angina, or patients may be completely asymptomatic, which increases the importance of early aggressive prevention. Neuropathy and autonomic denervation in diabetes result in atypical symptoms or the absence of symptoms [24].

Hypertension

Hypertension is strongly correlated with diabetes and leads to cardiac remodeling. Microvascular and macrovascular damage in diabetes may lead to the development of hypertension [25]. Accelerated atherosclerosis results in hypertension, which subsequently worsens cardiac disease. Chronic increases in afterload result in cardiac remodeling and myocyte hypertrophy. This can subsequently lead to diastolic dysfunction and symptomatic heart failure with preserved ejection fraction. This can also lead to disruption in normal coronary flow and further acceleration in atherosclerosis.

Diabetic Cardiomyopathy

Myocardial damage can arise from ischemic heart disease and coronary artery disease. In addition, further damage is caused by the entity of diabetic cardiomyopathy, or direct myocardial damage and increased fibrosis from increased inflammation and oxidative stress associated with the diabetic state that cannot be explained by coronary artery disease or hypertension. Advanced glycation end products deposit in the myocardium. Diabetic cardiomyopathy is characterized structurally by increased left ventricular mass, diastolic dysfunction, and, in latter stages, systolic dysfunction [26]. Pathologically, this is reflected by myocardial fibrosis, interstitial infiltration, and myocardial capillary disarray.

Population-based studies have demonstrated that those with diabetes mellitus and diastolic dysfunction are twice as likely to develop symptomatic heart failure and have worse mortality outcomes [27].

Heart Failure

The development of heart failure is multifactorial and includes all the above discussed mechanism. Coronary artery disease and hypertension lead to ischemic heart disease and can subsequently result in heart failure. Diabetes results in myocyte hypertrophy, myocardial damage from advanced glycation end products and increased inflammatory pathways, and abnormal endothelial function. All these mechanisms including coronary artery disease, hypertension, and diabetic cardiomyopathy contribute to symptomatic heart failure.

Epidemiology and Burden of Diabetes and Heart Disease

Coronary Artery Disease

There is a strong association between diabetes and coronary artery disease. Subjects with type 2 diabetes are at significantly increased risk of developing myocardial infarction and death (Table 2.1). Those with type 2 diabetes are at a 20% risk of developing a myocardial infarction over a 7-year period [28]. Diabetes is an independent risk factor for cardiovascular disease and increases risk in the population by 2 to 3 times [29]. In general, the presence of diabetes increases risk to such an extent that its presence alone is equivalent to a prior myocardial infarction [28].

Mortality is similarly increased, with 10% versus 3% mortality over a 12-year period among those with diabetes versus those without [30].

Additionally, there is gender disparity in risk. Females have increased risk for worse cardiovascular outcomes with diabetes, compared to males [31].

Heart Failure

Those with diabetes are at significantly increased risk of developing heart failure. In population studies, diabetes was found to be an independent predictor for the development of heart failure. Those with diabetes have a two times higher incidence of heart failure development than those without diabetes, even after adjusting for age and gender, and using multivariable cox regression analysis [32]. Risk ranges from 2 to 10 times compared to those without diabetes and may be higher for females and younger individuals [4, 33–39]. Additionally, increased risk of heart failure in diabetes is also correlated with longer duration of diabetes, poor glycemic control,

Table 2.1 Burden of heart disease and diabetes

Risk with diabetes	
Cardiovascular outcomes and burden	
Myocardial infarction, 7-year period	20%
Mortality, 12-year period	10%
Relative risk heart failure development	2–10×

[28, 29]
[30, 31]
[4, 33–39]

obesity, renal dysfunction, and additional cardiovascular comorbidities such as coronary artery disease and peripheral artery disease. Studies show that the prevalence of diabetic cardiomyopathy in the general population is approximately 1.1% [40].

Once patients with diabetes develop heart failure, they become at increased risk of poor outcomes, including hospitalization and mortality [41, 42]. Those with diabetes and heart failure with preserved ejection fraction had an even higher risk of heart failure hospitalization and mortality compared to those with reduced ejection fraction. Furthermore, those with pre-diabetes and heart failure are also at increased risk of worse outcomes.

Hypertension

Metabolic syndrome is a condition where diabetes, obesity, hypertension, and hyperlipidemia co-exist. Diabetes, in addition to being an independent risk factor for cardiovascular disease, is associated with many cardiovascular risk factors, including hypertension. Treatment for hypertension is also more aggressive among patients with diabetes, given increased cardiovascular risk when these two conditions exist concurrently.

Hyperlipidemia

Those with diabetes are more likely to have dyslipidemia. Those with type 2 diabetes tend to have hypertriglyceridemia and high LDL cholesterol, which may be secondary to insulin resistance and increased serum levels of insulin. Studies suggest treatment with aggressive lipid lowering, particularly with statin class medications for LDL reduction [43–45].

Management of Diabetes and Heart Disease

Glycemic Control

The cardiovascular disease outcomes, including myocardial infarction and death among those with type 2 diabetes, are directly related to glycemic control in addition to multifaceted risk factor reduction, and this principle remains the foundation for management of patients with diabetes [46]. Mechanistically, there is microvascular benefit with glycemic control, although macrovascular benefits have not been directly demonstrated. Therefore, for macrovascular disease prevention, including myocardial infarction and stroke, glycemic control should be combined with lifestyle modifications such as exercise, diet, lipid management, and tobacco cessation.

Multifactor risk reduction should include exercise, as well as aggressive blood pressure and dyslipidemia management. Exercise in observational studies has been shown to decrease cardiovascular mortality among those with diabetes [47].

Studies have shown that for each increase in 1% of HbA1c, there is a 1.2–1.4 relative odds of cardiovascular disease and all-cause mortality [48–50]. The mechanism of benefit is thought to be reduction in microvascular disease.

Pharmacologic Agents

While traditionally, metformin and insulin for aggressive glycemic control (target HbA1c ≤7%) have been the treatment of choice for those with diabetes, more recent data have supported benefits of specific classes of diabetes pharmacologic agents [51].

For those with concurrent heart failure with reduced ejection fraction and diabetes, treatment should focus on guideline-directed medical therapy for heart failure with reduced ejection fraction (HFrEF). Studies have demonstrated that regardless of diabetes status, guideline-directed medical therapy for HFrEF has similar beneficial effects in outcomes including hospitalization and mortality in patients.

Pharmacologic agents that act on the renin-angiotensin-aldosterone system, such as ACE inhibitors, angiotensin receptor blockers, and angiotensin receptor-neprilysin inhibitors, have beneficial effects in this population [4]. Additionally, the use of such agents in those with diabetes may portend long-term beneficial renal effects.

Beta-blockers also have an important role in the treatment of heart failure with reduced ejection fraction. Among those with diabetes, there is a similar benefit in reducing hospitalization and mortality. Furthermore, of the recommended beta-blockers for HFrEF, carvedilol, metoprolol succinate, and bisoprolol, carvedilol may be preferred due to greater effects on glycemic reduction [52].

Mineralocorticoid receptor antagonists (MRA), including spironolactone, also have proven benefit in HFrEF. Caution though should be implemented, as in the presence of diabetes and particularly renal dysfunction, these agents can cause hyperkalemia and should be avoided in this situation. MRAs may also have a benefit among those with heart failure with preserved ejection fraction [53].

SGLT2 Inhibitors

Sodium glucose cotransporter 2 (SGLT2) inhibitors act mainly by preventing reabsorption of urinary glucose in the proximal tubule. In addition to lifestyle modification and metformin, emerging data have demonstrated improved cardiac and renal outcomes for those with diabetes and cardiovascular disease. Specifically, trials have demonstrated benefit in those with diabetes and coronary artery disease and heart failure [54–56].

There has been recent robust data for the benefit of SGLT2 inhibitors for patients with diabetes and heart failure [57]. Specifically, heart failure hospitalization and cardiovascular mortality are reduced with this class of agents. This benefit is thought to be in addition to that provided by serum glucose reduction and is a pharmacologic agent class effect. Furthermore, there is also benefit in prevention of worsening renal disease in addition to glycemic control and cardiovascular benefit [58].

GLP1 Agonists

Glucagon-like peptide-1 receptor (GLP1) agonist is a novel class of antiglycemic agent that has also demonstrated favorable outcomes in diabetes and heart disease [59]. GLP1 agonists activate the GLP1 receptor, resulting in greater insulin synthesis and release of insulin. Benefits of GLP1 agonists, in addition to serum glucose reduction, also include weight loss and blood pressure. Studies have demonstrated that in those with type 2 diabetes, addition of a GLP1 agonist results in lower cardiovascular event rates and lower all-cause mortality [60].

Natriuretic Peptides

Natriuretic peptide deficiency is caused in part by insulin resistance and obesity. Natriuretic peptide deficiency leads to diabetes development, hypertension, and hypertrophy of the myocardium [61]. Genetic variants may play a role in levels of circulating natriuretic peptides, and further studies into the genetic variants in natriuretic peptide expression may provide insights into development of diabetes and heart failure [62].

Further studies are needed to determine if natriuretic peptide supplementation might result in prevention of diabetes and heart failure, given that low levels of circulating natriuretic peptides are associated with higher risk of diabetes development [63]. Post hoc analysis from the PARADIGM-HF trial showed that neprilysin inhibition, which raises natriuretic peptide levels, results in greater reduction in HbA1c [64]. Promising are studies showing infusion of BNP resulted in lower plasma glucose after loading [65].

Summary

In summary, cardiovascular disease and diabetes are closely related and major contributors to worldwide morbidity and mortality. Mechanism of cardiovascular disease in diabetes is multifactorial and includes microvascular and macrovascular damage, accelerated atherosclerosis, increased inflammatory pathways, direct myocardial damage, and development of heart failure. These two conditions are prevalent, and diabetes increases development and progression of heart disease. The foundation of treatment is glycemic control for microvascular benefit, but novel pharmacologic agents such as SGLT2 inhibitors and GLP1 agonists provide additional improvements in cardiovascular morbidity and mortality.

Disclosures Dr. Chen has patented designer peptides.

References

1. Horwich TB, Fonarow GC. Glucose, obesity, metabolic syndrome, and diabetes relevance to incidence of heart failure. J Am Coll Cardiol. 2010;55(4):283–93.
2. Dei Cas A, Khan SS, Butler J, Mentz RJ, Bonow RO, Avogaro A, et al. Impact of diabetes on epidemiology, treatment, and outcomes of patients with heart failure. JACC Heart Fail. 2015;3(2):136–45.
3. Ashrafian H, Frenneaux MP, Opie LH. Metabolic mechanisms in heart failure. Circulation. 2007;116(4):434–48.
4. Dunlay SM, Givertz MM, Aguilar D, Allen LA, Chan M, Desai AS, et al. Type 2 diabetes mellitus and heart failure: a scientific statement from the American Heart Association and the Heart Failure Society of America: this statement does not represent an update of the 2017 ACC/AHA/HFSA heart failure guideline update. Circulation. 2019;140(7):e294–324.
5. Vinnakota S, Chen HH. The importance of natriuretic peptides in cardiometabolic diseases. J Endocr Soc. 2020;4(6):bvaa052.
6. Lazo M, Young JH, Brancati FL, Coresh J, Whelton S, Ndumele CE, et al. NH2-terminal pro-brain natriuretic peptide and risk of diabetes. Diabetes. 2013;62(9):3189–93.
7. Jujic A, Nilsson PM, Engstrom G, Hedblad B, Melander O, Magnusson M. Atrial natriuretic peptide and type 2 diabetes development--biomarker and genotype association study. PLoS One. 2014;9(2):e89201.
8. Pfister R, Sharp S, Luben R, Welsh P, Barroso I, Salomaa V, et al. Mendelian randomization study of B-type natriuretic peptide and type 2 diabetes: evidence of causal association from population studies. PLoS Med. 2011;8(10):e1001112.
9. Bachmann KN, Deger SM, Alsouqi A, Huang S, Xu M, Ferguson JF, et al. Acute effects of insulin on circulating natriuretic peptide levels in humans. PLoS One. 2018;13(5):e0196869.
10. Cannone V, Boerrigter G, Cataliotti A, Costello-Boerrigter LC, Olson TM, McKie PM, et al. A genetic variant of the atrial natriuretic peptide gene is associated with cardiometabolic protection in the general community. J Am Coll Cardiol. 2011;58(6):629–36.
11. Coue M, Badin PM, Vila IK, Laurens C, Louche K, Marques MA, et al. Defective natriuretic peptide receptor signaling in skeletal muscle links obesity to type 2 diabetes. Diabetes. 2015;64(12):4033–45.
12. Neeland IJ, Winders BR, Ayers CR, Das SR, Chang AY, Berry JD, et al. Higher natriuretic peptide levels associate with a favorable adipose tissue distribution profile. J Am Coll Cardiol. 2013;62(8):752–60.
13. Jordan J, Birkenfeld AL, Melander O, Moro C. Natriuretic peptides in cardiovascular and metabolic crosstalk: implications for hypertension management. Hypertension. 2018;72(2):270–6.
14. Granger CB, Califf RM, Young S, Candela R, Samaha J, Worley S, et al. Outcome of patients with diabetes mellitus and acute myocardial infarction treated with thrombolytic agents. The Thrombolysis and Angioplasty in Myocardial Infarction (TAMI) Study Group. J Am Coll Cardiol. 1993;21(4):920–5.

15. Scognamiglio R, Negut C, Ramondo A, Tiengo A, Avogaro A. Detection of coronary artery disease in asymptomatic patients with type 2 diabetes mellitus. J Am Coll Cardiol. 2006;47(1):65–71.
16. Anand DV, Lim E, Lahiri A, Bax JJ. The role of non-invasive imaging in the risk stratification of asymptomatic diabetic subjects. Eur Heart J. 2006;27(8):905–12.
17. Yokoyama I, Momomura S, Ohtake T, Yonekura K, Nishikawa J, Sasaki Y, et al. Reduced myocardial flow reserve in non-insulin-dependent diabetes mellitus. J Am Coll Cardiol. 1997;30(6):1472–7.
18. Makimattila S, Virkamaki A, Groop PH, Cockcroft J, Utriainen T, Fagerudd J, et al. Chronic hyperglycemia impairs endothelial function and insulin sensitivity via different mechanisms in insulin-dependent diabetes mellitus. Circulation. 1996;94(6):1276–82.
19. Di Carli MF, Janisse J, Grunberger G, Ager J. Role of chronic hyperglycemia in the pathogenesis of coronary microvascular dysfunction in diabetes. J Am Coll Cardiol. 2003;41(8):1387–93.
20. Davi G, Catalano I, Averna M, Notarbartolo A, Strano A, Ciabattoni G, et al. Thromboxane biosynthesis and platelet function in type II diabetes mellitus. N Engl J Med. 1990;322(25):1769–74.
21. Saito I, Folsom AR, Brancati FL, Duncan BB, Chambless LE, McGovern PG. Nontraditional risk factors for coronary heart disease incidence among persons with diabetes: the Atherosclerosis Risk in Communities (ARIC) Study. Ann Intern Med. 2000;133(2):81–91.
22. Stec JJ, Silbershatz H, Tofler GH, Matheney TH, Sutherland P, Lipinska I, et al. Association of fibrinogen with cardiovascular risk factors and cardiovascular disease in the Framingham Offspring Population. Circulation. 2000;102(14):1634–8.
23. Moreno PR, Murcia AM, Palacios IF, Leon MN, Bernardi VH, Fuster V, et al. Coronary composition and macrophage infiltration in atherectomy specimens from patients with diabetes mellitus. Circulation. 2000;102(18):2180–4.
24. Langer A, Freeman MR, Josse RG, Armstrong PW. Metaiodobenzylguanidine imaging in diabetes mellitus: assessment of cardiac sympathetic denervation and its relation to autonomic dysfunction and silent myocardial ischemia. J Am Coll Cardiol. 1995;25(3):610–8.
25. Adler AI, Stratton IM, Neil HA, Yudkin JS, Matthews DR, Cull CA, et al. Association of systolic blood pressure with macrovascular and microvascular complications of type 2 diabetes (UKPDS 36): prospective observational study. BMJ. 2000;321(7258):412–9.
26. Lee MMY, McMurray JJV, Lorenzo-Almoros A, Kristensen SL, Sattar N, Jhund PS, et al. Diabetic cardiomyopathy. Heart. 2019;105(4):337–45.
27. From AM, Scott CG, Chen HH. The development of heart failure in patients with diabetes mellitus and pre-clinical diastolic dysfunction a population-based study. J Am Coll Cardiol. 2010;55(4):300–5.
28. Haffner SM, Lehto S, Ronnemaa T, Pyorala K, Laakso M. Mortality from coronary heart disease in subjects with type 2 diabetes and in nondiabetic subjects with and without prior myocardial infarction. N Engl J Med. 1998;339(4):229–34.
29. Kannel WB, McGee DL. Diabetes and cardiovascular disease. The Framingham study. JAMA. 1979;241(19):2035–8.
30. Stamler J, Vaccaro O, Neaton JD, Wentworth D. Diabetes, other risk factors, and 12-yr cardiovascular mortality for men screened in the Multiple Risk Factor Intervention Trial. Diabetes Care. 1993;16(2):434–44.
31. Huxley R, Barzi F, Woodward M. Excess risk of fatal coronary heart disease associated with diabetes in men and women: meta-analysis of 37 prospective cohort studies. BMJ. 2006;332(7533):73–8.
32. Klajda MD, Scott CG, Rodeheffer RJ, Chen HH, editors. Diabetes mellitus is an independent predictor for the development of heart failure: a population study, Mayo Clinic proceedings. Elsevier; 2020.
33. Nichols GA, Gullion CM, Koro CE, Ephross SA, Brown JB. The incidence of congestive heart failure in type 2 diabetes: an update. Diabetes Care. 2004;27(8):1879–84.

34. Bahrami H, Bluemke DA, Kronmal R, Bertoni AG, Lloyd-Jones DM, Shahar E, et al. Novel metabolic risk factors for incident heart failure and their relationship with obesity: the MESA (Multi-Ethnic Study of Atherosclerosis) study. J Am Coll Cardiol. 2008;51(18):1775–83.
35. Marwick TH, Ritchie R, Shaw JE, Kaye D. Implications of underlying mechanisms for the recognition and management of diabetic cardiomyopathy. J Am Coll Cardiol. 2018;71(3):339–51.
36. Ohkuma T, Komorita Y, Peters SAE, Woodward M. Diabetes as a risk factor for heart failure in women and men: a systematic review and meta-analysis of 47 cohorts including 12 million individuals. Diabetologia. 2019;62(9):1550–60.
37. Bertoni AG, Hundley WG, Massing MW, Bonds DE, Burke GL, Goff DC Jr. Heart failure prevalence, incidence, and mortality in the elderly with diabetes. Diabetes Care. 2004;27(3):699–703.
38. Iribarren C, Karter AJ, Go AS, Ferrara A, Liu JY, Sidney S, et al. Glycemic control and heart failure among adult patients with diabetes. Circulation. 2001;103(22):2668–73.
39. Barzilay JI, Kronmal RA, Gottdiener JS, Smith NL, Burke GL, Tracy R, et al. The association of fasting glucose levels with congestive heart failure in diabetic adults > or =65 years: the Cardiovascular Health Study. J Am Coll Cardiol. 2004;43(12):2236–41.
40. Dandamudi S, Slusser J, Mahoney DW, Redfield MM, Rodeheffer RJ, Chen HH. The prevalence of diabetic cardiomyopathy: a population-based study in Olmsted County, Minnesota. J Card Fail. 2014;20(5):304–9.
41. MacDonald MR, Petrie MC, Varyani F, Ostergren J, Michelson EL, Young JB, et al. Impact of diabetes on outcomes in patients with low and preserved ejection fraction heart failure: an analysis of the Candesartan in Heart failure: Assessment of Reduction in Mortality and morbidity (CHARM) programme. Eur Heart J. 2008;29(11):1377–85.
42. Kristensen SL, Preiss D, Jhund PS, Squire I, Cardoso JS, Merkely B, et al. Risk related to prediabetes mellitus and diabetes mellitus in heart failure with reduced ejection fraction: insights from prospective comparison of ARNI with ACEI to determine impact on global mortality and morbidity in heart failure trial. Circ Heart Fail. 2016;9(1):e002560.
43. Garg A, Grundy SM. Management of dyslipidemia in NIDDM. Diabetes Care. 1990;13(2):153–69.
44. O'Brien T, Nguyen TT, Zimmerman BR. Hyperlipidemia and diabetes mellitus. Mayo Clin Proc. 1998;73(10):969–76.
45. Haffner SM, Stern MP, Hazuda HP, Mitchell BD, Patterson JK. Cardiovascular risk factors in confirmed prediabetic individuals. Does the clock for coronary heart disease start ticking before the onset of clinical diabetes? JAMA. 1990;263(21):2893–8.
46. Bittner V, Bertolet M, Barraza Felix R, Farkouh ME, Goldberg S, Ramanathan KB, et al. Comprehensive cardiovascular risk factor control improves survival: the BARI 2D trial. J Am Coll Cardiol. 2015;66(7):765–73.
47. Gregg EW, Gerzoff RB, Caspersen CJ, Williamson DF, Narayan KM. Relationship of walking to mortality among US adults with diabetes. Arch Intern Med. 2003;163(12):1440–7.
48. Singer DE, Nathan DM, Anderson KM, Wilson PW, Evans JC. Association of HbA1c with prevalent cardiovascular disease in the original cohort of the Framingham Heart Study. Diabetes. 1992;41(2):202–8.
49. Khaw KT, Wareham N, Bingham S, Luben R, Welch A, Day N. Association of hemoglobin A1c with cardiovascular disease and mortality in adults: the European prospective investigation into cancer in Norfolk. Ann Intern Med. 2004;141(6):413–20.
50. Selvin E, Marinopoulos S, Berkenblit G, Rami T, Brancati FL, Powe NR, et al. Meta-analysis: glycosylated hemoglobin and cardiovascular disease in diabetes mellitus. Ann Intern Med. 2004;141(6):421–31.
51. American Diabetes Association. 6. Glycemic targets: standards of medical care in diabetes-2020. Diabetes Care. 2020;43(Suppl 1):S66–76.
52. Bakris GL, Fonseca V, Katholi RE, McGill JB, Messerli FH, Phillips RA, et al. Metabolic effects of carvedilol vs metoprolol in patients with type 2 diabetes mellitus and hypertension: a randomized controlled trial. JAMA. 2004;292(18):2227–36.

53. Pitt B, Pfeffer MA, Assmann SF, Boineau R, Anand IS, Claggett B, et al. Spironolactone for heart failure with preserved ejection fraction. N Engl J Med. 2014;370(15):1383–92.
54. Wiviott SD, Raz I, Bonaca MP, Mosenzon O, Kato ET, Cahn A, et al. Dapagliflozin and cardiovascular outcomes in type 2 diabetes. N Engl J Med. 2019;380(4):347–57.
55. Zinman B, Wanner C, Lachin JM, Fitchett D, Bluhmki E, Hantel S, et al. Empagliflozin, cardiovascular outcomes, and mortality in type 2 diabetes. N Engl J Med. 2015;373(22):2117–28.
56. Neal B, Perkovic V, Mahaffey KW, de Zeeuw D, Fulcher G, Erondu N, et al. Canagliflozin and cardiovascular and renal events in type 2 diabetes. N Engl J Med. 2017;377(7):644–57.
57. McMurray JJV, Solomon SD, Inzucchi SE, Kober L, Kosiborod MN, Martinez FA, et al. Dapagliflozin in patients with heart failure and reduced ejection fraction. N Engl J Med. 2019;381(21):1995–2008.
58. American Diabetes Association. 11. Microvascular complications and foot care: standards of medical care in diabetes-2020. Diabetes Care. 2020;43(Suppl 1):S135–S51.
59. Eng C, Kramer CK, Zinman B, Retnakaran R. Glucagon-like peptide-1 receptor agonist and basal insulin combination treatment for the management of type 2 diabetes: a systematic review and meta-analysis. Lancet. 2014;384(9961):2228–34.
60. Marso SP, Daniels GH, Brown-Frandsen K, Kristensen P, Mann JF, Nauck MA, et al. Liraglutide and cardiovascular outcomes in type 2 diabetes. N Engl J Med. 2016;375(4):311–22.
61. Wang TJ. Natriuretic peptide deficiency-when there is too little of a good thing. JAMA Cardiol. 2018;3(1):7–9.
62. Newton-Cheh C, Larson MG, Vasan RS, Levy D, Bloch KD, Surti A, et al. Association of common variants in NPPA and NPPB with circulating natriuretic peptides and blood pressure. Nat Genet. 2009;41(3):348–53.
63. Gruden G, Landi A, Bruno G. Natriuretic peptides, heart, and adipose tissue: new findings and future developments for diabetes research. Diabetes Care. 2014;37(11):2899–908.
64. Seferovic JP, Claggett B, Seidelmann SB, Seely EW, Packer M, Zile MR, et al. Effect of sacubitril/valsartan versus enalapril on glycaemic control in patients with heart failure and diabetes: a post-hoc analysis from the PARADIGM-HF trial. Lancet Diabetes Endocrinol. 2017;5(5):333–40.
65. Heinisch BB, Vila G, Resl M, Riedl M, Dieplinger B, Mueller T, et al. B-type natriuretic peptide (BNP) affects the initial response to intravenous glucose: a randomised placebo-controlled cross-over study in healthy men. Diabetologia. 2012;55(5):1400–5.

Chapter 3
Precision Medicine for Diabetes and Dyslipidemia

Ethan Alexander, Elizabeth Cristiano, and John M. Miles

Introduction

Cardiovascular disease (CVD) accounts for roughly one-quarter of deaths in the USA annually, and its largest component is coronary heart disease (CHD) [1]. The presence of diabetes mellitus (predominantly type 2 diabetes, or T2DM) increases the risk of cardiovascular death by two- to threefold [2–4]. Although conventional risk factors do not entirely explain this enormous increase in risk in patients with T2DM, dyslipidemia is a major contributor to this risk [5, 6]. Dyslipidemia is defined as triglyceride concentrations >200 mg/dl and/or HDL cholesterol levels <40 mg/dl, combined with an increase in small, dense LDL (sdLDL) particles [7]; using this definition, it is present in half or more of patients with T2DM [8]. In this chapter, we will review the pathogenesis and treatment of diabetic dyslipidemia.

Pathogenesis

Insulin resistance is central to the pathogenesis of dyslipidemia in nondiabetic individuals [9, 10] and is present in the majority of people with T2DM [11] as well as some individuals with type 1 diabetes [12, 13]. The dyslipidemia of diabetes is driven by hyperlipolysis in adipose tissue, leading to overproduction of VLDL [6]; it often precedes the development of hyperglycemia, and it has been suggested by McGarry that abnormalities in lipid metabolism play a causal role in the pathogenesis of type 2 diabetes [14]. In nondiabetic relatives of individuals with T2DM,

E. Alexander · E. Cristiano · J. M. Miles (✉)
Divisions of Endocrinology, Metabolism and Genetics, University of Kansas School of Medicine, Kansas City, KS, USA
e-mail: jmiles3@kumc.edu

R. Basu (ed.), *Precision Medicine in Diabetes*,
https://doi.org/10.1007/978-3-030-98927-9_3

hyperinsulinemia is accompanied by higher triglyceride concentrations and qualitative abnormalities in lipoprotein metabolism that include increased VLDL particle size and a shift toward smaller, dense HDL particles [15]. Using the euglycemic-hyperinsulinemic clamp and HOMA-IR techniques to assess insulin sensitivity in adults and children, several investigators have demonstrated that both the triglyceride/HDL-C ratio [16, 17] and the triglyceride/glucose product [18] correlate with insulin sensitivity.

While low-density lipoprotein cholesterol (LDL-C) typically lies within the normal reference range, the structure and size of the LDL particle is altered. The sdLDL particle is considered to be more atherogenic due to its lower affinity for the LDL-C receptor, leading to decreased metabolic clearance, as well as its susceptibility to oxidation and ease of trans-endothelial passage [19–21]. The LDL particle size shift to sdLDL is mediated by increased cholesterol ester transfer protein (CETP) function due to increased flux of triglyceride-rich lipoproteins, primarily VLDL; this leads to increased exchange of triglycerides in very-low-density lipoprotein (VLDL) for cholesterol in LDL-C and HDL-C [20, 21], perhaps contributing to reduced HDL-C. The triglycerides in both LDL-C and HDL-C are then hydrolyzed in the liver, effectively reducing particle size [20, 21]. Hypertriglyceridemia is due primarily to overproduction of VLDL (and apolipoprotein B100) [22], which in turn is caused by increased delivery of free fatty acids (FFA) to the liver [23]. Visceral adipose tissue is a major contributor to hepatic FFA supply [24]. In patients with type 2 diabetes, there is a relationship between increased visceral fat mass and both larger VLDL particles and smaller LDL and HDL particles [25].

Treatment

In spite of the proliferation of useful medications for the treatment of dyslipidemia, lifestyle modification remains a building block upon which effective treatment should be based. However, lifestyle modification alone is rarely sufficient; thus, the vast majority of patients will require pharmacological treatment. We will first discuss medications that primarily target LDL cholesterol. These include statins, PCSK9 inhibitors, ezetimibe, and bempedoic acid.

Statins

Statins are established as first-line therapy for diabetic dyslipidemia and play a crucial role in both primary and secondary cardiovascular prevention. The clinical practice guidelines of the Endocrine Society recommend routine statin therapy with an LDL-C target of 70 mg/dL for patients without established CVD and 55 mg/dL for those with established CVD [26]. The guidelines of the American

College of Cardiology and the American Heart Association advise the use of at least a moderate-intensity statin in patients with diabetes aged 40–75 and a high-intensity statin if the 10-year pooled-cohort atherosclerotic cardiovascular (ASCVD) risk calculator is significant or there are other risk factors for ASCVD [27–29]. The presence versus absence of dyslipidemia does not influence the recommendations in either guideline.

The mechanism by which statins lower LDL-C involves inhibition of hydroxymethylglutaryl-CoA (HMG-CoA) reductase, a key enzyme in the biochemical cholesterol synthesis pathway [30]. In addition to their well-known effects on LDL-C levels, statins have been shown to both lower triglycerides and raise HDL-C concentrations [31, 32]; this effect may be due in part to an increase in both pre-heparin and post-heparin plasma lipase activity [22]. However, effects of statins on LDL particle size are small [33] to negligible [34, 35]. Bempedoic acid, which is discussed below, inhibits another enzyme in this same biochemical pathway [36].

Secondary Prevention

The Scandinavian Simvastatin Survival Study (4S study) was a randomized, double-blind placebo-controlled trial involving over 4000 patients with previous coronary heart disease or ongoing angina followed for an average of 5.4 years; it compared simvastatin 40 mg daily to placebo in regard to outcomes that included cardiovascular and all-cause mortality [37]. In the placebo group, cardiovascular events were greater than twofold higher in people with diabetes than in nondiabetic individuals. Patients in the treatment arm had lower mean LDL-C, total cholesterol, and elevated HDL-C (−35%, −25%, and + 8%, respectively), together with a 42% decrease in cardiovascular death and a 30% reduction in all-cause mortality [37]. This study was the first to show that treatment of dyslipidemia in diabetic subjects significantly decreases cardiovascular events; in a subgroup analysis, reduction in events in patients with diabetes was greater than in the patients without diabetes (55% versus 32%, respectively), although the number of people with diabetes was small and the difference in all-cause mortality was not significant [37, 38].

There is substantial evidence from secondary prevention studies that high statin doses produce greater reduction in events than lower doses. In the PROVE IT-TIMI 22 trial, approximately 4200 patients with acute coronary syndrome were randomized to receive either pravastatin 40 mg daily or atorvastatin 80 mg daily [39]. The more intense treatment with atorvastatin produced lower LDL-C concentrations compared with pravastatin (62 mg/dL vs 95 mg/dL) and also resulted in a Kaplan-Meier estimate of a composite of cardiovascular events at 2 years that was 16% lower in those receiving high-intensity atorvastatin compared with pravastatin ($p = 0.005$) [39]. The benefit of high-intensity atorvastatin over pravastatin was equivalent in subjects with and without diabetes [39]. Another study used intravascular ultrasound and found that atorvastatin 80 mg daily, but not pravastatin 40 mg daily, halted the progression of atherosclerosis [40]. When interpreting these two studies, it is important to note that pravastatin 40 mg has been found to be equipotent to less than 10 mg atorvastatin with respect to lowering of LDL-C [41]. The TNT trial found that atorvastatin 80 mg was more effective in reducing events than atorvastatin 10 mg in patients with coronary heart disease [42]. Thus, in all three secondary prevention trials, the highest approved dose of atorvastatin was compared with the lowest available dose or an equivalent of even lower potency. These observations confirm that high-intensity statin therapy has greater effectiveness than moderate-intensity therapy, but they obscure the curvilinearity of the relationship between dose and risk reduction [6]. This is important because statin side effects tend to be dose-related [43, 44]; management of statin intolerance can be extremely difficult [45], requiring resources that are not consistently available to primary care physicians. If the incremental benefit of doubling a statin dose is small [46], one can make a case for moderate-dose statin therapy to minimize discontinuation of statin treatment [47], especially in a primary care setting.

Primary Prevention

Moderate-intensity statin therapy has been shown to provide considerable benefit in people with diabetes. The CARDS (Collaborative Atorvastatin Diabetes Study) trial compared the effect of atorvastatin 10 mg versus placebo for primary prevention of cardiovascular events in ~2800 diabetes subjects with a median follow-up of 3.9 years [48]. Participants had a mean hemoglobin A1c of 7.8% at baseline, normal LDL-C levels (averaging 117 mg/dl), and normal HDL-C concentrations (average 54 mg/dl). Mean triglyceride levels were 150 mg/dl, indicating the presence of hypertriglyceridemia in roughly half of the participants. Individuals receiving atorvastatin had an impressive 37% reduction in cardiovascular events and a 27% decrease in all-cause mortality compared with placebo. Atorvastatin produced virtually no change in HDL-C but significant decreases in LDL-C (−40%), triglycerides (−19%), and non-HDL cholesterol (−36%). The reduction in events in a population with relatively mild to absent lipid abnormalities argues in favor of moderate-intensity statin treatment in most if not all individuals with type 2 diabetes. Other studies have produced equivocal results. In the primary prevention ASCOT study in patients with hypertension, there was clear cardiovascular benefit of atorvastatin 10 mg when compared to placebo. However, significant benefit was not demonstrable in the subset of individuals with diabetes. The investigators acknowledged that the study was probably underpowered in the diabetes subgroup and that the drop-in rate in diabetic patients receiving placebo was relatively high [49, 50]. The ASPEN study also failed to demonstrate significant cardiovascular benefit from atorvastatin 10 mg in subjects with diabetes without established coronary heart disease [51]. However, rather high drop-in and dropout rates in that study compromise its interpretability [52]. A Cochrane review investigated the use of statins for the primary prevention of cardiovascular disease. The analysis included 18 randomized control trials, 14 of which had specific enrollment criteria, including trials looking at primary prevention in diabetes. This review found that there were significant reductions in all-cause mortality (OR 0.86, 95% CI 0.79 to 0.94), combined fatal and non-fatal myocardial infarction and stroke, as well as need for revascularization with statin therapy [53].

Do Statins Increase Newly Incident Diabetes?

The JUPITER trial was a randomized, double-blind, placebo-controlled primary prevention study in over 17,000 nondiabetic individuals comparing high-intensity rosuvastatin (20 mg) to placebo [54]. A secondary endpoint of the study was the development of new diabetes. Baseline hemoglobin A1c was 5.7% in both groups. After a median follow-up of 1.9 years, hemoglobin A1c was higher in the rosuvastatin group (5.9% versus 5.8%, $p = 0.001$). A diagnosis of new diabetes was more frequent in the rosuvastatin-treated subjects (3.0% vs 2.4%, $p = 0.01$), although the diagnoses were not adjudicated. As a result, the FDA subsequently added a warning to the label mentioning the risk of diabetes [55]. In the JUPITER trial, a post hoc analysis indicated that the increase in diabetes risk in rosuvastatin-treated participants was present in subjects with risk factors for diabetes, but not those in whom risk factors were absent [56]. Subsequent meta-analyses concluded that the relationship between statin use and new diabetes is equivocal [57] or absent [58]. A recent retrospective cohort study in ~6000 patients ≥70 years of age without a significant risk for developing diabetes showed no increase in newly incident diabetes with initiation of statin therapy [59]. In the same study, diabetes risk was increased in younger patients, many of whom had diabetes risk factors, with statin exposure [59]. In our view the effect of statins on diabetes appears to be small and is vastly outweighed by the cardiovascular benefits, as recently suggested by Bell [60].

PCSK-9 Inhibitors

Proprotein convertase subtilisin/kexin type 9 (PCSK9) is an important enzyme in the hepatic clearance of LDL-C. LDL-C binds to the LDL receptor in the liver and is internalized into the hepatocyte where it is metabolized [61]. Normally, the LDL receptor is recycled repeatedly to the cell surface in order to continue to clear LDL-C from the circulation [62]. Circulating PCSK9 binds to the LDL receptor on the hepatocyte and leads to receptor degradation, effectively limiting LDL-C clearance from the circulation [61–63]. It has been shown that gain of function mutations in PCSK9 are associated with increased cardiovascular risk, whereas loss of function mutations produce lower circulating LDL-C levels [62]. In addition to effects on LDL-C, PCSK9-mediated degradation of LDL receptors can have an impact on triglyceride-rich lipoprotein metabolism, since both VLDL and chylomicron remnants are cleared at the LDL receptor via binding to apolipoprotein E [64].

The Fourier trial tested evolocumab, the first available PCSK9 inhibitor, in the treatment of over 27,000 patients with cardiovascular disease taking a minimum of atorvastatin 20 mg daily or its equipotent equivalent [65]. Evolocumab reduced LDL-C concentrations to a median of 30 mg/dL compared with ~90 mg/dL in the placebo group. With relatively brief follow-up (2.2 years), evolocumab produced a relative risk reduction of 15% for the primary (MACE 5) endpoint and 20% for the secondary (MACE 3) endpoint versus placebo. There were significant reductions in key secondary composite endpoints in patients in the highest quartile for LDL-C concentration (126 mg/dL) and the lowest (73 mg/dL) [65]. Approximately 37% of participants in the study had diabetes, and the outcomes were similar in this subgroup [66]. There was no increase in newly diagnosed diabetes nor worsening of diabetes control associated with evolocumab treatment [66].

The ODYSSEY OUTCOMES Trial evaluated alirocumab in ~19,000 patients with acute coronary syndrome who were receiving a high-intensity statin [67]. With a median follow-up of 2.8 years, the primary composite endpoint (MACE 4) in alirocumab-treated patients was reduced by 14%. The greatest risk reduction occurred in patients whose baseline LDL levels were >100 mg/dl. A subgroup analysis showed no difference in endpoints among patients with diabetes, who represented 29% of participants. There was no difference in worsening diabetes or new-onset diabetes [67]. A separate study was conducted in subjects with type 1 and type 2 diabetes treated with insulin and alirocumab versus placebo; participants included individuals on varying doses of statins, some on no statin at all because of statin intolerance [68]. The average LDL-C decrease with alirocumab was 49% in both type 1 and type 2 patients, and there was no apparent adverse interaction between alirocumab and insulin [68]. A subsequent meta-analysis of 14 trials (1524 patients) in primarily T2DM patients with baseline hemoglobin A1c averaging 6.9% versus nondiabetic individuals found similar decreases in LDL-C and a similar safety profile in the two groups; the most common side effect was a local reaction at the injection site [68].

Epidemiological studies have shown that a low HDL particle number is associated with markers of insulin resistance and metabolic syndrome [69]. Using NMR measurements of HDL particle number and size, Ingueneau et al. recently studied 95 patients from an outpatient lipid clinic and found that PCSK9 inhibitors increased HDL-C by 7% and also HDL particle number, especially in patients not taking statins [70]. There was also an overall increase in HDL particle size, due primarily to an increase in medium-sized HDL particle number with little change in the number of small HDL and occurring in spite of a decrease in extra-large HDL particle number; this occurred because the latter were more than an order of magnitude less numerous than medium-sized particles [70]. Using the same technique, PCSK9 inhibitors were shown to increase overall VLDL particle size, primarily by decreasing the number of small, atherogenic VLDL remnants [71]. This effect can be explained by an effect of PCSK9 inhibitors on clearance of VLDL remnants at the LDL receptor, as mentioned above, and the effects on HDL may be secondary.

In summary, inhibitors of PCSK9 can reduce risk in patients with diabetes on statin therapy when additional LDL-C lowering is desired. Additional studies are needed to elucidate the mechanisms via which these agents exert their effects on the metabolism of multiple lipoproteins.

Ezetimibe

Ezetimibe is an oral medication whose mechanism of action is to inhibit cholesterol absorption into the enterocyte at the brush border in the intestines and can lower LDL-C by approximately 24% [72–74]. In the secondary prevention IMPROVE-IT trial, ezetimibe 10 mg once daily vs placebo was added to simvastatin 40 mg daily alone [72]. This trial enrolled over 18,000 patients and had a MACE 5 endpoint [72]. After 6 years of follow-up, the risk of myocardial infarction was 13% lower in the ezetimibe plus simvastatin group. In a subsequent diabetes subgroup ($n = 4933$) analysis of IMPROVE-IT, the investigators found that patients were more likely to present with non-ST segment elevation acute coronary syndrome as compared to nondiabetic patients ($p < 0.001$), and there were greater relative risk reductions in MI (24%) and ischemic stroke (39%) in this group than in nondiabetic subjects [75]. At study baseline, people with diabetes had higher triglyceride and lower HDL-C levels. Changes in these lipoprotein concentrations were not reported. Overall, analysis of data in this subgroup showed that adding ezetimibe to simvastatin in patients with diabetes added cardiovascular risk reduction. Ezetimibe added to atorvastatin produces greater improvement in LDL-C compared to doubling the atorvastatin dose [76]. In patients receiving maximally tolerated statin therapy, an ezetimibe/bempedoic acid combination resulted in greater reductions in LDL-C than bempedoic acid alone [77]. In summary, ezetimibe lowers LDL-C concentrations and reduces risk. The benefits of ezetimibe appear to occur in the absence of a change in HDL-C or LDL particle size [78]. Thus, a treatment that targets LDL-C and is complementary to statins is capable of reducing risk without improving the major elements of diabetic dyslipidemia. As a result, both the ACC/AHA and the Endocrine Society include ezetimibe as an option when LDL-C goal has not been achieved [26, 79].

Bempedoic Acid

Bempedoic acid is a small molecule that has recently been approved for the purpose of lowering LDL cholesterol. Its mechanism of action is to inhibit ATP citrate lyase in the liver, an enzyme in the same pathway but upstream from HMG-CoA reductase. The effectiveness of bempedoic acid in LDL-C lowering was evaluated in high-risk patients on maximally tolerated statins in the CLEAR Wisdom trial [80]. This study involved 779 patients (236 with T2DM) with cardiovascular disease and/or heterozygous familial hypercholesterolemia randomized 2:1 to 180 mg of bempedoic acid daily or placebo for 52 weeks. Primary outcomes were LDL-C change from baseline, and secondary endpoints included measurements of other lipoproteins and biomarkers. At the 12-week mark, mean LDL-C levels were significantly lower in the treatment group vs the placebo group (−15.1% vs 2.4%), and non-HDL, total cholesterol, apolipoprotein B, and hsCRP were all lower in the treatment group [80]. A meta-analysis of five trials ($n = 3629$) found that treatment with bempedoic acid resulted in a 34% reduction in new-onset diabetes or worsening of preexisting diabetes [81]. A second meta-analysis (11 trials, $n = 4392$) also found a reduction in new onset or worsening diabetes (RR 0.65) as well as a reduction in composite cardiovascular outcomes (RR 0.75) [82]. To our knowledge, there are no studies of the effects of bempedoic acid that have been conducted specifically in diabetic patients with dyslipidemia. Nonetheless, bempedoic acid used in conjunction with a maximally tolerated statin may be of use in diabetic patients who are not at their lipid goals.

Non-LDL Directed Medications

In the treatment of diabetic dyslipidemia, there is a potential role for medications that do not primarily target LDL-cholesterol metabolism. The clinical trials that have been conducted tend to be smaller than those with agents directed toward LDL-cholesterol, perhaps because some of them are considered nutraceuticals and to some extent have less proprietary interest behind them. These medications include fibrates and omega-3 fatty acids.

Fibrates

Although statins substantially reduce cardiovascular risk, they do not eliminate it; the majority of statin-treated patients still have events on this therapy [83]. Individuals with low HDL-C have increased risk in spite of statin treatment [84]. The fibrate class of medication made its first appearance over 50 years ago and is well-known to decrease triglycerides, raise HDL-C, and increase LDL particle size [34, 35, 85, 86]. The increase in LDL-C particle size with fibrate use is inversely correlated with the decrease in serum triglyceride level [87]. Fibrate medications should theoretically therefore be an ideal treatment, in combination with statins, for patients with dyslipidemia. In fact, fibrates should be considered complementary to statins, which lower triglycerides and raise HDL-C, but do not normalize them [88], and which have little to no effect on LDL particle size [33–35]. The effects of fibrates are mediated primarily via activation of the peroxisome proliferator-activated receptor-alpha (PPAR-α) transcription factor, increasing triglyceride clearance and raising HDL-C [89, 90].

Nonetheless, fibrates are not recommended by many experts in the management of patients with lipid disorders. The guidelines of the American College of Cardiology and the American Heart Association point out that the triglyceride-lowering properties of statins are similar to those of fibrates; use of fibrates is recommended only in patients with severe hypertriglyceridemia and not as an add-on to statin therapy [79]. On the other hand, the clinical practice guidelines of the

Endocrine Society indicate that fibrates may be used in high-risk T2DM patients with even mild hypertriglyceridemia and should be used in patients with diabetic retinopathy [26]. The ambivalence concerning fibrate use is in part because randomized, controlled trials have produced mixed results with respect to cardiovascular benefit when fibrates are given as monotherapy [91–94] or in combination with statins [95].

The Helsinki Heart Study was a primary prevention trial investigating cardiovascular benefits of gemfibrozil in middle-aged men. At 5 years, the rate of cumulative cardiac endpoints was 27.3 per 1000 in the treatment group (2051 men receiving 600 mg twice daily) and 41.4 per 1000 in the placebo group, $p < 0.05$. Gemfibrozil treatment resulted in a significant increase in HDL-C and reductions in triglycerides, LDL-C, and non-HDL cholesterol [91]. Only 3% of the participants had diabetes. VA-HIT was a secondary prevention study that also tested the potential benefit of gemfibrozil treatment [96]. This double-blind placebo-controlled trial compared 1200 mg of gemfibrozil daily to placebo in 2531 men with established coronary heart disease, an HDL-C of less than 40 mg/dl, and LDL-C ≤140 mg/dl [96]. The relative risk of a cardiovascular event was reduced by 22% in the gemfibrozil group compared to placebo ($p < 0.01$). There was a 41% decrease in coronary death ($P = 0.02$) in participants with diabetes. There was also a significant ($p < 0.05$) decrease in stroke in those with diabetes, but not in nondiabetic individuals. However, other large studies, including FIELD [91], the Bezafibrate Infarction Prevention study [93], and ACCORD [95], showed no benefit from addition of a fibrate. This explains why some organizations are at best lukewarm regarding the use of fibrates for prevention of cardiovascular events.

It has been pointed out that many of the subjects in the above trials did not have dyslipidemia [6] and therefore might not be expected to benefit from fibrate therapy. In fact, post hoc analyses of these studies have shown benefit in the subgroups with dyslipidemia [93]. Sacks pooled data from five large trials and in a post hoc analysis found a 35% reduction in cardiovascular events among individuals with dyslipidemia [97]. Table 3.1 shows mean lipid values in five major fibrate trials. It can be inferred from the data that many of the participants in these trials did not have dyslipidemia and would thus be less likely to benefit from a treatment that targets dyslipidemia.

A Cochrane Database Review evaluating fibrates for the primary prevention of cardiovascular events analyzed six eligible trials, four of which involved patients with T2DM, including over 16,000 patients [98]. The review found a 16% reduction

Table 3.1 Lipid values in five fibrate trials

Study (reference)	n	Total cholesterol	Triglycerides	HDL-C	LDL-C
89	4081	289	175	47	NA
91	3090	213	145	35	148
94	2531	175	160	32	111
92	9795	195	153	42	119
93	5518	175	162	38	101

in cardiovascular death, nonfatal MI, and nonfatal stroke [98]. Wang et al. published another Cochrane review evaluating fibrates for the secondary prevention of cardiovascular disease and stroke and included seven studies when clofibrate was excluded [99]. The analysis, which involved over 10,000 patients, found that fibrates did not decrease the risk of primary composite outcomes. However, the review found that fibrates did prevent myocardial infarction [99].

The effects of fenofibrate on renal function are of interest. In two large clinical trials, fenofibrate produced an acute, sustained increase in creatinine levels [94, 95]. In a washout substudy of the FIELD trial involving 661 patients, fenofibrate caused an acute rise in creatinine followed by a slower chronic increase compared to placebo, together with a decrease in urinary albumin ($p = 0.01$). With washout, creatinine was lower in those treated with fenofibrate compared with placebo, indicating preservation of eGFR [100]. There was great preservation of renal function in patients with dyslipidemia compared with non-dyslipidemic individuals [100]. These findings (an acute decrease in eGFR followed by preservation of renal function) would benefit from confirmation; they are strikingly similar to effects of SGLT2 medications on renal function and suggest reversal of hyperfiltration [101].

In summary, clinical trial results on the use of fibrates have been inconsistent and have been confounded by inclusion of participants without dyslipidemia. Post hoc analyses tend to suggest that subjects with dyslipidemia will benefit from addition of a fibrate medication to statin therapy. Additional studies are underway to investigate potential benefits of fibrates in patients with true dyslipidemia; hopefully, those results will provide further clarity on the subject. The FIELD trial results regarding effects of fenofibrate on renal function need confirmation but suggest that there may be off-target renal benefits of fibrate therapy. Taking the above data together, we tend to favor selective use of fibrates in high-risk patients with true dyslipidemia.

Omega-3 Fatty Acids

In 1999, the GISSI Prevenzione study was published, showing a significant decrease in a composite MACE 3 endpoint in post-myocardial infarction patients treated for 3.5 years with an omega-3 fatty acid supplement containing eicosapentaenoic acid (EPA) and docosahexaenoic acid (DHA) ethyl esters [102], generating considerable excitement about the potential for omega-3 fatty acids in cardiovascular risk reduction [103]. Subsequently, the JELIS trial demonstrated a 19% decrease in major coronary events in patients on low-dose statins who were given EPA 1.8 g daily (EPA) versus low-dose statin therapy alone [104]. Later research failed to confirm the findings in those studies [105–107], and interest in the idea that omega-3 fatty acids might confer cardiovascular protection faded to some extent.

In diabetic patients who are treated with statins, significant residual cardiovascular risk can remain, as discussed previously. Hypertriglyceridemia has been shown to be an independent risk factor for cardiovascular disease [108–110]. The REDUCE-IT trial was a 4.9-year study conducted to determine if 4 g/day icosapent ethyl, an ester of EPA, would reduce ischemic cardiovascular events versus placebo [111]. Over 8000 statin-treated patients with cardiovascular disease or diabetes with additional risk factors and elevated triglycerides were enrolled and randomized [111]. Icosapent ethyl resulted in a relative reduction in cardiovascular events (MACE 5) of 25% versus placebo. A subsequent analysis of the United States cohort of REDUCE-IT ($n = 3146$, of whom nearly 70% had diabetes) revealed a risk reduction of 31% [112]. Perhaps as a result, the 2020 Endocrine Society lipid management guidelines suggest that for diabetic patients on maximally tolerated statin therapy who have two additional risk factors for cardiovascular disease and triglyceride levels >150 mg/dL, 4 grams of EPA is added daily to reduce the risk of cardiovascular events [26]. Although the results of the clinical trials reviewed above have been inconsistent, a recent meta-analysis found significant benefit from omega-3 on total and fatal myocardial infarction and on total and fatal cardiovascular events [113].

The mechanism that accounts for the benefit in icosapent ethyl-treated patients in REDUCE-IT is unclear. Candidates include modulation of the immune system with reduced inflammatory response and alteration of cardiac sympathetic tone [114]. The role of lipoproteins is uncertain. Triglyceride levels decreased by only 18% in icosapent-treated subjects in REDUCE-IT, and risk reduction in subjects with baseline triglycerides 135–150 mg/dl was similar to that in those with baseline triglycerides >200 mg/dl; HDL-C did not change. A diet enriched in omega-3 fatty acids has been shown to decrease triglycerides and sdLDL [115]. An increase in LDL particle size has been shown with EPA treatment [116, 117], and omega-3 fatty acid treatment decreases HDL3 cholesterol (small particles) while not changing HDL2 (larger particles) [117, 118]. Thus, changes in lipoprotein particles that are not detected by standard clinical lipid tests may contribute to beneficial effects of omega-3 fatty acids.

Another possible mechanism for benefit from icosapent ethyl is an effect on platelet function. In the REDUCE-IT study, there was a nearly significant ($p = 0.06$) increase in serious bleeding events (2.6% vs 2.1% in the two groups). The potential for omega-3 fatty acid inhibition of platelet function was suggested many centuries ago; an ancient Norse document (*Historia Norvegiae*) written in 1170 AD describes the first encounter between Vikings and Inuit people in Greenland:

> On the other side of Greenland, toward the North, hunters have found some little people… when mortally wounded their blood will hardly stop running [119].

Prolonged bleeding times have since been demonstrated in the Inuit, who have a diet high in omega-3 fatty acids and a very low incidence of cardiovascular disease [120]. The potential for a contribution of altered platelet function in REDUCE-IT has been reviewed in detail recently [121]. In support of a cardioprotective role for impaired platelet function, a population-based study in Sweden recently found that although patients with von Willebrand disease do have cardiovascular disease, cardiovascular mortality was reduced in this condition by 60% compared with the general population [122]. However, clinically significant bleeding is generally not observed when omega-3 fatty acids are given at a dose of 4 g/day [123].

In summary, omega-3 fatty acids, especially EPA, appear to have a role for cardiovascular risk reduction in selected high-risk patients with hypertriglyceridemia.

Diabetes-Specific Medications

Because cardiovascular events dominate mortality in T2DM, it is critically important to emphasize diabetes medications that have favorable effects on cardiovascular outcomes and de-emphasize treatments that might have deleterious effects. For many years, the only available medications for diabetes treatment were in the insulin provision category, including sulfonylureas and insulin itself. Evidence has accumulated to indicate that insulin provision therapy may raise blood pressure. This evidence is direct for insulin itself [124, 125] and indirect for sulfonylureas [6]. The likely cause is weight gain [6, 124, 125]. Insulin treatment has also been associated with an increase in newly incident heart failure and worsening of heart failure outcomes [126]. In our view, it is appropriate to de-emphasize insulin provision treatment in most T2DM patients, where insulin resistance due to overweight and obesity is prominent [127].

Metformin

Metformin is recommended as first-line treatment in international guidelines on T2DM [128]. The reason for this is the rather dramatic reduction in myocardial infarction resulting from metformin treatment reported in the UK Prospective Diabetes Study [129]. The chief strength of this study was a two-decade follow-up – unheard of in modern clinical trials. Metformin decreases energy intake [130], lowers triglycerides [131, 132], raises (in some studies) HDL-C [133], increases LDL particle size [134], and lowers blood pressure [6]. It also is associated with improved heart failure outcomes [126, 135]. Metformin and statins have much in common. Both are treatments for which there is arguably no substitute. Both are safe, inexpensive, and effective, and both have side effects that can interfere with treatment. The gastrointestinal side effects of metformin, in our experience, can usually be managed without discontinuation of the drug.

GLP-1 Receptor Agonists

GLP-1 receptor agonists (GLP-1Ras) have assumed a prominent role in the treatment of type 2 diabetes since their introduction more than 15 years ago. Most are given by subcutaneous injection, although an oral form is available [136]. GLP-1 is secreted by the enteroendocrine cells of the gut in response to postprandial glycemic excursion and helps potentiate insulin secretion from the pancreas and limit the impact of glucagon secretion [137]. Although the effects on insulin and glucagon secretion are most often cited as the principal mechanism of action of these agents, they also delay gastric emptying, decrease satiety, and decrease energy intake [137, 138] [139]; these effects may be more important in the use of these medications than the effects on insulin and glucagon secretion.

The SUSTAIN-6 study was conducted in ~3300 patients with uncontrolled T2DM and a history of cardiovascular events. Semaglutide given over a median follow-up of 2.1 years resulted in a 26% decrease in MACE-4 events [140]. The LEADER study of cardiovascular effects of liraglutide, published in the same year, also showed cardiovascular benefit with a 13% decrease in events over a 3.8-year follow-up [141]. A study of albiglutide versus placebo in 9300 patients with T2DM found a 22% decrease in cardiovascular events over a 1.9-year period of observation [142]. A more recent trial in 9900 T2DM patients with cardiovascular disease conducted over 5.4 years demonstrated a 12% decrease in MACE 3 events with dulaglutide 1.5 mg weekly treatment [143].

The lipid-lowering properties of GLP-1RAs have received little attention; lipids are not reported consistently in the large clinical trials mentioned above. A recent study found an increase in LDL particle size after 4 months of treatment with liraglutide [144]. We were able to find six published studies that provide triglyceride data at baseline and at follow-up [140, 145–149]. Figure 3.1 shows the relationship between median baseline triglyceride concentrations and the decrease in triglycerides that was observed during the study. There was a strong correlation between the degree of hypertriglyceridemia and the magnitude of triglyceride lowering observed ($r = 0.90$, $p = 0.01$). There was also an association between the average amount of weight loss and decrease in triglycerides, but it was not significant in this small data set ($r = 0.50$, $p =$ NS, not shown). These results suggest that the lipid effects of GLP-1RAs depend on the magnitude of the lipid abnormality.

Thiazolidinediones

The thiazolidinedione class of diabetes medications was developed in Japan in the 1980s, in large part because of the lipid-lowering properties of some of the agents. Pioglitazone has robust triglyceride-lowering and HDL-C-raising effects [150]. In addition, it increases LDL particle size [151] and lowers blood pressure. It has been shown in clinical trials to reduce stroke [152]. It produced equivocal results in the PROACTIVE study, which missed a significant effect on the primary composite cardiovascular endpoint ($p = 0.095$) but did result in a significant 16% reduction in the principal secondary endpoint, $p = 0.027$ [153]. We use pioglitazone as a third-line treatment in selected diabetic patients with dyslipidemia on condition they are treated with either metformin or a GLP-1RA or both, in order to mitigate weight gain.

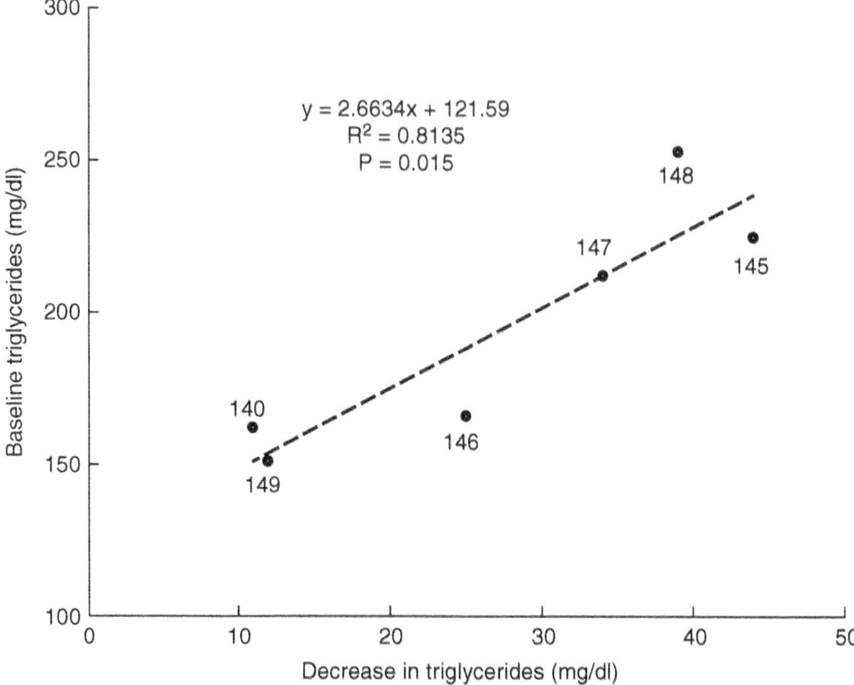

Fig. 3.1 Relationship between average baseline triglyceride concentrations and the decrease in triglyceride level observed in response to treatment with a GLP-1 receptor agonist in six studies. The number next to each data point corresponds to the reference for the study

Summary

Cardiovascular events dominate outcomes in T2DM, and dyslipidemia, which affects over half of all patients, is a major contributor. A variety of lipid-specific medications, beginning with statins, are useful in management, and the use of multiple agents has a place in treatment. In addition, aggressive diabetes pharmacotherapy, with an emphasis on medications that have been shown to improve dyslipidemia in T2DM, is warranted.

Acknowledgments We thank W. S. Harris for helpful comments.

References

1. Ahmad FB, Anderson RN. The leading causes of death in the US for 2020. JAMA. 2021;325(18):1829–30.
2. Stamler J, Vaccaro O, Neaton JD, Wentworth D. Diabetes, other risk factors, and 12-yr cardiovascular mortality for men screened in the multiple risk factor intervention trial. Diabetes Care. 1993;16(2):434–44.

3. Gu K, Cowie CC, Harris MI. Mortality in adults with and without diabetes in a national cohort of the U.S. population, 1971-1993. Diabetes Care. 1998;21(7):1138–45.
4. Raghavan S, Vassy JL, Ho YL, Song RJ, Gagnon DR, Cho K, Wilson PWF, Phillips LS. Diabetes mellitus-related all-cause and cardiovascular mortality in a National Cohort of adults. J Am Heart Assoc. 2019;8(4):e011295.
5. Ginsberg HN. REVIEW: efficacy and mechanisms of action of statins in the treatment of diabetic dyslipidemia. J Clin Endocrinol Metab. 2006;91(2):383–92.
6. Anabtawi A, Moriarty PM, Miles JM. Pharmacologic treatment of dyslipidemia in diabetes: a case for therapies in addition to statins. Curr Cardiol Rep. 2017;19(7):62.
7. Third Report of the National Cholesterol Education Program (NCEP) expert panel on detection, evaluation, and treatment of high blood cholesterol in adults (Adult Treatment Panel III) final report. Circulation. 2002;106(25):3143–421.
8. Taskinen MR, Borén J. New insights into the pathophysiology of dyslipidemia in type 2 diabetes. Atherosclerosis. 2015;239(2):483–95.
9. Grundy SM. Hypertriglyceridemia, insulin resistance, and the metabolic syndrome. Am J Cardiol. 1999;83(9b):25f–9f.
10. Chapman MJ, Ginsberg HN, Amarenco P, Andreotti F, Borén J, Catapano AL, Descamps OS, Fisher E, Kovanen PT, Kuivenhoven JA, et al. Triglyceride-rich lipoproteins and high-density lipoprotein cholesterol in patients at high risk of cardiovascular disease: evidence and guidance for management. Eur Heart J. 2011;32(11):1345–61.
11. Howard BV, Mayer-Davis EJ, Goff D, Zaccaro DJ, Laws A, Robbins DC, Saad MF, Selby J, Hamman RF, Krauss RM, et al. Relationships between insulin resistance and lipoproteins in nondiabetic African Americans, Hispanics, and non-Hispanic whites: the insulin resistance atherosclerosis study. Metab Clin Exp. 1998;47(10):1174–9.
12. Bjornstad P, Snell-Bergeon JK, Rewers M, Jalal D, Chonchol MB, Johnson RJ, Maahs DM. Early diabetic nephropathy: a complication of reduced insulin sensitivity in type 1 diabetes. Diabetes Care. 2013;36(11):3678–83.
13. Priya G, Kalra S. A review of insulin resistance in type 1 diabetes: is there a place for adjunctive metformin? Diabetes Therapy: Research, Treatment and Education of Diabetes and Related Disorders. 2018;9(1):349–61.
14. McGarry JD. What if Minkowski had been ageusic? An alternative angle on diabetes. Science. 1992;258:766–70.
15. Tilly-Kiesi M, Knudsen P, Groop L, Taskinen MR. Hyperinsulinemia and insulin resistance are associated with multiple abnormalities of lipoprotein subclasses in glucose-tolerant relatives of NIDDM patients. Botnia Study Group. J Lipid Res. 1996;37(7):1569–78.
16. Karelis AD, Pasternyk SM, Messier L, St-Pierre DH, Lavoie JM, Garrel D, Rabasa-Lhoret R. Relationship between insulin sensitivity and the triglyceride-HDL-C ratio in overweight and obese postmenopausal women: a MONET study. Applied physiology, nutrition, and metabolism = Physiologie appliquee, nutrition et metabolisme. 2007;32(6):1089–96.
17. Iwani NA, Jalaludin MY, Zin RM, Fuziah MZ, Hong JY, Abqariyah Y, Mokhtar AH, Wan Nazaimoon WM. Triglyceride to HDL-C ratio is associated with insulin resistance in overweight and obese children. Scientific reports. 2017;7:40055.
18. Guerrero-Romero F, Simental-Mendía LE, González-Ortiz M, Martínez-Abundis E, Ramos-Zavala MG, Hernández-González SO, Jacques-Camarena O, Rodríguez-Morán M. The product of triglycerides and glucose, a simple measure of insulin sensitivity. Comparison with the euglycemic-hyperinsulinemic clamp. J Clin Endocrinol Metab. 2010;95(7):3347–51.
19. Feingold KR, Grunfeld C, Pang M, Doerrler W, Krauss RM. LDL subclass phenotypes and triglyceride metabolism in non-insulin-dependent diabetes. Arteriosclerosis Thrombosis: A Journal of Vascular Biology. 1992;12(12):1496–502.
20. Bays H, Conard S, Leiter LA, Bird S, Jensen E, Hanson ME, Shah A, Tershakovec AM. Are post-treatment low-density lipoprotein subclass pattern analyses potentially misleading?. Lipids Health Dis. 2010;9:136.
21. Klop B, Elte JW, Cabezas MC. Dyslipidemia in obesity: mechanisms and potential targets. Nutrients. 2013;5(4):1218–40.

22. Isley WL, Miles JM, Patterson BW, Harris WS. The effect of high-dose simvastatin on triglyceride-rich lipoprotein metabolism in patients with type 2 diabetes mellitus. J Lipid Res. 2006;47(1):193–200.
23. Lewis GF, Uffelman KD, Szeto LW, Weller B, Steiner G. Interaction between free fatty acids and insulin in the acute control of very low density lipoprotein production in humans. J Clin Invest. 1995;95(1):158–66.
24. Muthusamy K, Nelson R, Singh E, Vlazny D, Smailovic A, Miles J. Effect of insulin infusion on spillover of meal-derived fatty acids. J Clin Endocrinol Metab. 2012;97:4201–5.
25. Sam S, Haffner S, Davidson MH, D'Agostino RB Sr, Feinstein S, Kondos G, Perez A, Mazzone T. Relationship of abdominal visceral and subcutaneous adipose tissue with lipoprotein particle number and size in type 2 diabetes. Diabetes. 2008;57(8):2022–7.
26. Newman CB, Blaha MJ, Boord JB, Cariou B, Chait A, Fein HG, Ginsberg HN, Goldberg IJ, Murad MH, Subramanian S, et al. Lipid management in patients with endocrine disorders: an endocrine society clinical practice guideline. J Clin Endocrinol Metab. 2020;105(12).
27. Arnett DK, Blumenthal RS, Albert MA, Buroker AB, Goldberger ZD, Hahn EJ, Himmelfarb CD, Khera A, Lloyd-Jones D, McEvoy JW, et al. 2019 ACC/AHA guideline on the primary prevention of cardiovascular disease: a report of the American College of Cardiology/American Heart Association task force on clinical practice guidelines. Circulation. 2019;140(11):e596–646.
28. Goff DC Jr, Lloyd-Jones DM, Bennett G, Coady S, D'Agostino RB, Gibbons R, Greenland P, Lackland DT, Levy D, O'Donnell CJ, et al. 2013 ACC/AHA guideline on the assessment of cardiovascular risk: a report of the American College of Cardiology/American Heart Association task force on practice guidelines. Circulation. 2014;129(25 Suppl 2):S49–73.
29. Muntner P, Colantonio LD, Cushman M, Goff DC Jr, Howard G, Howard VJ, Kissela B, Levitan EB, Lloyd-Jones DM, Safford MM. Validation of the atherosclerotic cardiovascular disease pooled cohort risk equations. JAMA. 2014;311(14):1406–15.
30. Istvan ES. Structural mechanism for statin inhibition of 3-hydroxy-3-methylglutaryl coenzyme a reductase. Am Heart J. 2002;144(6 Suppl):S27–32.
31. Schaefer EJ, McNamara JR, Tayler T, Daly JA, Gleason JL, Seman LJ, Ferrari A, Rubenstein JJ. Comparisons of effects of statins (atorvastatin, fluvastatin, lovastatin, pravastatin, and simvastatin) on fasting and postprandial lipoproteins in patients with coronary heart disease versus control subjects. Am J Cardiol. 2004;93(1):31–9.
32. Jones PH, Davidson MH, Stein EA, Bays HE, McKenney JM, Miller E, Cain VA, Blasetto JW. Comparison of the efficacy and safety of rosuvastatin versus atorvastatin, simvastatin, and pravastatin across doses (STELLAR* trial). Am J Cardiol. 2003;92(2):152–60.
33. Wakatsuki A, Okatani Y, Ikenoue N. Effects of combination therapy with estrogen plus simvastatin on lipoprotein metabolism in postmenopausal women with type IIa hypercholesterolemia. Atherosclerosis. 2000;150(1):103–11.
34. Lemieux I, Laperrière L, Dzavik V, Tremblay G, Bourgeois J, Després JP. A 16-week fenofibrate treatment increases LDL particle size in type IIA dyslipidemic patients. Atherosclerosis. 2002;162(2):363–71.
35. Grundy SM, Vega GL, Yuan Z, Battisti WP, Brady WE, Palmisano J. Effectiveness and tolerability of simvastatin plus fenofibrate for combined hyperlipidemia (the SAFARI trial). Am J Cardiol. 2005;95(4):462–8.
36. Markham A. Bempedoic acid: first approval. Drugs. 2020;80(7):747–53.
37. Haffner SM, Alexander CM, Cook TJ, Boccuzzi SJ, Musliner TA, Pedersen TR, Kjekshus J, Pyorala K. Reduced coronary events in simvastatin-treated patients with coronary heart disease and diabetes or impaired fasting glucose levels: subgroup analyses in the Scandinavian simvastatin survival study. Arch Intern Med. 1999;159(22):2661–7.
38. Haffner SM. The Scandinavian simvastatin survival study (4S) subgroup analysis of diabetic subjects: implications for the prevention of coronary heart disease. Diabetes Care. 1997;20(4):469–71.

39. Cannon CP, Braunwald E, McCabe CH, Rader DJ, Rouleau JL, Belder R, Joyal SV, Hill KA, Pfeffer MA, Skene AM. Intensive versus moderate lipid lowering with statins after acute coronary syndromes. N Engl J Med. 2004;350(15):1495–504.
40. Nissen SE, Tuzcu EM, Schoenhagen P, Brown BG, Ganz P, Vogel RA, Crowe T, Howard G, Cooper CJ, Brodie B, et al. Effect of intensive compared with moderate lipid-lowering therapy on progression of coronary atherosclerosis: a randomized controlled trial. JAMA. 2004;291(9):1071–80.
41. Naci H, Brugts JJ, Fleurence R, Ades AE. Dose-comparative effects of different statins on serum lipid levels: a network meta-analysis of 256,827 individuals in 181 randomized controlled trials. Eur J Prev Cardiol. 2013;20(4):658–70.
42. Deedwania P, Barter P, Carmena R, Fruchart JC, Grundy SM, Haffner S, Kastelein JJ, LaRosa JC, Schachner H, Shepherd J, et al. Reduction of low-density lipoprotein cholesterol in patients with coronary heart disease and metabolic syndrome: analysis of the treating to new targets study. Lancet. 2006;368(9539):919–28.
43. Backes JM, Venero CV, Gibson CA, Ruisinger JF, Howard PA, Thompson PD, Moriarty PM. Effectiveness and tolerability of every-other-day rosuvastatin dosing in patients with prior statin intolerance. Ann Pharmacother. 2008;42(3):341–6.
44. Jacobson TA. Statin safety: lessons from new drug applications for marketed statins. Am J Cardiol. 2006;97(8a):44c–51c.
45. Backes JM, Ruisinger JF, Gibson CA, Moriarty PM. Statin-associated muscle symptoms-managing the highly intolerant. J Clin Lipidol. 2017;11(1):24–33.
46. Bays H, Stein EA. Pharmacotherapy for dyslipidaemia--current therapies and future agents. Expert Opin Pharmacother. 2003;4(11):1901–38.
47. Cohen JD, Brinton EA, Ito MK, Jacobson TA. Understanding statin use in America and gaps in patient education (USAGE): an internet-based survey of 10,138 current and former statin users. J Clin Lipidol. 2012;6(3):208–15.
48. Colhoun HM, Betteridge DJ, Durrington PN, Hitman GA, Neil HA, Livingstone SJ, Thomason MJ, Mackness MI, Charlton-Menys V, Fuller JH. Primary prevention of cardiovascular disease with atorvastatin in type 2 diabetes in the collaborative atorvastatin diabetes study (CARDS): multicentre randomised placebo-controlled trial. Lancet. 2004;364(9435):685–96.
49. Sever PS, Dahlof B, Poulter NR, Wedel H, Beevers G, Caulfield M, Collins R, Kjeldsen SE, Kristinsson A, McInnes GT, et al. Prevention of coronary and stroke events with atorvastatin in hypertensive patients who have average or lower-than-average cholesterol concentrations, in the Anglo-Scandinavian cardiac outcomes trial--lipid lowering arm (ASCOT-LLA): a multicentre randomised controlled trial. Lancet. 2003;361(9364):1149–58.
50. Sever PS, Poulter NR, Dahlof B, Wedel H, Collins R, Beevers G, Caulfield M, Kjeldsen SE, Kristinsson A, McInnes GT, et al. Reduction in cardiovascular events with atorvastatin in 2,532 patients with type 2 diabetes: Anglo-Scandinavian cardiac outcomes trial--lipid-lowering arm (ASCOT-LLA). Diabetes Care. 2005;28(5):1151–7.
51. Knopp RH, d'Emden M, Smilde JG, Pocock SJ. Efficacy and safety of atorvastatin in the prevention of cardiovascular end points in subjects with type 2 diabetes: the atorvastatin study for prevention of coronary heart disease endpoints in non-insulin-dependent diabetes mellitus (ASPEN). Diabetes Care. 2006;29(7):1478–85.
52. Gazi IF, Mikhailidis DP. Efficacy and safety of atorvastatin in the prevention of cardiovascular end points in subjects with type 2 diabetes: the Atorvastatin Study for Prevention of Coronary Heart Disease Endpoints in Non-Insulin-Dependent Diabetes Mellitus (ASPEN): response to Knopp. Diabetes Care. 2006;29(11):2561; author reply –2.
53. Taylor F, Huffman MD, Macedo AF, Moore TH, Burke M, Davey Smith G, Ward K, Ebrahim S. Statins for the primary prevention of cardiovascular disease. Cochrane Database Sys Rev. 2013;2013(1):Cd004816.
54. Ridker PM, Danielson E, Fonseca FA, Genest J, Gotto AM Jr, Kastelein JJ, Koenig W, Libby P, Lorenzatti AJ, MacFadyen JG, et al. Rosuvastatin to prevent vascular events in men and women with elevated C-reactive protein. N Engl J Med. 2008;359(21):2195–207.

55. FDA. FDA drug safety communication: important safety label changes to cholesterol-lowering statin drugs. https://www.fda.gov/drugs/drug-safety-and-availability/fda-drug-safety-communication-important-safety-label-changes-cholesterol-lowering-statin-drugs. 2012.
56. Ridker PM, Pradhan A, MacFadyen JG, Libby P, Glynn RJ. Cardiovascular benefits and diabetes risks of statin therapy in primary prevention: an analysis from the JUPITER trial. Lancet. 2012;380(9841):565–71.
57. Rajpathak SN, Kumbhani DJ, Crandall J, Barzilai N, Alderman M, Ridker PM. Statin therapy and risk of developing type 2 diabetes: a meta-analysis. Diabetes Care. 2009;32(10): 1924–9.
58. Cai T, Abel L. Associations between statins and adverse events in primary prevention of cardiovascular disease: systematic review with pairwise, network, and dose-response meta-analyses. 2021;374:n1537.
59. Lavie G, Hoshen M, Leibowitz M, Benis A, Akriv A, Balicer R, Reges O. Statin therapy for primary prevention in the elderly and its association with new-onset diabetes, cardiovascular events, and all-cause mortality. Am J Med. 2021;134(5):643–52.
60. Bell DSH, Goncalves E. Diabetogenic effects of cardioprotective drugs. 2021;23(4):877–85.
61. Brown MS, Anderson RG, Goldstein JL. Recycling receptors: the round-trip itinerary of migrant membrane proteins. Cell. 1983;32(3):663–7.
62. Handelsman Y, Lepor NE. PCSK9 inhibitors in lipid management of patients with diabetes mellitus and high cardiovascular risk: a review. J Am Heart Associat. 2018;7(13).
63. Seidah NG, Awan Z, Chrétien M, Mbikay M. PCSK9: a key modulator of cardiovascular health. Circ Res. 2014;114(6):1022–36.
64. Lagace TA. PCSK9 and LDLR degradation: regulatory mechanisms in circulation and in cells. Curr Opin Lipidol. 2014;25(5):387–93.
65. Sabatine MS, Giugliano RP, Keech AC, Honarpour N, Wiviott SD, Murphy SA, Kuder JF, Wang H, Liu T, Wasserman SM, et al. Evolocumab and clinical outcomes in patients with cardiovascular disease. N Engl J Med. 2017;376(18):1713–22.
66. Sabatine MS, Leiter LA, Wiviott SD, Giugliano RP, Deedwania P, De Ferrari GM, Murphy SA, Kuder JF, Gouni-Berthold I, Lewis BS, et al. Cardiovascular safety and efficacy of the PCSK9 inhibitor evolocumab in patients with and without diabetes and the effect of evolocumab on glycaemia and risk of new-onset diabetes: a prespecified analysis of the FOURIER randomised controlled trial. Lancet Diabetes Endocrinol. 2017;5(12):941–50.
67. Schwartz GG, Steg PG, Szarek M, Bhatt DL. Alirocumab and cardiovascular outcomes after acute coronary syndrome. 2018;379(22):2097–107.
68. Leiter LA, Cariou B, Müller-Wieland D, Colhoun HM, Del Prato S. Efficacy and safety of alirocumab in insulin-treated individuals with type 1 or type 2 diabetes and high cardiovascular risk: The ODYSSEY DM-INSULIN randomized trial. 2017;19(12):1781–92.
69. Mani P, Ren HY, Neeland IJ, McGuire DK, Ayers CR, Khera A, Rohatgi A. The association between HDL particle concentration and incident metabolic syndrome in the multi-ethnic Dallas Heart Study. Diabetes Metabol Synd. 2017;11(Suppl 1):S175–9.
70. Ingueneau C, Hollstein T, Grenkowitz T, Ruidavets JB, Kassner U, Duparc T, Combes G, Perret B, Genoux A, Schumann F, et al. Treatment with PCSK9 inhibitors induces a more anti-atherogenic HDL lipid profile in patients at high cardiovascular risk. Vascular Pharmacol. 2020;135:106804.
71. Hollstein T, Vogt A, Grenkowitz T, Stojakovic T, März W, Laufs U, Bölükbasi B, Steinhagen-Thiessen E, Scharnagl H, Kassner U. Treatment with PCSK9 inhibitors reduces atherogenic VLDL remnants in a real-world study. Vascular Pharmacol. 2019;116:8–15.
72. Cannon CP, Blazing MA, Giugliano RP, McCagg A, White JA, Theroux P, Darius H, Lewis BS, Ophuis TO, Jukema JW, et al. Ezetimibe added to statin therapy after acute coronary syndromes. N Engl J Med. 2015;372(25):2387–97.
73. Kosoglou T, Statkevich P, Johnson-Levonas AO, Paolini JF, Bergman AJ, Alton KB. Ezetimibe: a review of its metabolism, pharmacokinetics and drug interactions. Clin Pharmacokinet. 2005;44(5):467–94.

74. Nutescu EA, Shapiro NL. Ezetimibe: a selective cholesterol absorption inhibitor. Pharmacotherapy. 2003;23(11):1463–74.
75. Giugliano RP, Cannon CP, Blazing MA, Nicolau JC, Corbalán R, Špinar J, Park JG, White JA, Bohula EA, Braunwald E. Benefit of adding ezetimibe to statin therapy on cardiovascular outcomes and safety in patients with versus without diabetes mellitus: results from IMPROVE-IT (improved reduction of outcomes: Vytorin efficacy international trial). Circulation. 2018;137(15):1571–82.
76. Conard S, Bays H, Leiter LA, Bird S, Lin J, Hanson ME, Shah A, Tershakovec AM. Ezetimibe added to atorvastatin compared with doubling the atorvastatin dose in patients at high risk for coronary heart disease with diabetes mellitus, metabolic syndrome or neither. Diabetes Obes Metab. 2010;12(3):210–8.
77. Ballantyne CM, Laufs U, Ray KK, Leiter LA, Bays HE, Goldberg AC, Stroes ES, MacDougall D, Zhao X, Catapano AL. Bempedoic acid plus ezetimibe fixed-dose combination in patients with hypercholesterolemia and high CVD risk treated with maximally tolerated statin therapy. Eur J Prev Cardiol. 2020;27(6):593–603.
78. Tribble DL, Farnier M, Macdonell G, Perevozskaya I, Davies MJ, Gumbiner B, Musliner TA. Effects of fenofibrate and ezetimibe, both as monotherapy and in coadministration, on cholesterol mass within lipoprotein subfractions and low-density lipoprotein peak particle size in patients with mixed hyperlipidemia. Metab Clin Exp. 2008;57(6):796–801.
79. Grundy SM, Stone NJ, Bailey AL, Beam C, Birtcher KK, Blumenthal RS, Braun LT, de Ferranti S, Faiella-Tommasino J, Forman DE, et al. 2018 AHA/ACC/AACVPR/AAPA/ABC/ACPM/ADA/AGS/APhA/ASPC/NLA/PCNA guideline on the Management of Blood Cholesterol: a report of the American College of Cardiology/American Heart Association task force on clinical practice guidelines. Circulation. 2019;139(25):e1082–e143.
80. Goldberg AC, Leiter LA, Stroes ESG, Baum SJ, Hanselman JC, Bloedon LT, Lalwani ND, Patel PM, Zhao X, Duell PB. Effect of Bempedoic acid vs placebo added to maximally tolerated statins on low-density lipoprotein cholesterol in patients at high risk for cardiovascular disease: the CLEAR wisdom randomized clinical trial. JAMA. 2019;322(18):1780–8.
81. Masson W, Lobo M, Lavalle-Cobo A, Masson G, Molinero G. Effect of bempedoic acid on new onset or worsening diabetes: a meta-analysis. Diabetes Res Clin Pract. 2020;168:108369.
82. Wang X, Zhang Y, Tan H, Wang P, Zha X, Chong W, Zhou L, Fang F. Efficacy and safety of bempedoic acid for prevention of cardiovascular events and diabetes: a systematic review and meta-analysis. 2020;19(1):128.
83. Libby P. The forgotten majority: unfinished business in cardiovascular risk reduction. J Am Coll Cardiol. 2005;46(7):1225–8.
84. Sacks FM, Tonkin AM, Shepherd J, Braunwald E, Cobbe S, Hawkins CM, Keech A, Packard C, Simes J, Byington R, et al. Effect of pravastatin on coronary disease events in subgroups defined by coronary risk factors: the Prospective pravastatin pooling project. Circulation. 2000;102(16):1893–900.
85. Vakkilainen J, Steiner G, Ansquer JC, Perttunen-Nio H, Taskinen MR. Fenofibrate lowers plasma triglycerides and increases LDL particle diameter in subjects with type 2 diabetes. Diabetes Care. 2002;25(3):627–8.
86. Shipman KE, Strange RC, Ramachandran S. Use of fibrates in the metabolic syndrome: a review. World J Diabetes. 2016;7(5):74–88.
87. Davidson MH, Bays HE, Stein E, Maki KC, Shalwitz RA, Doyle R. Effects of fenofibrate on atherogenic dyslipidemia in hypertriglyceridemic subjects. Clin Cardiol. 2006;29(6):268–73.
88. McTaggart F, Jones P. Effects of statins on high-density lipoproteins: a potential contribution to cardiovascular benefit. Cardiovasc Drugs Ther. 2008;22(4):321–38.
89. Remick J, Weintraub H, Setton R, Offenbacher J, Fisher E, Schwartzbard A. Fibrate therapy: an update. Cardiol Rev. 2008;16(3):129–41.
90. Fruchart JC, Hermans MP, Fruchart-Najib J, Kodama T. Selective peroxisome proliferator-activated receptor alpha modulators (SPPARMα) in the metabolic syndrome: is Pemafibrate light at the end of the tunnel? Curr Atheroscler Rep. 2021;23(1):3.

91. Frick MH, Elo O, Haapa K, Heinonen OP, Heinsalmi P, Helo P, Huttunen JK, Kaitaniemi P, Koskinen P, Manninen V, et al. Helsinki heart study: primary-prevention trial with gemfibrozil in middle-aged men with dyslipidemia. Safety of treatment, changes in risk factors, and incidence of coronary heart disease. N Engl J Med. 1987;317(20):1237–45.
92. Rubins HB, Robins SJ, Collins D, Fye CL, Anderson JW, Elam MB, Faas FH, Linares E, Schaefer EJ, Schectman G, et al. Gemfibrozil for the secondary prevention of coronary heart disease in men with low levels of high-density lipoprotein cholesterol. Veterans affairs high-density lipoprotein cholesterol intervention trial study group. N Engl J Med. 1999;341(6):410–8.
93. Group BS. Secondary prevention by raising HDL cholesterol and reducing triglycerides in patients with coronary artery disease. Circulation. 2000;102(1):21–7.
94. Keech A, Simes RJ, Barter P, Best J, Scott R, Taskinen MR, Forder P, Pillai A, Davis T, Glasziou P, et al. Effects of long-term fenofibrate therapy on cardiovascular events in 9795 people with type 2 diabetes mellitus (the FIELD study): randomised controlled trial. Lancet. 2005;366(9500):1849–61.
95. Ginsberg HN, Elam MB, Lovato LC, Crouse JR 3rd, Leiter LA, Linz P, Friedewald WT, Buse JB, Gerstein HC, Probstfield J, et al. Effects of combination lipid therapy in type 2 diabetes mellitus. N Engl J Med. 2010;362(17):1563–74.
96. Robins SJ, Collins D, Wittes JT, Papademetriou V, Deedwania PC, Schaefer EJ, McNamara JR, Kashyap ML, Hershman JM, Wexler LF, et al. Relation of gemfibrozil treatment and lipid levels with major coronary events: VA-HIT: a randomized controlled trial. JAMA. 2001;285(12):1585–91.
97. Sacks FM, Carey VJ, Fruchart JC. Combination lipid therapy in type 2 diabetes. N Engl J Med. 2010;363(7):692–4. author reply 4-5.
98. Jakob T, Nordmann AJ, Schandelmaier S, Ferreira-Gonzalez I, Briel M. Fibrates for primary prevention of cardiovascular disease events. Cochrane Database Systemat Rev. 2016;11:Cd009753.
99. Wang D, Liu B, Tao W, Hao Z, Liu M. Fibrates for secondary prevention of cardiovascular disease and stroke. Cochrane Database Systemat Rev. 2015;10:Cd009580.
100. Davis TM, Ting R, Best JD, Donoghoe MW, Drury PL, Sullivan DR, Jenkins AJ, O'Connell RL, Whiting MJ, Glasziou PP, et al. Effects of fenofibrate on renal function in patients with type 2 diabetes mellitus: the Fenofibrate intervention and event lowering in diabetes (FIELD) study. Diabetologia. 2011;54(2):280–90.
101. Cersosimo E, Miles JM. Hormonal, metabolic and hemodynamic adaptations to glycosuria in type 2 diabetes patients treated with sodium-glucose co-transporter inhibitors. Curr Diabetes Rev. 2019;15(4):314–27.
102. Marchioli R, Barzi F, Bomba E, Chieffo C, Di Gregorio D, Di Mascio R, Franzosi MG, Geraci E, Levantesi G, Maggioni AP, et al. Early protection against sudden death by n-3 polyunsaturated fatty acids after myocardial infarction: time-course analysis of the results of the Gruppo Italiano per lo studio della Sopravvivenza nell'Infarto Miocardico (GISSI)-Prevenzione. Circulation. 2002;105(16):1897–903.
103. Leaf A. On the reanalysis of the GISSI-Prevenzione. Circulation. 2002;105(16):1874–5.
104. Yokoyama M, Origasa H, Matsuzaki M, Matsuzawa Y, Saito Y, Ishikawa Y, Oikawa S, Sasaki J, Hishida H, Itakura H, et al. Effects of eicosapentaenoic acid on major coronary events in hypercholesterolaemic patients (JELIS): a randomised open-label, blinded endpoint analysis. Lancet. 2007;369(9567):1090–8.
105. Galan P, Kesse-Guyot E, Czernichow S, Briancon S, Blacher J, Hercberg S. Effects of B vitamins and omega 3 fatty acids on cardiovascular diseases: a randomised placebo controlled trial. BMJ. 2010;341:c6273.
106. Bosch J, Gerstein HC, Dagenais GR, Díaz R, Dyal L, Jung H, Maggiono AP, Probstfield J, Ramachandran A, Riddle MC, et al. N-3 fatty acids and cardiovascular outcomes in patients with dysglycemia. N Engl J Med. 2012;367(4):309–18.

107. Rizos EC, Ntzani EE, Bika E, Kostapanos MS, Elisaf MS. Association between omega-3 fatty acid supplementation and risk of major cardiovascular disease events: a systematic review and meta-analysis. JAMA. 2012;308(10):1024–33.
108. Nichols GA, Philip S, Reynolds K, Granowitz CB, Fazio S. Increased cardiovascular risk in Hypertriglyceridemic patients with statin-controlled LDL cholesterol. J Clin Endocrinol Metab. 2018;103(8):3019–27.
109. Navar AM. The evolving story of triglycerides and coronary heart disease risk. JAMA. 2019;321(4):347–9.
110. Nelson AJ, Navar AM, Mulder H, Wojdyla D, Philip S, Granowitz C, Peterson ED, Pagidipati NJ. Association between triglycerides and residual cardiovascular risk in patients with type 2 diabetes mellitus and established cardiovascular disease (From the Bypass Angioplasty Revascularization Investigation 2 Diabetes [BARI 2D] Trial). Am J Cardiol. 2020;132:36–43.
111. Bhatt DL, Steg PG, Miller M, Brinton EA, Jacobson TA, Ketchum SB, Doyle RT Jr, Juliano RA, Jiao L, Granowitz C, et al. Cardiovascular risk reduction with Icosapent ethyl for hypertriglyceridemia. N Engl J Med. 2019;380(1):11–22.
112. Bhatt DL, Miller M, Brinton EA, Jacobson TA, Steg PG, Ketchum SB, Doyle RT Jr, Juliano RA, Jiao L, Granowitz C, et al. REDUCE-IT USA: results from the 3146 patients randomized in the United States. Circulation. 2020;141(5):367–75.
113. Bernasconi AA, Wiest MM, Lavie CJ, Milani RV, Laukkanen JA. Effect of Omega-3 dosage on cardiovascular outcomes: an updated meta-analysis and meta-regression of interventional trials. Mayo Clin Proc. 2021;96(2):304–13.
114. Darwesh AM, Sosnowski DK, Lee TY, Keshavarz-Bahaghighat H, Seubert JM. Insights into the cardioprotective properties of n-3 PUFAs against ischemic heart disease via modulation of the innate immune system. Chemico-Biological Interactions. 2019;308:20–44.
115. Griffin MD, Sanders TA, Davies IG, Morgan LM, Millward DJ, Lewis F, Slaughter S, Cooper JA, Miller GJ, Griffin BA. Effects of altering the ratio of dietary n-6 to n-3 fatty acids on insulin sensitivity, lipoprotein size, and postprandial lipemia in men and postmenopausal women aged 45-70 y: the OPTILIP study. Am J Clin Nutr. 2006;84(6):1290–8.
116. Tani S, Nagao K, Matsumoto M, Hirayama A. Highly purified eicosapentaenoic acid may increase low-density lipoprotein particle size by improving triglyceride metabolism in patients with hypertriglyceridemia. Circulat J Off J Japanese Circulat Soc. 2013;77(9):2349–57.
117. Mori TA, Burke V, Puddey IB, Watts GF, O'Neal DN, Best JD, Beilin LJ. Purified eicosapentaenoic and docosahexaenoic acids have differential effects on serum lipids and lipoproteins, LDL particle size, glucose, and insulin in mildly hyperlipidemic men. Am J Clin Nutr. 2000;71(5):1085–94.
118. Tani S, Matsuo R, Yagi T, Matsumoto N. Administration of eicosapentaenoic acid may alter high-density lipoprotein heterogeneity in statin-treated patients with stable coronary artery disease: a 6-month randomized trial. J Cardiol. 2020;75(3):282–8.
119. McGovern TH. Cows, harp seals and churchbells: adaption and extinction in Norse Greenland. Human Ecol. 1980;8:245–75.
120. Dyerberg J, Bang HO. Haemostatic function and platelet polyunsaturated fatty acids in Eskimos. Lancet. 1979;2(8140):433–5.
121. Sheikh O, Vande Hei AG, Battisha A, Hammad T, Pham S, Chilton R. Cardiovascular, electrophysiologic, and hematologic effects of omega-3 fatty acids beyond reducing hypertriglyceridemia: as it pertains to the recently published REDUCE-IT trial. Cardiovasc Diabetol. 2019;18(1):84.
122. Holm E, Osooli M. Cardiovascular disease-related hospitalization and mortality among persons with von Willebrand disease: a nationwide register study in Sweden. 2019;25(1):109–15.
123. Jeansen S, Witkamp RF, Garthoff JA, van Helvoort A, Calder PC. Fish oil LC-PUFAs do not affect blood coagulation parameters and bleeding manifestations: analysis of 8 clinical studies with selected patient groups on omega-3-enriched medical nutrition. Clin Nutr. 2018;37(3):948–57.

124. Yki-Jarvinen H, Ryysy L, Kauppila M, Kujansuu E, Lahti J, Marjanen T, Niskanen L, Rajala S, Salo S, Seppala M, et al. Effect of obesity on the response to insulin therapy in noninsulin-dependent diabetes mellitus. J Clin Endocrinol Metab. 1997;82:4037–43.
125. Genev N, Lau I, Willey K, Molyneaux L, Xu Z, Zilkens R, Wyndham R, Yue D. Does insulin therapy have a hypertensive effect in type 2 diabetes?. J Cardiovasc Pharmacol. 1998;32:39–41.
126. Nichols GA, Koro CE, Gullion CM, Ephross SA, Brown JB. The incidence of congestive heart failure associated with antidiabetic therapies. Diabet/Metab Res Rev. 2005;21(1):51–7.
127. Groop L. Pathogenesis of type 2 diabetes: the relative contribution of insulin resistance and impaired insulin secretion. Inter J Clin Pract Supple. 2000;11(3):3–13.
128. Davies MJ, D'Alessio DA, Fradkin J, Kernan WN, Mathieu C. Management of hyperglycemia in type 2 diabetes, 2018. A Consensus Report by the American Diabetes Association (ADA) and the European Association for the Study of Diabetes (EASD). 2018;41(12):2669–701.
129. Holman R, Paul S, Bethel M, Matthews D, Neil H. 10-year follow-up of intensive glucose control in type 2 diabetes. N Engl J Med. 2008;359:1577–89.
130. Makimattila S, Nikkila K, Yki-Jarvinen H. Causes of weight gain during insulin therapy with and without metformin in patients with Type II diabetes mellitus. Diabetologia. 1999;42:406–12.
131. Nagi DK, Yudkin JS. Effects of metformin on insulin resistance, risk factors for cardiovascular disease, and plasminogen activator inhibitor in NIDDM subjects. A study of two ethnic groups. Diabetes Care. 1993;16(4):621–9.
132. DeFronzo RA, Goodman AM. Efficacy of metformin in patients with non-insulin-dependent diabetes mellitus. The multicenter metformin study group. N Engl J Med. 1995;333(9):541–9.
133. Giugliano D, Quatraro A, Consoli G, Minei A, Ceriello A, De Rosa N, D'Onofrio F. Metformin for obese, insulin-treated diabetic patients: improvement in glycaemic control and reduction of metabolic risk factors. Eur J Clin Pharmacol. 1993;44(2):107–12.
134. Ohira M, Miyashita Y, Ebisuno M, Saiki A, Endo K, Koide N, Oyama T, Murano T, Watanabe H, Shirai K. Effect of metformin on serum lipoprotein lipase mass levels and LDL particle size in type 2 diabetes mellitus patients. Diabetes Res Clin Pract. 2007;78(1):34–41.
135. Eurich DT, Majumdar SR, McAlister FA, Tsuyuki RT, Johnson JA. Improved clinical outcomes associated with metformin in patients with diabetes and heart failure. Diabetes Care. 2005;28(10):2345–51.
136. Buse JB, Bode BW, Mertens A, Cho YM, Christiansen E, Hertz CL, Nielsen MA, Pieber TR. Long-term efficacy and safety of oral semaglutide and the effect of switching from sitagliptin to oral semaglutide in patients with type 2 diabetes: a 52-week, randomized, open-label extension of the PIONEER 7 trial. BMJ Open Diabetes Res Care. 2020;8(2).
137. Drucker DJ. Mechanisms of action and therapeutic application of glucagon-like Peptide-1. Cell Metab. 2018;27(4):740–56.
138. O'Neil PM, Birkenfeld AL, McGowan B, Mosenzon O, Pedersen SD, Wharton S, Carson CG, Jepsen CH, Kabisch M, Wilding JPH. Efficacy and safety of semaglutide compared with liraglutide and placebo for weight loss in patients with obesity: a randomised, double-blind, placebo and active controlled, dose-ranging, phase 2 trial. Lancet. 2018;392(10148):637–49.
139. Ahrén B, Atkin SL. Semaglutide induces weight loss in subjects with type 2 diabetes regardless of baseline BMI or gastrointestinal adverse events in the SUSTAIN 1 to 5 trials. 2018;20(9):2210–9.
140. Marso SP, Bain SC, Consoli A, Eliaschewitz FG, Jódar E, Leiter LA, Lingvay I, Rosenstock J, Seufert J, Warren ML, et al. Semaglutide and cardiovascular outcomes in patients with type 2 diabetes. N Engl J Med. 2016;375(19):1834–44.
141. Marso SP, Daniels GH, Brown-Frandsen K, Kristensen P, Mann JF, Nauck MA, Nissen SE, Pocock S, Poulter NR, Ravn LS, et al. Liraglutide and cardiovascular outcomes in type 2 diabetes. N Engl J Med. 2016;375(4):311–22.
142. Hernandez AF, Green JB, Janmohamed S, D'Agostino RB Sr, Granger CB, Jones NP, Leiter LA, Rosenberg AE, Sigmon KN, Somerville MC, et al. Albiglutide and cardiovascular out-

comes in patients with type 2 diabetes and cardiovascular disease (harmony outcomes): a double-blind, randomised placebo-controlled trial. Lancet. 2018;392(10157):1519–29.
143. Gerstein HC, Colhoun HM, Dagenais GR, Diaz R, Lakshmanan M, Pais P, Probstfield J, Riesmeyer JS, Riddle MC, Rydén L, et al. Dulaglutide and cardiovascular outcomes in type 2 diabetes (REWIND): a double-blind, randomised placebo-controlled trial. Lancet. 2019;394(10193):121–30.
144. Nikolic D, Giglio RV, Rizvi AA, Patti AM, Montalto G, Maranta F, Cianflone D, Stoian AP, Rizzo M. Liraglutide reduces carotid intima-media thickness by reducing small dense low-density lipoproteins in a real-world setting of patients with type 2 diabetes: a novel anti-Atherogenic effect. Diabetes Therapy: Research, Treatment and Education of Diabetes and Related Disorders. 2021;12(1):261–74.
145. Klonoff DC, Buse JB, Nielsen LL, Guan X, Bowlus CL, Holcombe JH, Wintle ME, Maggs DG. Exenatide effects on diabetes, obesity, cardiovascular risk factors and hepatic biomarkers in patients with type 2 diabetes treated for at least 3 years. Curr Med Res Opin. 2008;24(1):275–86.
146. Drucker DJ, Buse JB, Taylor K, Kendall DM, Trautmann M, Zhuang D, Porter L. Exenatide once weekly versus twice daily for the treatment of type 2 diabetes: a randomised, open-label, non-inferiority study. Lancet. 2008;372(9645):1240–50.
147. Zinman B, Gerich J, Buse JB, Lewin A, Schwartz S, Raskin P, Hale PM, Zdravkovic M, Blonde L. Efficacy and safety of the human glucagon-like peptide-1 analog liraglutide in combination with metformin and thiazolidinedione in patients with type 2 diabetes (LEAD-4 met+TZD). Diabetes Care. 2009;32(7):1224–30.
148. Blonde L, Pencek R, MacConell L. Association among weight change, glycemic control, and markers of cardiovascular risk with exenatide once weekly: a pooled analysis of patients with type 2 diabetes. Cardiovasc Diabetol. 2015;14(12).
149. Husain M, Birkenfeld AL, Donsmark M, Dungan K, Eliaschewitz FG, Franco DR, Jeppesen OK, Lingvay I, Mosenzon O, Pedersen SD, et al. Oral Semaglutide and cardiovascular outcomes in patients with type 2 diabetes. N Engl J Med. 2019;381(9):841–51.
150. Betteridge DJ. Effects of pioglitazone on lipid and lipoprotein metabolism. Diabetes Obes Metab. 2007;9(5):640–7.
151. Deeg MA, Buse JB, Goldberg RB, Kendall DM, Zagar AJ, Jacober SJ, Khan MA, Perez AT, Tan MH. Pioglitazone and rosiglitazone have different effects on serum lipoprotein particle concentrations and sizes in patients with type 2 diabetes and dyslipidemia. Diabetes Care. 2007;30(10):2458–64.
152. Kernan WN, Viscoli CM, Furie KL, Young LH, Inzucchi SE, Gorman M, Guarino PD, Lovejoy AM, Peduzzi PN, Conwit R, et al. Pioglitazone after ischemic stroke or transient ischemic attack. N Engl J Med. 2016;374(14):1321–31.
153. Dormandy JA, Charbonnel B, Eckland DJ, Erdmann E, Massi-Benedetti M, Moules IK, Skene AM, Tan MH, Lefebvre PJ, Murray GD, et al. Secondary prevention of macrovascular events in patients with type 2 diabetes in the PROactive study (PROspective pioglitAzone clinical trial in macroVascular events): a randomised controlled trial. Lancet. 2005;366(9493):1279–89.

Chapter 4
Imaging in Precision Medicine for Diabetes

Oana Patricia Zaharia, Vera B. Schrauwen-Hinderling, and Michael Roden

Role of Noninvasive Imaging Techniques in Precision Diabetology

People with diabetes mellitus present heterogeneous metabolic features and – in contrast to current paradigms – with large variation in both insulin resistance and beta-cell dysfunction [1]. Indeed, differences in metabolic regulation exist among individuals even in those with comparable glycemic control [2].Moreover, differences in tissue-specific metabolism and diabetes-related comorbidities and complications are present already at diagnosis of diabetes [3, 4]. These features may represent primordial factors for identifying subtypes (subgroups, clusters) of diabetes mellitus and contribute to diagnostic procedures and therapeutic decisions. Recent advances in comprehensive phenotyping allowed to propose subgroups of patients of non-autoimmune diabetes with different susceptibility to

O. P. Zaharia · M. Roden (✉)
Department of Endocrinology and Diabetology, Medical Faculty and University Hospital Düsseldorf, Heinrich-Heine-University Düsseldorf, Düsseldorf, Germany

Institute for Clinical Diabetology, German Diabetes Center, Leibniz Institute for Diabetes Research at Heinrich-Heine-University, Düsseldorf, Germany

German Center for Diabetes Research, Partner Düsseldorf, München-Neuherberg, Germany
e-mail: michael.roden@ddz.de

V. B. Schrauwen-Hinderling
Institute for Clinical Diabetology, German Diabetes Center, Leibniz Institute for Diabetes Research at Heinrich-Heine-University, Düsseldorf, Germany

German Center for Diabetes Research, Partner Düsseldorf, München-Neuherberg, Germany

Department of Radiology and Nuclear Medicine/Nutrition and Movement Sciences, NUTRIM School of Nutrition and Translational Research in Metabolism Maastricht University Medical Center, Maastricht, The Netherlands

R. Basu (ed.), *Precision Medicine in Diabetes*,
https://doi.org/10.1007/978-3-030-98927-9_4

diabetes-related sequelae, which could help pave the road for precise, targeted prevention and treatment [3, 5–8].

Precision medicine in diabetes [5, 9], which we prefer to term precision diabetology, holds promise to improve prevention and treatment of this multifactorial disease on various levels. Imaging tools can help discriminate subgroups of patients with specific structural, functional, or molecular abnormalities, who are otherwise classified under the broad umbrella of type 1 diabetes or type 2 diabetes, and provide the basis for optimal preventive or therapeutic measures [8, 10].

Questions remain regarding the clinical utility of these data and how best to incorporate them into routine diabetes care [11, 12]. In addition to advances in clinical decision-making tools, there is also a need to integrate other types of "omics" ((epi)genomics, metabolomics, lipidomics, proteomics, or transcriptomics) but also diverse imaging techniques to provide a full landscape of the correlations between disease pathways, phenotypes, and treatment response. To this end, it is required to provide an optimized framework encompassing established -omics and biomarkers, together with imaging and spectroscopic data, allowing for in vivo metabolic flux analysis (fluxomics) and to incorporate this data into clinical records for evaluation of validity, efficacy, and cost-effectiveness [13]. In addition, more research efforts are required to build the clinical evidence and roadmap for achieving consensus and developing guidelines [14] in the pursuit of precision medicine for optimal disease management outcome.

This chapter will focus on noninvasive in vivo imaging tools for assessing tissue-specific abnormalities and alterations of fluxomics in the context of diabetes mellitus and its role for its targeted prevention, diagnosis, and treatment.

Imaging Tools for Assessing Body Composition and Adipose Tissue Compartments

Obesity is associated with an increased risk of developing insulin resistance and type 2 diabetes [15], and the large majority of people with type 2 diabetes are overweight or obese. Differences in adipose tissue compartments might enable an early identification of people at risk of diabetes-related complications, as not only the amount but also the distribution of adipose tissue is expected to play an essential role in the pathogenesis and disease progression of diabetes [16]. A classification of the different adipose tissue compartments and the ectopic fat depots to be further addressed in this chapter is presented in Fig. 4.1 [17].

Particularly, visceral adipose tissue (VAT) has been suggested to play an important role in the pathogenesis of insulin resistance, abnormal glucose metabolism ("prediabetes"), and type 2 diabetes. This is based on the observation of a stronger correlation of insulin resistance with VAT than with total fat mass [18–20]. However, the quantification of VAT volume is dependent on body height, and therefore, normalization to body size or to total adipose tissue is necessary. When evaluating several indices derived from VAT volume, VAT/m^3 appears to provide a good marker

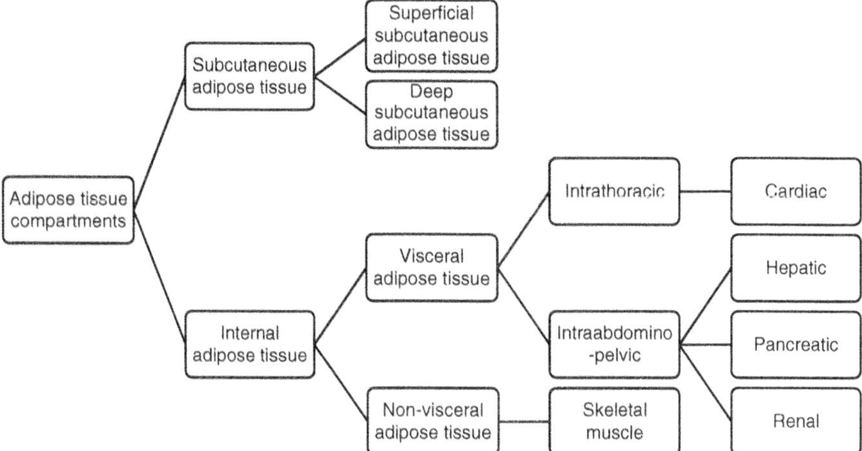

Fig. 4.1 Adipose tissue compartments. Proposed classification of adipose tissue compartments based on imaging. (Adapted from [17])

of metabolic disturbances as it was identified to correlate best with insulin sensitivity and glycemic control [18].

Furthermore, recent data provide evidence for differences in metabolic activity between deep subcutaneous adipose tissue (DSAT) and superficial subcutaneous adipose tissue (SSAT) [21], which are separated by Scarpa's fascia [22]. This structure is particularly visible using ultrasound imaging techniques [21].

SSAT volume negatively associates with levels of glycated hemoglobin (HbA_{1c}) and positively with high-density lipoprotein (HDL) cholesterol concentration in type 2 diabetes [23], therefore rather suggesting that SSAT volume is a marker of metabolic health [24] (Fig. 4.2). In contrast, DSAT volume showed a positive association with insulin resistance, similar to visceral VAT volume [22]. Furthermore, DSAT volume, similarly to VAT, might be a good predictor of fasting insulin levels [19]. These imaging parameters may add to the in-depth metabolic characterization of patients with diabetes allowing a more precise stratification [3, 6, 7, 25].

Assessment of whole-body adiposity can be performed by different techniques including bioimpedance, hydrostatic weighing, air displacement plethysmography, densitometry (DXA), computed tomography (CT), and magnetic resonance imaging (MRI). Of note, the different techniques assess different aspects of adipose tissue. Hydrostatic weighing and air displacement only provide whole-body density from which fat percentage can be deduced. If detailed information of adipose tissue distribution is desired without exposure to ionizing radiation, MRI is the most reliable choice.

Air displacement plethysmography uses whole-body densitometry to determine body volume and can accommodate a wide range of populations. This method is specifically relevant for humans with contraindications for other noninvasive measuring tools such as MRI [26]. Based on tissue density, body composition (body fat

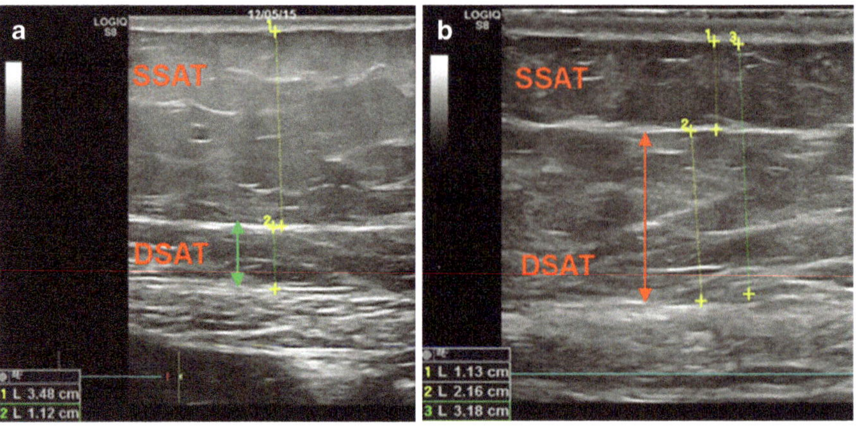

Fig. 4.2 Subcutaneous adipose tissue compartments. Subcutaneous adipose tissue compartments (deep and superficial subcutaneous adipose tissue, DSAT and SSAT) in volunteers with normal glucose tolerance (**a**) and with type 2 diabetes (**b**). (Modified from [21])

and fat-free mass) can be estimated by air displacement plethysmography and hydrostatic weighing.

Dual-energy X-ray absorptiometry (DXA) is a means of measuring body composition using spectral imaging. However, as it is a projection method, anterior-posterior information is lost. Nevertheless, thanks to the association of data within big data bases and new algorithms, the differential estimate of subcutaneous and intra-abdominal visceral fat content is possible [27].

In CT, the contrast between adipose tissue and non-adipose tissue is less pronounced, and as the technique uses X-rays, it is not indicated for all applications. An advantage of CT with respect to MRI is that image homogeneity is superior, which makes the threshold-based image segmentation much easier for CT. Studies using CT to assess metabolic syndrome and diabetes revealed that accumulation of visceral adipose tissue and fat distribution are relevant markers of metabolic risk.

MRI based on T1-weighted, T2-weighted, or Dixon images provide high contrast between adipose tissue and non-adipose tissue, making segmentation possible. This provides a reliable basis for interindividual comparison of the body fat distribution and allows a fast and reliable quantification of total body adipose tissue and the distribution of different adipose tissue components as subcutaneous and visceral fat in different body regions.

The coefficients of variation for adipose tissue measurements by MRI are 3–18% compared to CT where the variations are around 2% [28–30]. The signal intensity of MRI pixels from the same tissue may vary from region to region due to magnetic field heterogeneity. There may also be some sequence-related artifacts with MRI, such as chemical shift and blood flow artifacts. These effects collectively lower the accuracy and precision of MRI adipose tissue estimates, particularly as image analysis requires establishing the irregular boundaries between VAT and other tissues and organs.

Imaging Tools for Assessing Skeletal Muscle Tissue Structure and Metabolism

When obesity develops, triglycerides are primarily stored in adipose tissue, but with increasing adipose tissue dysfunction, triglycerides, fatty acids, and glycerol are also distributed to non-adipose tissues such as skeletal muscle cells, hepatocytes, or cardiomyocytes, where triglycerides accumulate within small lipid droplets in the cytoplasm. This phenomenon is known as "ectopic" fat storage. The lipid accumulation in muscle tissue could further refine the precise characterization of humans with diabetes.

Intramyocellular Lipid Content

Accumulation of intramyocellular lipids (IMCL) is associated with insulin resistance in muscle, and interestingly, this IMCL accumulation appears to be a very early event in the development of insulin resistance, as IMCL is already found to be increased in insulin-resistant offspring of patients with diabetes, which are healthy but have an increased risk to develop type 2 diabetes [31]. Increased IMCL accumulate, when the supply of fatty acids to skeletal muscle exceeds the capacity and need for muscular fat oxidation. On the other hand, accumulated fatty acids and their derivatives in IMCL may interfere with muscle insulin signaling. The imbalance between supply and oxidation of fatty acids can be induced by a positive energy balance due to overnutrition or physical inactivity or a reduced capacity for muscular fat oxidation (i.e., reduced mitochondrial oxidative capacity), as observed in the elderly [16, 32]. Strikingly, this negative relationship between IMCL and insulin sensitivity, however, has not been found in well-trained endurance athletes, who exhibit high IMCL, yet are highly insulin sensitive [33, 34]. This has been termed the "athlete's paradox," and it was shown that there is a U-shaped relationship between IMCL content and oxidative capacity (which is low in diabetic patients and is increased as an adaptation to physical exercise training in endurance trained individuals) [35]. While initial observations focused on intramuscular triglycerides and their impact on insulin resistance [36], it soon became clear that not the triglycerides per se, but rather bioactive lipid species, in particular diacylglycerols (DAG) and ceramides, have a role in mediating lipid-induced insulin resistance via inhibition of insulin signaling by increasing insulin receptor substrate (IRS)-1 tyrosine phosphorylation or by decreasing AKT activity, respectively [37, 38].Biochemical quantification of lipid content in muscle biopsies does not confer a true quantification of IMCL as contamination of the biopsy specimen by lipids from adipose tissue that infiltrates muscle (also called extramyocellular lipid (EMCL) is almost impossible to prevent, leading to large variation in IMCL determination. It has been demonstrated that magnetic resonance spectroscopy (MRS) techniques are capable of distinguishing IMCL from EMCL in vivo, thereby offering the potential to derive more reliable IMCL measures [39–41].The origin of the separation of the IMCL and EMCL signals in the 1H-MR spectrum is a magnetic susceptibility effect, which results in the separation of the IMCL and EMCL resonances of up to 0.2 ppm [41, 42]. The magnitude of this separation depends on the relative orientation of the adipose tissue layers of EMCL to the main magnetic field, and therefore, maximal separation (and therefore most reliable quantification) is reached in muscles where the muscle fibers run parallel to the leg and when the leg is placed parallel to the main magnetic field [41]. Therefore, IMCL content is often investigated in the tibialis anterior and the soleus muscle where fiber orientation is favorable. In line, the quantification in the vastuslateralis muscle is more challenging, due to the variable direction of muscle fibers, which results in a lesser separation of the IMCL and EMCL resonances. As pointed out above, the EMCL signal originates from adipose tissue that is "marbelling" skeletal muscle. Of note, in contrast to IMCL, the quantification of this EMCL signal by MR spectroscopy is not realistic, as the adipose tissue signal is highly variable, depending on the placement of the region of interest (voxel). In order to quantify such adipose tissue that infiltrates muscle, MRI imaging or CT is better suitable. Based on images with good contrast between adipose tissue and muscle tissue, segmentation of the images can be performed, and the volume of adipose tissue (EMCL) can be determined. Therefore, while EMCL can be quantified by imaging methods (MRI and CT) based on segmentation, this is not valid for IMCL determination, which depends on MR spectroscopy, as on an MRI or CT image, the partial volume effect prevents the quantification of IMCL without EMCL contamination [43].

Assessment of Mitochondrial Function in Skeletal Muscle

In order to investigate energy metabolism, phosphorous MRS can be used, and a decreased mitochondrial function was reported as an early hallmark of type 2 diabetes mellitus [44] in skeletal muscle by phosphorous spectroscopy, either by using saturation transfer [44] or PCr recovery measurements [45]. The saturation transfer measurements quantify the ATP synthetic flux, however, tend to overestimate the flux because the unidirectional flux (rather than the net flux) is determined and the measurement is not restricted to mitochondrial ATP synthesis, but also includes cytoplasmatic components, making the interpretation as a marker of mitochondrial function rather difficult [46]. PCr recovery measurements assume that the kinetic of PCr resynthesis reflects mitochondrial capacity, as it is largely fuelled by aerobic metabolism. These assumptions were validated, and generally, PCr recovery is accepted to be a robust measure of skeletal muscle oxidative capacity and therefore in vivo mitochondrial function [47].Initial reports on decreased in mitochondrial function in diabetes that were found with saturation transfer were confirmed by PCr recovery measurements [48].

Assessment of Metabolic Fluxes

Monitoring specific metabolites can make it possible to draw conclusions about the rate-limiting steps in series of reactions. To this end, ^{31}P MRS is commonly used. An elegant example of how this principle was used is the classical studies that show that insulin resistance in skeletal muscle results in lower concentrations of glucose-6 phosphate during insulin-stimulated glucose disposal [39, 49]. These results indicate that glucose transport and phosphorylation rather than the subsequent glycogen synthesis is responsible for muscle insulin resistance [50]. Thus, real-time monitoring of intracellular metabolites under standardized situations allows for gaining mechanistic insights and may in the future help identify specific abnormalities in (pre)diabetes subgroups [8].

Recently, ^{1}H-MRS was shown to be able to quantify acetylcarnitine concentrations directly in vivo in skeletal muscle and to be negatively correlated with insulin sensitivity [51]. A recent study in people with type 2 diabetes shows that carnitine supplementation can increase acetylcarnitine concentrations in muscle and at the same time improve insulin sensitivity. While these results are promising, the biological mechanisms involved and the exact interpretation of acetylcarnitine need to be investigated in more detail in future studies, and it will need to investigate which subgroups of patients can profit most from carnitine supplementation.

Imaging Tools for Assessing Hepatic Tissue Function and Metabolism

Hepatocellular Lipid Content

Metabolic disorders, such as obesity and diabetes mellitus, also tightly associate with increased risk and accelerated progression of non-alcoholic fatty liver disease (NAFLD), which comprises various pathologies ranging from simple fatty liver (hepatic steatosis or non-alcoholic fatty liver disease, NAFL) over non-alcoholic steatohepatitis (NASH) to fibrosis and cirrhosis [1, 52, 53]. NAFL is one important example of ectopic triglyceride accumulation and coexists with insulin resistance, and associates with adipose tissue dysfunction, defined by local inflammation, excessive lipolysis, and altered adipocytokine secretion [1, 52, 53]. Moreover, obese individuals feature altered adaptation of hepatic mitochondria to higher lipid flux [54] with subsequent intracellular accumulation of diacylglycerols and/or ceramides [55, 56], which may underlie the association between hepatocellular lipids (HCL)and insulin resistance [1, 57, 58].

There is strong evidence that NAFL is associated with insulin resistance and an important risk factor for diabetes mellitus. In fact, individuals with NAFL were as insulin resistant as age- and BMI-matched patients with type 2 diabetes [59]. Next to an increased risk to develop diabetes, NAFL also predisposes to the progression of liver disease, specifically to inflammation and fibrosis. To this end, early detection of increased liver fat content is crucial, and here, MR spectroscopy methods can be used, but also MRI imaging is a valuable tool, as in the liver, there are no adipose tissue infiltrations and all fat signal can be interpreted as signal from lipid droplets in hepatocytes (= truly ectopic intracellular fat).

Especially fat- and water-selective MRI methods are currently widely applied to determine hepatic fat content. Compared to ultrasound sonography, which detects hyperintense liver tissue as NAFL only when steatosis is severe (above a liver fat content of about 10%), MRI is much more sensitive and can be useful in detecting an even slightly increased liver fat content. When compared to MR spectroscopy, MRI has the advantage of being fast and easy in analysis (vendors provide reconstructed maps of proton density fat fraction (PDFF) based on the water and fat MRI images) and to cover the whole liver, while MRS is restricted to a volume of interest of a few cm3. Thus, MRI is superior to single-voxel MRS for detecting inhomogeneous fat accumulation within the liver (focal steatosis). The easy and noninvasive screening for NAFL is important to identify individuals with NAFL and monitor them more stringently for progression to either diabetes or NASH.

MR spectroscopy has the advantage that next to only fat content, more information can be deduced, and, for example, the fatty acid composition in terms of relative percentage of saturated fatty acids (SFA), mono-unsaturated FA (MUFA), and poly-unsaturated FA(PUFA) can be determined. It was recently shown that the SFA content is a marker for de novo lipogenesis (DNL) [60], and therefore, people with NAFL and high SFA may be treated in order to specifically decrease DNL, for example, by dietary means (decreasing fructose intake and lowering the glycemic index of the diet). Therefore, the determination of fatty acid composition by means of MRS may add to a more stratified NAFL management.

Progression of NAFLD

An advantage of determining liver fat with MRI or MRS is that it can be combined with noninvasive measurements that give indications of progression of NAFL, for example, magnetic resonance elastography (MRE) regarding the development of fibrosis. MRE yields information about the stiffness of tissue by assessing the propagation of mechanical waves through the tissue with a special MRI technique. MRE is mainly being used clinically for the assessment of patients with chronic liver diseases and is emerging as a safe, reliable, and noninvasive alternative to liver biopsy for staging hepatic fibrosis [61] (Fig. 4.3).

It has been shown that humans with diabetes can be allocated to specific clusters that present differences in the presence and severity of NAFLD [3, 62]. Specifically, patients with severe insulin-resistant diabetes present with high HCL and are more

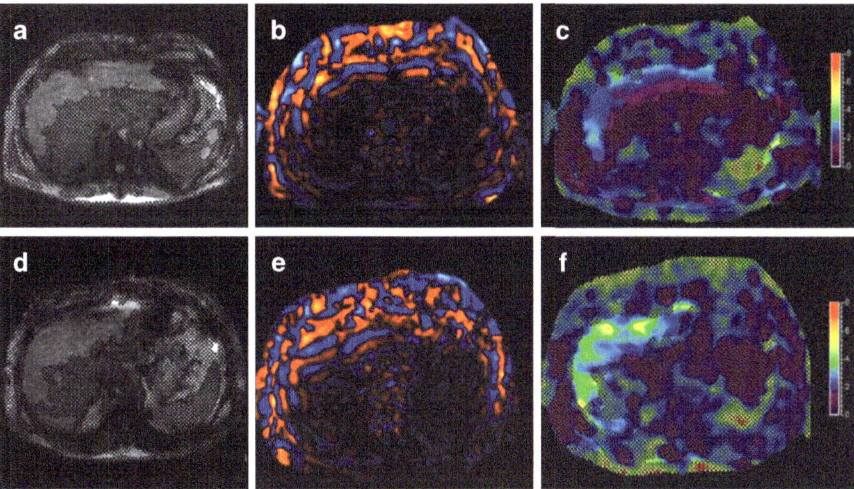

Fig. 4.3 Magnetic resonance elastography of the liver. Images (**a**–**c**) show physiological liver parameters, while images (**d**–**f**) show manifestations of NAFLD. Panels (**a** and **d**) show magnitude image, panels (**b** and **e**) show wave image, and panels (**c** and **f**) show liver stiffness

likely to exhibit NAFLD progression during the early course of diabetes. Genetic variants may further contribute to the susceptibility toward NAFLD progression for certain subgroups [62]. Therefore, it is of increased relevance to identify early changes in HCL and liver fibrosis and initiate early treatment in patients with diabetes that are at high risk for NAFLD.

Mitochondrial Function

Mitochondrial function can be also investigated by quantifying the flux through the TCA cycle, by applying ^{13}C MR spectroscopy in the muscle and liver, in combination with infusion of ^{13}C-labelled acetate. Using these measurements, it was shown that mitochondrial flux was decreased in insulin resistance [32, 63]. Subsequent studies revealed that increased HCL relates to upregulated mitochondrial respiration and increased acetyl-CoA flux [64], whereas in vivo ^{13}C MRS found no relevant alterations in rates of hepatic mitochondrial oxidation and pyruvate cycling at least in non-obese NAFLD [65]. The differences between these studies may result from the quality of metabolic control and duration of obesity or diabetes.

In the liver, type 2 diabetes mellitus was associated with lower absolute concentrations of ATP, as compared to age- and BMI-matched groups [66–68]. Future research needs to investigate how absolute ATP concentrations are related to mitochondrial function in the liver.

Measurement of Metabolic Fluxes

The principle of using a ^{13}C-labelled substrate and following the signal by MRS into other tissues or monitoring the conversion into other metabolites can also be used in a broader sense. A feasibility study demonstrated that it is possible to "follow" ^{13}C-labelled fatty acids that were consumed with a meal to the liver by determining the ^{13}C enrichment of the hepatic lipid signal over time [51]. Refinement of the technical aspects of such measurements paves the way to a broader application. This has the potential to quantify the importance of the various pathways that contribute to the development of fatty liver in individuals in order to cluster and treat them accordingly.

The challenge of the relatively low sensitivity of the MR signal can be addressed by hyperpolarizing metabolites and injecting them as tracers. Hyperpolarization increases the MR visibility manyfold for a short time. Immediately after injection, the metabolite can be detected and can be followed while it is converted to other metabolites. Thereby, metabolic conversions can be visualized, and fluxes can be determined. A caveat of these experiments is that plasma concentrations of the hyperpolarized metabolite typically change quite strongly, which will also influence kinetics, rendering the experiment not completely physiological. However, experiments yielded certainly valuable information. For example, in this way, it was shown that pyruvate is converted to acetylcarnitine in the heart, thereby buffering acetyl-CoA concentrations [69].

Imaging Tools for Assessing Cardiovascular Function and Metabolism

Cardiac imaging refers to noninvasive imaging of the heart using ultrasound, MRI, CT, or imaging with PET or SPECT including myocardial perfusion imaging.

Transthoracic echocardiography uses ultrasonic waves for continuous heart chamber and blood movement visualization. It is the most commonly used imaging tool for diagnosing heart disease, as it allows noninvasive visualization of the heart and the blood flow through the heart, using a technique known as Doppler. Transesophageal echocardiography uses a specialized probe and is only indicated for specific examinations.

MRI is able to measure the size, shape, function, and tissue characteristics of the heart. It is more reproducible than echocardiography with lower inter-observer variability. Additional benefits from cardiac MRI include the ability to detect fibrosis using late gadolinium enhancement, and MRS techniques may identify myocellular lipid infiltrations. Disadvantages of MRI include lengthy protocols and the potential for claustrophobia.

Certain subgroups of patients with diabetes have exhibited nominally increased cardiac risk [7], specifically for major adverse cardiac events [70]. A targeted prevention and diagnosis may be therefore of high clinical relevance in the context of precision diabetology.

Myocardial Lipid Contents

Recent experimental data suggest that adiposity, next to elevating the well-known cardiovascular health risks such as increasing blood pressure and increasing the risk for plaque formation, can also directly affect the heart by promoting ectopic deposition of triglyceride, a process known as myocardial steatosis. Using proton magnetic resonance spectroscopy (1H MRS) as an in vivo tool to measure myocardial lipid content constitutes a reproducible technique for the measurement of myocardial triglyceride levels [42]. Increased myocardial triglyceride content was accompanied by elevated left ventricular mass and suppressed septal wall thickening as measured by cardiac imaging [42] (Fig. 4.4). However, the importance of cardiac steatosis for clinically diminishment in cardiac function remains to be elucidated. This holds promise especially for subgroups of persons with diabetes at excessive cardiovascular risk [70].

Myocardial Mitochondrial Function

Also in the heart, decreased mitochondrial function was suggested to be involved in diabetic cardiomyopathy and heart failure (as reviewed in [71] and in line with a diminished mitochondrial capacity, the energy status of the heart (determined as PCr/ATP) was found to be decreased in diabetes in some, but not all studies [72–74]).

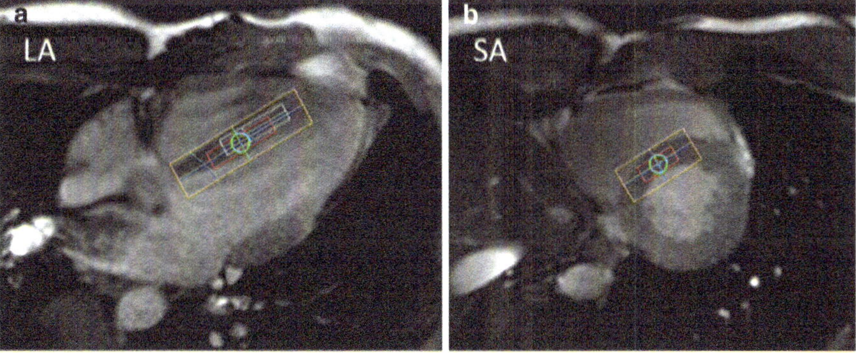

Fig. 4.4 MRS quantification of cardiac lipids. Image (**a**) shows the placement of the voxel on the long axis of the interventricular septum (LA). Image (**b**) shows the short axis (SA). (Red Box, Voxel; White Box, Voxel position for fat; Orange Box, Shim volume)

Diabetes-Associated Vascular Disease

Noninvasive techniques provide information on macrovascular anatomy, as well as on functional parameters concerning blood flow in large vessels, tissue perfusion, and microcirculation, all of which may be affected in humans with diabetes. Ultrasonography (US) is mainly used to assess the atherosclerotic burden in non-coronary arteries. Doppler US has been successfully employed for an early and accurate characterization of the vasculopathy of lower limb arteries [75], thus contributing to the prevention or delay of foot complications, especially amputation. Moreover, the measurement of the carotid intima-media thickness (IMT) by US has been demonstrated a useful marker of the progression of atherosclerosis throughout the body and an excellent predictor of cardiovascular events even in diabetic population [76, 77]. Furthermore, carotid IMT can be used to evaluate the efficacy of new treatments and is often referred to as a primary outcome in cardiovascular research in patients with diabetes [78–80].

Endothelial dysfunction is frequent in patients with diabetes mellitus and is associated with the burden of cardiovascular risk in long-standing diabetes [81]. Endothelial dysfunction is characterized by a reduced flow-mediated vasodilation due to decreased nitric oxide (NO) bioavailability [82]. Vasodilation is mainly driven by NO production from the endothelium which is susceptible to changes in the glucometabolic milieu. Several mechanisms of endothelial dysfunction have been reported in relation to diabetes, including impaired release of NO as well as signal transduction and substrate availability, enhanced release of endothelium-derived constricting factors, and decreased sensitivity of the vascular smooth muscle to NO signaling [83]. Investigation of the flow-mediated dilatation of the brachial artery is a noninvasive technique to measure endothelial NO release during reactive hyperemia after blood flow restriction of the brachial artery [81] (Fig. 4.5). Endothelium-independent nitroglycerin-mediated dilatation can assess further mechanisms involved in early atherosclerotic changes [84].

In the presence of endothelial dysfunction, there is a blunting and delay of the hyperemic response, which can be measured noninvasively using a variety of MRI methods. Recent developments in non-contrast, proton MRI ensure for dynamic quantification of blood flow and oxygenation, for example, by detecting the blood oxygenation-level dependent signal that reflects a combined effect of blood flow and capillary bed oxygen content; arterial spin labeling for quantification of regional perfusion; phase contrast to quantify arterial flow waveforms and macrovascular blood flow velocity and rate; high-resolution MRI for luminal flow-mediated dilation; and dynamic MR oximetry to quantify oxygen saturation. Overall, results suggest that these dynamic and quantitative MRI methods can detect endothelial dysfunction both in the presence of overt cardiovascular disease and in subclinical settings [85].

Moreover, metabolic abnormalities that are common in diabetes, particularly hyperglycemia, increased free fatty acids, and insulin resistance [1] can further

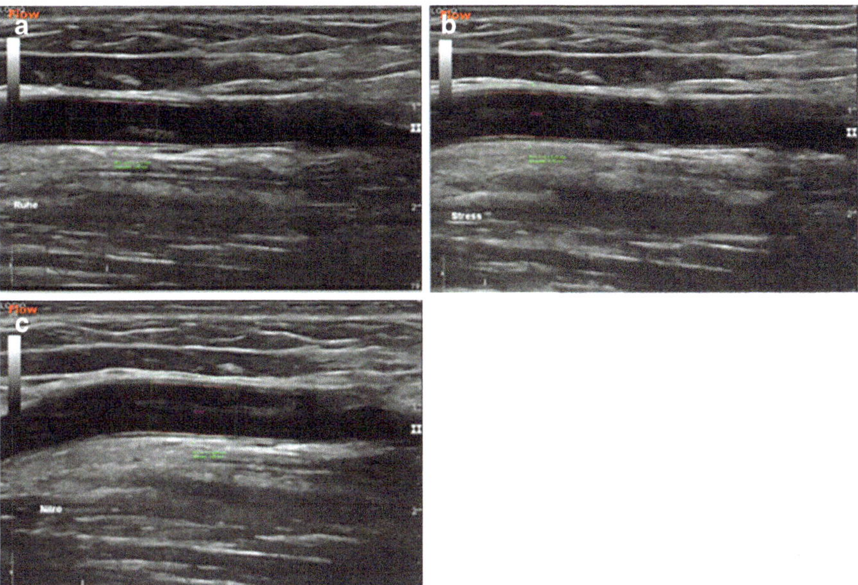

Fig. 4.5 Flow-mediated and nitroglycerin-mediated dilation of the brachial artery. Image (**a**) shows a baseline image of the brachial artery, Image (**b**) shows the arterial section after 5 minutes of compression, and Image (**c**) shows the brachial artery after administration of nitroglycerin spray

contribute to the alteration of the endothelial function and structure. Consequently, it is of great clinical relevance to identify patient groups at risk and implement early detection methods of endothelial dysfunction in patients with diabetes.

Blood supply to the pancreas may be of specific relevance in diabetes. Recently studies using MRI in experimental studies on rodent diabetes models [86] evaluated pancreatic vascular volume, microvascular flow, and permeability as possible pathophysiological backgrounds for the development of diabetes and the heterogeneity of clinical manifestations [87].

In addition, novel imaging techniques have been investigating in the characterization of atherosclerotic plaques by MRI among others by using negative contrast agents (decreasing signal intensity) based on superparamagnetic iron oxides: SPIO (superparamagnetic iron oxide) and USPIO (ultrasmall superparamagnetic iron oxide) [88, 89].

Further new approach for in vivo visualization of inflammatory processes by MRI uses biochemically inert nanoemulsions of perfluorocarbons (PFCs). PFCs can serve as "positive" contrast agent for detection of inflammation by ^{19}F-MRI, permitting a spatial resolution close to the anatomical 1H image and an excellent degree of specificity due to lack of any 19F background. Since PFCs are nontoxic, this approach may have a broad application in the imaging and diagnosis of numerous inflammatory states [90] with relevance for atherosclerosis and cardiovascular complications in diabetes.

Imaging Tools for Assessing Pancreatic Steatosis in the Context of Diabetes

Radiotracers could potentially be used to target beta cell mass in relation to beta cell function. This assessment is essential for further elucidating the pathophysiology of diabetes in order to monitor disease progression. PET/SPECT imaging biomarkers are under development that have the potential to change the way we look at the pathophysiology of islet function in the context of diabetes. Among these, radiolabelled exendin-4 has the highest sensitivity and specificity for beta cells. The in vivo specificity of [^{18}F]FP-dihydrotetrabenazine for beta cells suggests this tracer can serve as a good biomarker of human beta cell mass. [^{11}C]5-hydroxytryptamine(HTP) may reflect total endocrine rather than beta cell mass. The combination of [^{11}C]5-HTP and radiolabeled exendin-4 imaging may increase specificity for beta cell function and mass [91].

The role of the amount of pancreatic fat and its association with beta cell function in humans also remains controversially discussed. 1H-MRS and MRI techniques are used to noninvasively quantify pancreatic fat compartments.

Pancreatic Steatosis

Also in the pancreas, lipids can accumulate, and potentially lipotoxic mechanisms were suggested inducing apoptosis and hampering insulin secretion. While accumulation of fat droplets in the pancreatic cells is indeed possible, if pancreatic fat is determined by in vivo imaging techniques (MRI or MRS-based), the fat content likely reflects a mixture of signal from parenchymal lipid droplets and from adipocytes either from single, infiltrated adipocyte or from partial volume effects from surrounding adipose tissue. The latter are minimized by the use of erosion filters [92], but cannot be excluded completely. Fatty infiltrations are generally more prominent when total visceral fat is increased and can be a potential confounder. Nevertheless, some interesting correlations of such pancreatic fat with functional outcomes, such as insulin secretion and glucose intolerance [93–95], were reported in some but not all [96] studies. Potentially, the determination of pancreatic fat may convey a tool to further characterize diabetic patients and cluster patients with a similar phenotype; however, the specific added value of pancreatic fat requires further study.

Similar to VAT, peripancreatic, interlobular, and intralobular adipose tissue may alter beta cell function through the release of adipocytokines. On the other hand, lipid accumulation in beta cells could result in parenchymal or intracellular pancreatic steatosis, activating cellular mechanisms in analogy to hepatic steatosis. Distinguishing between these compartments in vivo could therefore aid in the accurate assessment of the specific effects of individual fat depots on beta cell function and lead to a more precise characterization of diabetes subphenotypes. This may be of interest specifically for insulin-deficient diabetes subgroups.

Imaging Tools for Assessing and Monitoring Diabetic Nephropathy

Patients with severe insulin-resistant diabetes have been shown to present with advanced diabetic neuropathy, even at the time of diagnosis [3, 7]. Noninvasive quantitative measurement of fibrosis in chronic kidney disease (CKD) would be desirable diagnostically and therapeutically especially for patients at risk. In that respect, MRE may also be used to monitor progression of kidney fibrosis [97]. Since decreased kidney perfusion decreases tissue stiffness, combined three-dimensional MRE shear stiffness measurements with MR arterial spin labeling kidney blood flow rates represent a new tool to evaluate fibrosis in diabetic nephropathy [97]. MRI with arterial spin labeling blood flow rates can noninvasively measure decreasing kidney cortical tissue perfusion and correlate with increasing fibrosis. Differing from the liver, MRE shear stiffness surprisingly decreases with worsening CKD, likely related to decreased tissue turgor from lower blood flow rates [97].

Imaging Tools for Assessing and Monitoring Diabetic Retinopathy

Diabetic retinopathy is a common microvascular complication of diabetes mellitus. Fundus photography can be used to document retinal disease over time and may be increasingly helpful in screening of diabetic patients for retinopathy (Fig. 4.6). It has the advantage of being cost- and time-effective and is noninvasive and easy to

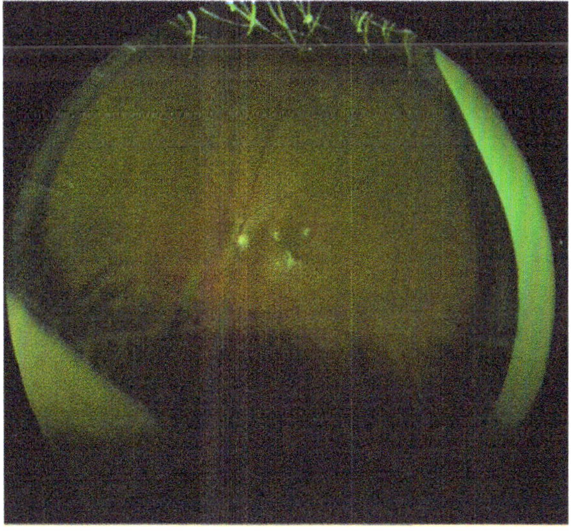

Fig. 4.6 Fundus photography of diabetic retinopathy. Fundus photography of mild diabetic retinopathy showing hard exudates

implement in a clinical setting. B-scan ultrasonography can be helpful in patients with media opacity, such as vitreous hemorrhage or cataract.

Optical coherence tomography angiography (OCTA) has been developed to visualize the retinal microvasculature and choriocapillaris based on the motion contrast of circulating blood cells. OCTA enables quantification of microvascular alterations in the retinal capillary network, in addition to the detection of classical features associated with diabetic retinopathy, including microaneurysms, intraretinal microvascular abnormalities, and neovascularization [98]. Furthermore, OCTA can identify preclinical microvascular abnormalities preceding the onset of clinically detectable diabetic retinopathy. This is particularly relevant for patients with severe insulin-deficient diabetes who have been shown to present with higher prevalence of diabetic retinopathy [7]. Advancement of OCTA technology in clinical research will ultimately lead to enhancement of targeted management and prevention of visual impairment in patients with diabetes.

In patients with diabetic retinopathy, fluorescein angiography can show microaneurysms, which manifest as punctate areas of hyperfluorescence [99]. Patchy areas of hypofluorescence can signify ischemia in retinal capillaries. Fluorescein can also show abnormal blood vessels in the eye such as intraretinal microvascular abnormalities or retinal neovascularization and can leak out of incompetent blood vessels. Retinal neovascularization also can cause fluorescein leakage, and fluorescein angiography is a useful test to confirm the diagnosis of neovascularization in proliferative diabetic retinopathy but also for the diagnosis of macular edema [100, 101].

As these technologies have continued to evolve, their importance in the diagnosis and management of diabetic retinopathy has become increasingly evident.

Concluding Remarks

Precision medicine in diabetes requires accurate profiling of individuals belonging to a given sub(pheno)type (subgroup, cluster), by integrating imaging data to the advances already made in clinical classifications. Presently, there is a diverse array of imaging techniques at the disposal of clinicians and researchers aiding the comprehensive assessment of metabolic features in humans with diabetes. Most relevant to current translational objectives in precision diabetology are the potential implications of imaging techniques for preventive and therapeutic strategies for the management of diabetes and its complications.

References

1. Roden M, Shulman GI. The integrative biology of type 2 diabetes. Nature. 2019;576:51–60.
2. Faerch K, Hulman A, Solomon TP. Heterogeneity of pre-diabetes and type 2 diabetes: implications for prediction, prevention and treatment responsiveness. Curr Diabetes Rev. 2016;12:30–41.

3. Zaharia OP, Strassburger K, Strom A, Bonhof GJ, Karusheva Y, Antoniou S, Bodis K, Markgraf DF, Burkart V, Mussig K, Hwang JH, Asplund O, Groop L, Ahlqvist E, Seissler J, Nawroth P, Kopf S, Schmid SM, Stumvoll M, Pfeiffer AFH, Kabisch S, Tselmin S, Haring HU, Ziegler D, Kuss O, Szendroedi J, Roden M. Risk of diabetes-associated diseases in subgroups of patients with recent-onset diabetes: a 5-year follow-up study. Lancet Diabetes Endocrinol. 2019;7:684–94.
4. Sarría-Santamera A, Orazumbekova B, Maulenkul T, Gaipov A, Atageldiyeva K. The identification of diabetes mellitus subtypes applying cluster analysis techniques: a systematic review. Int J Environ Res Public Health. 2020;17:9523.
5. Chung WK, Erion K, Florez JC, Hattersley AT, Hivert M-F, Lee CG, McCarthy MI, Nolan JJ, Norris JM, Pearson ER, Philipson L, McElvaine AT, Cefalu WT, Rich SS, Franks PW. Precision medicine in diabetes: a consensus report from the American Diabetes Association (ADA) and the European Association for the Study of diabetes (EASD). Diabetologia. 2020;63:1671–93.
6. Ahlqvist E, Prasad RB, Groop L. Subtypes of type 2 diabetes determined from clinical parameters. Diabetes. 2020;69:2086–93.
7. Ahlqvist E, Storm P, Karajamaki A, Martinell M, Dorkhan M, Carlsson A, Vikman P, Prasad RB, Aly DM, Almgren P, Wessman Y, Shaat N, Spegel P, Mulder H, Lindholm E, Melander O, Hansson O, Malmqvist U, Lernmark A, Lahti K, Forsen T, Tuomi T, Rosengren AH, Groop L. Novel subgroups of adult-onset diabetes and their association with outcomes: a data-driven cluster analysis of six variables. Lancet Diabetes Endocrinol. 2018;6:361–9.
8. Wagner R, Heni M, Tabák AG, Machann J, Schick F, Randrianarisoa E, Hrabě de Angelis M, Birkenfeld AL, Stefan N, Peter A, Häring HU, Fritsche A. Pathophysiology-based subphenotyping of individuals at elevated risk for type 2 diabetes. Nat Med. 2021;27:49–57.
9. Fitipaldi H, McCarthy MI, Florez JC, Franks PW. A global overview of precision medicine in type 2 diabetes. Diabetes. 2018;67:1911–22.
10. Florez JC. Precision medicine in diabetes: is it time? Diabetes Care. 2016;39:1085–8.
11. Merino J, Udler MS, Leong A, Meigs JB. A decade of genetic and Metabolomic contributions to type 2 diabetes risk prediction. Curr Diab Rep. 2017;17:135.
12. Dennis JM, Shields BM, Henley WE, Jones AG, Hattersley AT. Disease progression and treatment response in data-driven subgroups of type 2 diabetes compared with models based on simple clinical features: an analysis using clinical trial data. Lancet Diabetes Endocrinol. 2019;7:442–51.
13. Floyd JS, Psaty BM. The application of genomics in diabetes: barriers to discovery and implementation. Diabetes Care. 2016;39:1858–69.
14. Schully SD, Lam TK, Dotson WD, Chang CQ, Aronson N, Birkeland ML, Brewster SJ, Boccia S, Buchanan AH, Calonge N, Calzone K, Djulbegovic B, Goddard KA, Klein RD, Klein TE, Lau J, Long R, Lyman GH, Morgan RL, Palmer CG, Relling MV, Rubinstein WS, Swen JJ, Terry SF, Williams MS, Khoury MJ. Evidence synthesis and guideline development in genomic medicine: current status and future prospects. Genetics in Medicine: Official Journal of the American College of Medical Genetics. 2015;17:63–7.
15. Kahn SE, Hull RL, Utzschneider KM. Mechanisms linking obesity to insulin resistance and type 2 diabetes. Nature. 2006;444:840–6.
16. Machann J, Thamer C, Schnoedt B, Haap M, Haring HU, Claussen CD, Stumvoll M, Fritsche A, Schick F. Standardized assessment of whole body adipose tissue topography by MRI. Journal of Magnetic Resonance Imaging: An Official Journal of the International Society for Magnetic Resonance in Medicine. 2005;21:455–62.
17. Shen W, Wang Z, Punyanita M, Lei J, Sinav A, Kral JG, Imielinska C, Ross R, Heymsfield SB. Adipose tissue quantification by imaging methods: a proposed classification. Obes Res. 2003;11:5–16.
18. Machann J, Stefan N, Wagner R, Fritsche A, Bell JD, Whitcher B, Häring H-U, Birkenfeld AL, Nikolaou K, Schick F, Thomas EL. Normalized indices derived from visceral adipose mass assessed by magnetic resonance imaging and their correlation with markers for insulin resistance and prediabetes. Nutrients. 2020;12.

19. Smith SR, Lovejoy JC, Greenway F, Ryan D, De Jonge L, De la Bretonne J. Contributions of total body fat, abdominal subcutaneous adipose tissue compartments, and visceral adipose tissue to the metabolic complications of obesity. Metab Clin Exp. 2001;50:425–35.
20. Van der Kooy K, Seidell JC. Techniques for the measurement of visceral fat: a practical guide. Int J Obes. 1993;17:187.
21. Bódis K, Jelenik T, Lundbom J, Markgraf DF, Strom A, Zaharia O-P, Karusheva Y, Burkart V, Müssig K, Kupriyanova Y, Ouni M, Wolkersdorfer M, Hwang J-H, Ziegler D, Schürmann A, Roden M, Szendroedi J, Group GDSs. Expansion and impaired mitochondrial efficiency of deep subcutaneous adipose tissue in recent-onset type 2 diabetes. J Clin Endocrinol Metabol. 2019:dgz267.
22. Kelley DE, Thaete FL, Troost F, Huwe T, Goodpaster BH. Subdivisions of subcutaneous abdominal adipose tissue and insulin resistance. Am J Phys Endocrinol Metab. 2000;278:E941–8.
23. Golan R, Shelef I, Rudich A, Gepner Y, Shemesh E, Chassidim Y, Harman-Boehm I, Henkin Y, Schwarzfuchs D, Ben Avraham S, Witkow S, Liberty IF, Tangi-Rosental O, Sarusi B, Stampfer MJ, Shai I. Abdominal superficial subcutaneous fat: a putative distinct protective fat subdepot in type 2 diabetes. Diabetes Care. 2012;35:640–7.
24. Lundbom J, Hakkarainen A, Lundbom N, Taskinen MR. Deep subcutaneous adipose tissue is more saturated than superficial subcutaneous adipose tissue. Int J Obes. 2013;37:620–2.
25. Zou X, Zhou X, Zhu Z, Ji L. Novel subgroups of patients with adult-onset diabetes in Chinese and US populations. Lancet Diabetes Endocrinol. 2019;7:9–11.
26. Ginde SR, Geliebter A, Rubiano F, Silva AM, Wang J, Heshka S, Heymsfield SB. Air displacement plethysmography: validation in overweight and obese subjects. Obes Res. 2005;13:1232–7.
27. Bazzocchi A, Ponti F, Albisinni U, Battista G, Guglielmi G. DXA: technical aspects and application. Eur J Radiol. 2016;85:1481–92.
28. Elbers J, Haumann G, Asscheman H, Seidell J, Gooren LJ. Reproducibility of fat area measurements in young, non-obese subjects by computerized analysis of magnetic resonance images. Int J Obes. 1997;21:1121–9.
29. Seidell JC, Bakker C, van der Kooy K. Imaging techniques for measuring adipose-tissue distribution--a comparison between computed tomography and 1.5-T magnetic resonance. Am J Clin Nutr. 1990;51:953–7.
30. Ross R, Léger L, Morris D, de Guise J, Guardo R. Quantification of adipose tissue by MRI: relationship with anthropometric variables. J Appl Physiol (1985). 1992;72:787–95.
31. Jacob S, Machann J, Rett K, Brechtel K, Volk A, Renn W, Maerker E, Matthaei S, Schick F, Claussen CD, Häring HU. Association of increased intramyocellular lipid content with insulin resistance in lean nondiabetic offspring of type 2 diabetic subjects. Diabetes. 1999;48:1113–9.
32. Petersen KF, Befroy D, Dufour S, Dziura J, Ariyan C, Rothman DL, DiPietro L, Cline GW, Shulman GI. Mitochondrial dysfunction in the elderly: possible role in insulin resistance. Science (New York, NY). 2003;300:1140–2.
33. Goodpaster BH, He J, Watkins S, Kelley DE. Skeletal muscle lipid content and insulin resistance: evidence for a paradox in endurance-trained athletes. J Clin Endocrinol Metab. 2001;86:5755–61.
34. van Loon LJ, Goodpaster BH. Increased intramuscular lipid storage in the insulin-resistant and endurance-trained state. Pflugers Archiv Europ J Physiol. 2006;451:606–16.
35. Thamer C, Machann J, Bachmann O, Haap M, Dahl D, Wietek B, Tschritter O, Niess A, Brechtel K, Fritsche A, Claussen C, Jacob S, Schick F, Häring HU, Stumvoll M. Intramyocellular lipids: anthropometric determinants and relationships with maximal aerobic capacity and insulin sensitivity. J Clin Endocrinol Metab. 2003;88:1785–91.
36. Phillips DI, Caddy S, Ilic V, Fielding BA, Frayn KN, Borthwick AC, Taylor R. Intramuscular triglyceride and muscle insulin sensitivity: evidence for a relationship in nondiabetic subjects. Metabolism. 1996;45:947–50.

37. Szendroedi J, Yoshimura T, Phielix E, Koliaki C, Marcucci M, Zhang D, Jelenik T, Muller J, Herder C, Nowotny P, Shulman GI, Roden M. Role of diacylglycerol activation of PKCtheta in lipid-induced muscle insulin resistance in humans. Proc Natl Acad Sci U S A. 2014;111:9597–602.
38. Petersen MC, Shulman GI. Mechanisms of insulin action and insulin resistance. Physiol Rev. 2018;98:2133–223.
39. Cline GW, Petersen KF, Krssak M, Shen J, Hundal RS, Trajanoski Z, Inzucchi S, Dresner A, Rothman DL, Shulman GI. Impaired glucose transport as a cause of decreased insulin-stimulated muscle glycogen synthesis in type 2 diabetes. N Engl J Med. 1999;341:240–6.
40. Schick F, Eismann B, Jung WI, Bongers H, Bunse M, Lutz O. Comparison of localized proton NMR signals of skeletal muscle and fat tissue in vivo: two lipid compartments in muscle tissue. Magn Reson Med. 1993;29:158–67.
41. Boesch C, Slotboom J, Hoppeler H, Kreis R. In vivo determination of intra-myocellular lipids in human muscle by means of localized 1H-MR-spectroscopy. Magn Reson Med. 1997;37:484–93.
42. Szczepaniak LS, Dobbins RL, Metzger GJ, Sartoni-D'Ambrosia G, Arbique D, Vongpatanasin W, Unger R, Victor RG. Myocardial triglycerides and systolic function in humans: in vivo evaluation by localized proton spectroscopy and cardiac imaging. Magn Reson Med. 2003;49:417–23.
43. Schrauwen-Hinderling VB, Hesselink MKC, Schrauwen P, Kooi ME. Intramyocellular lipid content in human skeletal muscle. Obesity. 2006;14:357–67.
44. Petersen KF, Dufour S, Shulman GI. Decreased insulin-stimulated ATP synthesis and phosphate transport in muscle of insulin-resistant offspring of type 2 diabetic parents. PLoS Med. 2005;2:e233.
45. Phielix E, Schrauwen-Hinderling VB, Mensink M, Lenaers E, Meex R, Hoeks J, Kooi ME, Moonen-Kornips E, Sels JP, Hesselink MK, Schrauwen P. Lower intrinsic ADP-stimulated mitochondrial respiration underlies in vivo mitochondrial dysfunction in muscle of male type 2 diabetic patients. Diabetes. 2008;57:2943–9.
46. Schmid AI, Schrauwen-Hinderling VB, Andreas M, Wolzt M, Moser E, Roden M. Comparison of measuring energy metabolism by different (31) P-magnetic resonance spectroscopy techniques in resting, ischemic, and exercising muscle. Magn Reson Med. 2012;67:898–905.
47. Kemp GJ, Ahmad RE, Nicolay K, Prompers JJ. Quantification of skeletal muscle mitochondrial function by 31P magnetic resonance spectroscopy techniques: a quantitative review. Acta physiologica (Oxford, England). 2015;213:107–44.
48. Schrauwen-Hinderling VB, Kooi ME, Hesselink MK, Jeneson JA, Backes WH, van Echteld CJ, van Engelshoven JM, Mensink M, Schrauwen P. Impaired in vivo mitochondrial function but similar intramyocellular lipid content in patients with type 2 diabetes mellitus and BMI-matched control subjects. Diabetologia. 2007;50:113–20.
49. Rothman DL, Magnusson I, Cline G, Gerard D, Kahn CR, Shulman RG, Shulman GI. Decreased muscle glucose transport/phosphorylation is an early defect in the pathogenesis of non-insulin-dependent diabetes mellitus. Proc Natl Acad Sci. 1995;92:983.
50. Roden M, Price TB, Perseghin G, Petersen KF, Rothman DL, Cline GW, Shulman GI. Mechanism of free fatty acid-induced insulin resistance in humans. J Clin Invest. 1996;97:2859–65.
51. Lindeboom L, Nabuurs CI, Hesselink MK, Wildberger JE, Schrauwen P, Schrauwen-Hinderling VB. Proton magnetic resonance spectroscopy reveals increased hepatic lipid content after a single high-fat meal with no additional modulation by added protein. Am J Clin Nutr. 2015;101:65–71.
52. Tilg H, Moschen AR, Roden M. NAFLD and diabetes mellitus. Nat Rev Gastroenterol Hepatol. 2017;14:32–42.
53. Gancheva S, Jelenik T, Alvarez-Hernandez E, Roden M. Interorgan metabolic crosstalk in human insulin resistance. Physiol Rev. 2018;98:1371–415.

54. Koliaki C, Szendroedi J, Kaul K, Jelenik T, Nowotny P, Jankowiak F, Herder C, Carstensen M, Krausch M, Knoefel WT, Schlensak M, Roden M. Adaptation of hepatic mitochondrial function in humans with non-alcoholic fatty liver is lost in steatohepatitis. Cell Metab. 2015;21:739–46.
55. Kolak M, Westerbacka J, Velagapudi VR, Wagsater D, Yetukuri L, Makkonen J, Rissanen A, Hakkinen AM, Lindell M, Bergholm R, Hamsten A, Eriksson P, Fisher RM, Oresic M, Yki-Jarvinen H. Adipose tissue inflammation and increased ceramide content characterize subjects with high liver fat content independent of obesity. Diabetes. 2007;56:1960–8.
56. Apostolopoulou M, Gordillo R, Koliaki C, Gancheva S, Jelenik T, De Filippo E, Herder C, Markgraf D, Jankowiak F, Esposito I, Schlensak M, Scherer PE, Roden M. Specific hepatic sphingolipids relate to insulin resistance, oxidative stress, and inflammation in nonalcoholic steatohepatitis. Diabetes Care. 2018;41:1235–43.
57. Grunnet LG, Laurila E, Hansson O, Almgren P, Groop L, Brons C, Poulsen P, Vaag A. The triglyceride content in skeletal muscle is associated with hepatic but not peripheral insulin resistance in elderly twins. J Clin Endocrinol Metab. 2012;97:4571–7.
58. Mantovani A, Byrne CD, Bonora E, Targher G. Nonalcoholic fatty liver disease and risk of incident type 2 diabetes: a meta-analysis. Diabetes Care. 2018;41:372–82.
59. Brouwers B, Schrauwen-Hinderling VB, Jelenik T, Gemmink A, Havekes B, Bruls Y, Dahlmans D, Roden M, Hesselink MKC, Schrauwen P. Metabolic disturbances of non-alcoholic fatty liver resemble the alterations typical for type 2 diabetes. Clin Sci (London, England: 1979). 2017;131:1905–17.
60. Roumans KHM, Lindeboom L, Veeraiah P, Remie CME, Phielix E, Havekes B, Bruls YMH, Brouwers MCGJ, Ståhlman M, Alssema M, Peters HPF, de Mutsert R, Staels B, Taskinen M-R, Borén J, Schrauwen P, Schrauwen-Hinderling VB. Hepatic saturated fatty acid fraction is associated with de novo lipogenesis and hepatic insulin resistance. Nat Commun. 2020;11:1891.
61. Mariappan YK, Glaser KJ, Ehman RL. Magnetic resonance elastography: a review. Clin Anat. 2010;23:497–511.
62. Zaharia OP, Strassburger K, Knebel B, Kupriyanova Y, Karusheva Y, Wolkersdorfer M, Bódis K, Markgraf DF, Burkart V, Hwang JH, Kotzka J, Al-Hasani H, Szendroedi J, Roden M. Role of Patatin-like phospholipase domain-containing 3 gene for hepatic lipid content and insulin resistance in diabetes. Diabetes Care. 2020;43:2161–8.
63. Jucker BM, Dufour S, Ren J, Cao X, Previs SF, Underhill B, Cadman KS, Shulman GI. Assessment of mitochondrial energy coupling in vivo by 13C/31P NMR. Proc Natl Acad Sci U S A. 2000;97:6880–4.
64. Sunny NE, Parks EJ, Browning JD, Burgess SC. Excessive hepatic mitochondrial TCA cycle and gluconeogenesis in humans with nonalcoholic fatty liver disease. Cell Metab. 2011;14:804–10.
65. Petersen KF, Befroy DE, Dufour S, Rothman DL, Shulman GI. Assessment of hepatic mitochondrial oxidation and pyruvate cycling in NAFLD by (13)C magnetic resonance spectroscopy. Cell Metab. 2016;24:167–71.
66. Szendroedi J, Chmelik M, Schmid AI, Nowotny P, Brehm A, Krssak M, Moser E, Roden M. Abnormal hepatic energy homeostasis in type 2 diabetes. Hepatology. 2009;50:1079–86.
67. Gancheva S, Bierwagen A, Kaul K, Herder C, Nowotny P, Kahl S, Giani G, Klueppelholz B, Knebel B, Begovatz P, Strassburger K, Al-Hasani H, Lundbom J, Szendroedi J, Roden M. German diabetes study G: variants in genes controlling oxidative metabolism contribute to lower hepatic ATP independent of liver fat content in type 1 diabetes. Diabetes. 2016;65:1849–57.
68. Wolf P, Fellinger P, Pfleger L, Smajis S, Beiglböck H, Gajdošík M, Anderwald CH, Trattnig S, Luger A, Winhofer Y, Krššák M, Krebs M. Reduced hepatocellular lipid accumulation and energy metabolism in patients with long standing type 1 diabetes mellitus. Sci Rep. 2019;9:2576.

69. Schroeder MA, Atherton HJ, Dodd MS, Lee P, Cochlin LE, Radda GK, Clarke K, Tyler DJ. The cycling of acetyl-coenzyme a through acetylcarnitine buffers cardiac substrate supply: a hyperpolarized 13C magnetic resonance study. Circ Cardiovasc Imaging. 2012;5:201–9.
70. Kahkoska AR, Geybels MS, Klein KR, Kreiner FF, Marx N, Nauck MA, Pratley RE, Wolthers BO, Buse JB. Validation of distinct type 2 diabetes clusters and their association with diabetes complications in the DEVOTE, LEADER and SUSTAIN-6 cardiovascular outcomes trials. Diabetes Obes Metab. 2020;22:1537–47.
71. Schrauwen-Hinderling VB, Kooi ME, Schrauwen P. Mitochondrial function and diabetes: consequences for skeletal and cardiac muscle metabolism. Antioxid Redox Signal. 2016;24:39–51.
72. Rijzewijk LJ, Jonker JT, van der Meer RW, Lubberink M, de Jong HW, Romijn JA, Bax JJ, de Roos A, Heine RJ, Twisk JW, Windhorst AD, Lammertsma AA, Smit JW, Diamant M, Lamb HJ. Effects of hepatic triglyceride content on myocardial metabolism in type 2 diabetes. J Am Coll Cardiol. 2010;56:225–33.
73. Scheuermann-Freestone M, Clarke K. Abnormal cardiac high-energy phosphate metabolism in a patient with type 2 diabetes mellitus. J Cardiometab Syndr. 2006;1:366–8.
74. Scheuermann-Freestone M, Madsen PL, Manners D, Blamire AM, Buckingham RE, Styles P, Radda GK, Neubauer S, Clarke K. Abnormal cardiac and skeletal muscle energy metabolism in patients with type 2 diabetes. Circulation. 2003;107:3040–6.
75. Rahman A, Moizuddin M, Ahmad M, Salim M. Vasculopathy in patients with diabetic foot using Doppler ultrasound. Pak J Med Sci. 2009;25:428–33.
76. Yoshida M, Mita T, Yamamoto R, Shimizu T, Ikeda F, Ohmura C, Kanazawa A, Hirose T, Kawamori R, Watada H. Combination of the Framingham risk score and carotid intima-media thickness improves the prediction of cardiovascular events in patients with type 2 diabetes. Diabetes Care. 2012;35:178–80.
77. Katakami N, Kaneto H, Shimomura I. Carotid ultrasonography: a potent tool for better clinical practice in diagnosis of atherosclerosis in diabetic patients. J Diabetes Investig. 2014;5:3–13.
78. Esposito K, Giugliano D, Nappo F, Marfella R. Regression of carotid atherosclerosis by control of postprandial hyperglycemia in type 2 diabetes mellitus. Circulation. 2004;110:214–9.
79. Katakami N, Yamasaki Y, Hayaishi-Okano R, Ohtoshi K, Kaneto H, Matsuhisa M, Kosugi K, Hori M. Metformin or gliclazide, rather than glibenclamide, attenuate progression of carotid intima-media thickness in subjects with type 2 diabetes. Diabetologia. 2004;47:1906–13.
80. Davidson M, Meyer PM, Haffner S, Feinstein S, D'Agostino R Sr, Kondos GT, Perez A, Chen Z, Mazzone T. Increased high-density lipoprotein cholesterol predicts the pioglitazone-mediated reduction of carotid intima-media thickness progression in patients with type 2 diabetes mellitus. Circulation. 2008;117:2123–30.
81. Flammer AJ, Anderson T, Celermajer DS, Creager MA, Deanfield J, Ganz P, Hamburg NM, Luscher TF, Shechter M, Taddei S, Vita JA, Lerman A. The assessment of endothelial function: from research into clinical practice. Circulation. 2012;126:753–67.
82. Versari D, Daghini E, Virdis A, Ghiadoni L, Taddei S. Endothelial dysfunction as a target for prevention of cardiovascular disease. Diabetes Care. 2009;32(Suppl 2):S314–21.
83. De Vriese AS, Verbeuren TJ, Van de Voorde J, Lameire NH, Vanhoutte PM. Endothelial dysfunction in diabetes. Br J Pharmacol. 2000;130:963–74.
84. Kawano N, Emoto M, Mori K, Yamazaki Y, Urata H, Tsuchikura S, Motoyama K, Morioka T, Fukumoto S, Shoji T, Koyama H, Okuno Y, Nishizawa Y, Inaba M. Association of endothelial and vascular smooth muscle dysfunction with cardiovascular risk factors, vascular complications, and subclinical carotid atherosclerosis in type 2 diabetic patients. J Atheroscler Thromb. 2012;19:276–84.
85. Englund EK, Langham MC. Quantitative and dynamic MRI measures of peripheral vascular function. Front Physiol. 2020;11:120.

86. Medarova Z, Greiner DL, Ifediba M, Dai G, Bolotin E, Castillo G, Bogdanov A, Kumar M, Moore A. Imaging the pancreatic vasculature in diabetes models. Diabetes Metab Res Rev. 2011;27:767–72.
87. De Paepe M, Corriveau M, Tannous W, Seemayer T, Colle E. Increased vascular permeability in pancreas of diabetic rats: detection with high resolution protein A-gold cytochemistry. Diabetologia. 1992;35:1118–24.
88. McAteer MA, Sibson NR, von Zur MC, Schneider JE, Lowe AS, Warrick N, Channon KM, Anthony DC, Choudhury RP. In vivo magnetic resonance imaging of acute brain inflammation using microparticles of iron oxide. Nat Med. 2007;13:1253–8.
89. Morishige K, Kacher DF, Libby P, Josephson L, Ganz P, Weissleder R, Aikawa M. High-resolution magnetic resonance imaging enhanced with superparamagnetic nanoparticles measures macrophage burden in atherosclerosis. Circulation. 2010;122:1707–15.
90. Flögel U, Ding Z, Hardung H, Jander S, Reichmann G, Jacoby C, Schubert R, Schrader J. In vivo monitoring of inflammation after cardiac and cerebral ischemia by 19F magnetic resonance imaging. Circulation. 2008;118:140.
91. Eriksson O, Laughlin M, Brom M, Nuutila P, Roden M, Hwa A, Bonadonna R, Gotthardt M. In vivo imaging of beta cells with radiotracers: state of the art, prospects and recommendations for development and use. Diabetologia. 2016;59:1340–9.
92. Al-Mrabeh A, Hollingsworth KG, Steven S, Tiniakos D, Taylor R. Quantification of intrapancreatic fat in type 2 diabetes by MRI. PLoS One. 2017;12:e0174660.
93. Heni M, Machann J, Staiger H, Schwenzer NF, Peter A, Schick F, Claussen CD, Stefan N, Häring HU, Fritsche A. Pancreatic fat is negatively associated with insulin secretion in individuals with impaired fasting glucose and/or impaired glucose tolerance: a nuclear magnetic resonance study. Diabetes Metab Res Rev. 2010;26:200–5.
94. Tushuizen ME, Bunck MC, Pouwels PJ, Bontemps S, van Waesberghe JH, Schindhelm RK, Mari A, Heine RJ, Diamant M. Pancreatic fat content and beta-cell function in men with and without type 2 diabetes. Diabetes Care. 2007;30:2916–21.
95. Lim EL, Hollingsworth KG, Aribisala BS, Chen MJ, Mathers JC, Taylor R. Reversal of type 2 diabetes: normalisation of beta cell function in association with decreased pancreas and liver triacylglycerol. Diabetologia. 2011;54:2506–14.
96. Begovatz P, Koliaki C, Weber K, Strassburger K, Nowotny B, Nowotny P, Müssig K, Bunke J, Pacini G, Szendrödi J, Roden M. Pancreatic adipose tissue infiltration, parenchymal steatosis and beta cell function in humans. Diabetologia. 2015;58:1646–55.
97. Brown RS, Sun MRM, Stillman IE, Russell TL, Rosas SE, Wei JL. The utility of magnetic resonance imaging for noninvasive evaluation of diabetic nephropathy. Nephrology Dialysis Transplantation. 2020;35:970–8.
98. Sun Z, Yang D, Tang Z, Ng DS, Cheung CY. Optical coherence tomography angiography in diabetic retinopathy: an updated review. Eye. 2020.
99. Salz DA, Witkin AJ. Imaging in diabetic retinopathy. Middle East Afr J Ophthalmol. 2015;22:145–50.
100. Wessel MM, Nair N, Aaker GD, Ehrlich JR, D'Amico DJ, Kiss S. Peripheral retinal ischaemia, as evaluated by ultra-widefield fluorescein angiography, is associated with diabetic macular oedema. Br J Ophthalmol. 2012;96:694–8.
101. Muqit MM, Marcellino GR, Henson DB, Young LB, Patton N, Charles SJ, Turner GS, Stanga PE. Optos-guided pattern scan laser (Pascal)-targeted retinal photocoagulation in proliferative diabetic retinopathy. Acta Ophthalmol. 2013;91:251–8.

Chapter 5
Implementation of Precision Genetic Approaches for Type 1 and 2 Diabetes

Ronald C. W. Ma and Juliana C. N. Chan

Introduction

The genomic revolution and discoveries in the genetics of type 1 (T1D) and type 2 diabetes (T2D) have been a major driving force in the development and realization of the potential of precision medicine in diabetes. Although delivering precision medicine does not need to include genetic markers, it is very much the advances in genetic research in diabetes which have spearheaded the movement to develop a precision medicine approach to diabetes management. The advent of genomic technology, sequencing of the human genome and the rise of genome-wide association studies (GWAS) in diabetes and related traits have led to the identification of novel gene regions as well as genetic markers that can be used for risk prediction. Furthermore, these findings have given rise to the development of different tools, including polygenic risk scores (PRS), which are accessible and ready for incorporation into clinical practice.

For example, genome-wide association studies (GWAS), with its agnostic and hypothesis-generating approach, have led to the identification 78 loci for T1D [1] and more than 300 loci for T2D [2, 3]. The functional validation and fine-mapping for the causal variants and genes are still underway for many of the regions, but the identification of these association signals has led to the development of PRS based on findings from GWAS studies. Furthermore, other "omics" discoveries have

R. C. W. Ma (✉) · J. C. N. Chan
Department of Medicine and Therapeutics, The Chinese University of Hong Kong, Hong Kong, China

Hong Kong Institute of Diabetes and Obesity, The Chinese University of Hong Kong, Hong Kong, China

Li Ka Shing Institute of Health Sciences, The Chinese University of Hong Kong, Hong Kong, China
e-mail: rcwma@cuhk.edu.hk; jchan@cuhk.edu.hk

R. Basu (ed.), *Precision Medicine in Diabetes*,
https://doi.org/10.1007/978-3-030-98927-9_5

vastly expanded our knowledge of biomarkers associated with diabetes and its related traits and complications, hence providing great opportunities to utilize these additional biomarkers to improve care.

Whilst precision approach to diabetes management does not necessarily involve genetics or other biomarkers, genetics do offer different opportunities especially before the appearance of clinical phenotypes to provide a more individualized and tailored approach for prevention and treatment purposes. Other "biomarkers" which might be of use for precision medicine include approaches that incorporate clinical risk factors, risk scores, algorithms, imaging data as well as a variety of "omics" technology including proteomics, metabolomics, epigenomics, miRNA markers and others, to guide clinical care. In addition to individual genetic markers that have been found to be associated with diabetes or diabetes-related outcomes, approaches to construct PRS, or genome-wide PRS (gwPRS), are additional approaches that are becoming feasible and more popular (Fig. 5.1).

The American Diabetes Association (ADA), for example, has recently launched a Precision Medicine in Diabetes Initiative (PMDI) and, in its first consensus report for the initiative, has provided a framework for considering how precision medicine can be implemented in diabetes [4]. The Consensus report conceptualizes the pillars of precision medicine as applied to diabetes management and can serve as a useful framework for reviewing the current state of knowledge with regard to precision

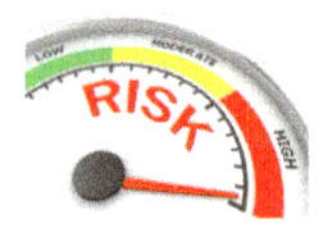

"Traditional" biomarkers (e.g. HbA1c, microalbuminuria) with clinical subphenotypes (e.g. C peptide, autoantibodies)

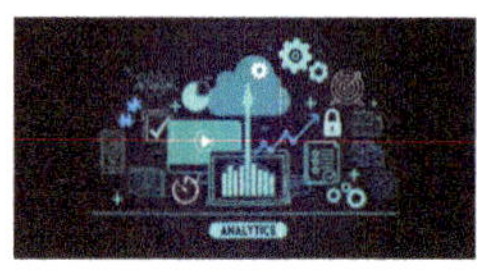

Risk models/equations using clinical markers (e.g. UKPDS Risk Engine, RECODe, JADE algorithms and technology)

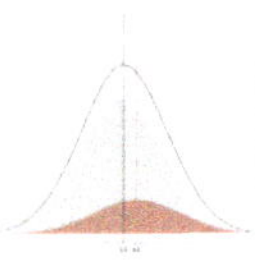

Genetic polymorphisms (e.g. SNPs from GWAS, polygenic risk scores)

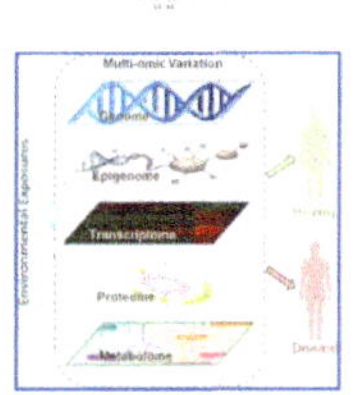

"Novel" biomarkers (e.g. omics including proteomics, metabolomics and transcriptomics) and other data analytics (e.g. continuous glucose monitoring, heart rate, blood pressure from wearables, imaging data, retinal vessels on fundus photos etc).

Fig. 5.1 Examples of tools and approaches for delivering precision medicine in diabetes. (Last figure reprinted from Advance in Genetics, Vol. 93, Yan V. Sun and Yi-Juan Hu, Chap. 3- Integrative analysis of multi-omics data for discovery and functional studies of human complex diseases, Pages 147–190, copyright (2016), with permission from Elsevier)

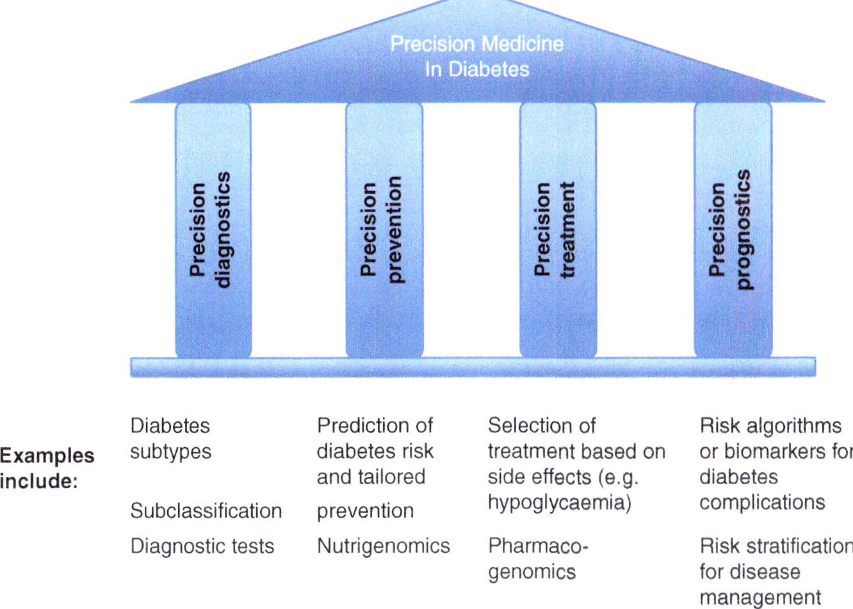

Fig. 5.2 The pillars of precision medicine as applied to Precision Medicine in Diabetes

medicine in diabetes, as well as thinking ahead in terms of implementation of precision medicine. As illustrated in Fig. 5.2, these pillars of precision medicine include the following:

- (i) Precision diagnosis – using a broad range of information to facilitate more precise diagnosis and sub-classification of diabetes.
- (ii) Precision prevention – predicting the onset of diabetes by incorporating information for designing tailor-made prevention strategies such as modifying diet/exercise according to biological makeup. This may also include precision monitoring, which is focused on implementing strategies to monitor patterns of glucose excursion and other risk factor control based on the individual's makeup.
- (iii) Precision treatment – selecting and modifying doses of medications based on personalized clinical information, biological characteristics and treatment responses.
- (iv) Precision prognostics – predicting the onset and progression of diabetes complications based on biomarkers and treatment responses for formulating personalized strategies.

In addition to these individualized biomedical information relevant to the prediction, prevention and personalized care in diabetes, clinical acumen including the recognition of secondary causes of diabetes (e.g. endocrine disorders, pancreatic diseases [5]), other population-relevant factors (e.g. chronic low-grade infections [6]), external factors that can affect glucose metabolism (e.g. concomitant medications [7]) and, importantly, the cognitive-psychosocial factors [8] that underlie a patient's values and perspectives in determining behaviours are additional factors needed in the holistic evaluation and management of patients who have or are at risk of having diabetes.

These premises set out the framework by which precision medicine can be considered and implemented in diabetes care. In particular, the PMDI has outlined some of the key steps in the implementation of precision medicine in diabetes, as will be discussed in more detail in the closing section of this chapter. The PMDI is currently undertaking multiple systematic reviews to generate the evidence and identify gaps in knowledge with regard to precision medicine in diabetes. For the remaining parts of the chapter, we will use this framework to discuss some emerging examples of how precision medicine in diabetes may be implemented. We will discuss this in the context of traditional classification of T1D versus T2D, though as will be appreciated later in the discussion, the development and implementation of precision medicine in diabetes also lend itself towards renewed efforts to gain novel insights and may potentially facilitate better classification and sub-phenotyping of diabetes itself.

Potential for Precision Medicine in Type 1 Diabetes (T1D)

Precision Diagnosis in T1D

Whilst the diagnosis of T1D in children and adolescents is usually straightforward, the recognition of adult-onset T1D is comparatively more challenging. Given the large majority of adults with newly diagnosed diabetes have T2D, the small proportion who have underlying autoimmune diabetes are sometimes missed, leading to delayed initiation of insulin and suboptimal glucose control. Whilst different biomarkers including anti-glutamic acid decarboxylase (Anti-GAD) or other autoantibodies have been used in the diagnosis of T1D, they also have their limitations, including false positivity, and potential for misdiagnosis in a population that is in general at low risk for T1D [9]. The development of PRS for T1D, based on findings from GWAS, provides opportunities to identify those at risk and has been found to be of help to differentiate adults with T1D versus T2D and identify individuals who require early insulin therapy [10].

Precision Prevention in T1D

One of the major breakthroughs in our understanding of the pathophysiology of T1D is its progressive nature. The onset of beta-cell destruction, insulin deficiency and hyperglycaemia is often preceded years earlier by gradual appearance of markers of autoimmunity, including anti-islet antibodies. This has given rise to a large number of clinical trials to investigate the possibility to delay the onset or progression of T1D, for example, in at-risk individuals with family history of T1D. These are summarized in several excellent reviews, and the details are beyond the scope of this chapter [11]. Suffice to say, the use of agents to modify the potential development and progression of T1D is a prime example of implementing precision prevention in T1D. The most successful example to date is use of the Anti-CD3 antibody, teplizumab, which was associated with a 60% reduction in development of T1D in at-risk relatives in a phase 2 trial [12]. Future efforts to use non-pharmacological measures (e.g. vitamin D or other agents) and drugs to delay development of T1D, guided by individual genotypes or biomarkers, appear promising. For example, a recent study incorporating genetic, clinical and immunological factors was found to dramatically improve T1D prediction at 2–8 years compared to autoantibodies alone. This multicomponent strategy may be used to facilitate population-based newborn screening program to prevent ketoacidosis in childhood and identification of high-risk subjects for prevention trials [13].

Precision Monitoring in T1D

Optimal management of T1D, or any type of diabetes, for that matter, requires stable control of blood glucose and prevention of hypoglycaemia. This is particularly challenging among patients with T1D, especially those with long disease duration who often have minimal residual islet function with reduced secretion of both insulin and glucagon and autonomic dysfunction putting them at high risk of hypoglycaemia unawareness. Advances in diabetes technology have led to major improvement in glucose monitoring, with availability of different continuous glucose monitoring systems (CGMS), as well as ambulatory CGM. These provide opportunities for patients to receive more detailed, and more importantly, real-time feedback of interstitial glucose values, to guide patient and clinician interventions to address postprandial glucose excursions, optimize treatment targets and facilitate prevention of hypoglycaemia. Using risk factors or algorithms to identify individuals who are at high risk of severe hypoglycaemia and thus at need of additional monitoring would likely be most cost-effective and most beneficial.

Precision Treatment in T1D

All patients with T1D are treated with insulin following diagnosis. Nevertheless, there are emerging strategies to facilitate subtype classification, for example, according to whether there is residual C-peptide production. These subtypes may be matched to different treatment strategies, including intensive insulin therapy, or selection of patients for continuous subcutaneous insulin infusion (CSII) or, more recently, hybrid-closed loop insulin infusion pumps [14]. For example, a machine-learning artificial intelligence platform has been developed to guide insulin dosage for patients with T1D and may be used to improve glycaemic outcomes [15].

There is also the possibility of matching specific treatments based on better understanding of an individual's underlying pathophysiology. This has been highlighted by a recent case of T1D with recurrent respiratory infections, which was later found to carry a gain-of-function mutation in the signal transducer and activator of transcription 1 (STAT1) gene. Treatment with ruxolitinib, an inhibitor of Janus kinase (JAK) 1 and 2 and the STAT signaling pathway, was associated with remission of T1D as well as his chronic mucocutaneous candidiasis [16]. Although an unusual case, this case highlights the possibility of using immunomodulating agents to modify the natural history of T1D.

Another example of precision treatment in T1D is the use of cell replacement therapy. Although islet cell transplantation is the mainstay approach, stem cell-based therapies are emerging as potential options in the future. These alternative sources of beta-cells include those derived from embryonic stem cells, human pluripotent stem cells and induced pluripotent stem cells (iPSCs), among others, and can include cells obtained from the patient and expanded ex vivo before being returned to the patient, although ongoing autoimmune destruction may remain a challenge. A detailed discussion of cell replacement in T1D is beyond the scope of this chapter, and readers can refer to several excellent review articles [17, 18] for additional details. The use of patient-specific cell lines may have applications in T1D or other forms of diabetes and related complications.

Precision Prognostics in T1D

There is considerable heterogeneity in the development of complications in patients with T1D, such as retinopathy, nephropathy and neuropathy. Whilst hyperglycaemia is a shared pathogenetic factor, other pathways may also be implicated in these complications. Thus, the ability to predict future risk of specific complications will facilitate risk stratification for management based on these personalized risks of diabetes-related complications. Several studies have sought to identify genetic variants associated with diabetes complications, though few have attained genome-wide association threshold, or have been consistently replicated [19–21]. Some successful examples from recent large consortia-based studies have identified variants associated with diabetic kidney disease in T1D, including a common missense mutation in the collagen type IV alpha 3 chain (COL4A3) gene [22]. In addition, the haptoglobin genotype has been demonstrated to be associated with risk of cardiovascular complications in T1D. In the Epidemiology of Diabetes Complications Study, individuals with the haptoglobin 2/2 genotype had approximately twofold increased risk of incident coronary artery disease (CAD) compared to those with haptoglobin 1/1 genotype during 18 years of follow-up [23]. Incorporating these genetic markers, with or without additional inclusion of clinical risk factors, for the prediction of future complications, may facilitate better risk stratification for intensive treatment.

Potential for Precision Medicine in Type 2 Diabetes (T2D)

Similar to what has been described for T1D, comparable strategies can be adapted to deliver precision medicine in T2D. Nevertheless, the current classification of diabetes into T1D, T2D and other forms of diabetes, including monogenic diabetes, is itself subject to revision following increasing understanding of the underlying biology and emergence of strategies of sub-classification based on underlying pathophysiology or complication risk [24–26].

Precision Diagnosis in T2D

Although a diagnosis of T2D in adults is by far the most common type of diabetes, diagnosis has traditionally been achieved through exclusion of other forms of diabetes. As mentioned earlier, a T1D PRS has been found to be more useful to differentiate between T1D, T2D and maturity-onset diabetes of the young (MODY) in young adults presenting with diabetes, compared to, for example, a PRS constructed based on genetic variants for T2D [10]. Furthermore, using a MODY calculator, supplemented by molecular testing, to exclude monogenic forms of diabetes is also important, especially among those with young-onset diabetes. In the original study involving 594 subjects with MODY, 278 with T1D and 319 with T2D, use of the prediction model based on clinical characteristics improved considerably the sensitivity and specificity for identifying MODY compared with standard criteria of diagnosis before age 25 and an affected parent [27]. A diagnosis of MODY would have significant treatment implications, as patients with glucokinase (GCK)-MODY (MODY 2) would in general not require glucose-lowering treatment, the introduction of a new class of GCK activator may offer new opportunity for correcting this metabolic defect [28]. On the other hand, individuals with hepatic nuclear factor (HNF)-1A (MODY 3) or HNF-4A MODY (MODY 1) would respond well to low-dose sulphonylurea treatment [29].

In addition to using algorithms with or without biomarkers to diagnose T2D, it has also become possible to utilize these strategies to identify subtypes of T2D according to underlying pathophysiology or by clustering of clinical features. In one of the best-known examples from Sweden, the use of clinical data from 8980 patients with newly diagnosed diabetes from the Swedish All New Diabetics in Scania (ANDIS) cohort, data-driven cluster analysis using K-means clustering and hierarchical clustering led to the identification of five individual clusters of patients with diabetes. Importantly, these different clusters (or "subtypes") of diabetes had different prognosis. Individuals with "severe insulin-deficient diabetes" had the highest risk of incident diabetic retinopathy, whereas those with "severe insulin-resistant diabetes" were mostly likely to develop chronic kidney disease (CKD) compared to the other subtypes [25]. The clinical and prognostic significance of these diabetes subtypes has subsequently been replicated in various studies from different populations. An alternative "soft clustering" approach, based on GRS for five different pathophysiological pathways associated with T2D (e.g. beta-cell, pro-insulin, obesity, lipodystrophy, liver/lipid), has likewise facilitated the classification of individuals with T2D according to underlying pathophysiology and the opportunity to better tailor treatment according to underlying pathophysiological defects [26].

Precision Prevention in T2D

Driven by the identification of genetic variants associated with T2D, different research studies have explored the potential to use PRS for T2D to identify individuals at increased risk of T2D and to investigate strategies to empower prevention of T2D. Incremental improvement in the development of PRS for T2D has improved the ability to stratify risk. The use of phenotypes may also increase the validity of PRS. For example, in the InterAct study, the relative risk of a T2D PRS was greater among young and lean individuals. The 10-year cumulative incidence of T2D rose from 0.25% to 0.89% across extreme quartiles of the genetic score in normal-weight individuals, compared to 4.22% to 7.99% in obese individuals. Given the overriding effect of obesity at any level of genetic risk, this result suggests that population-based approach to create a health-enabling environment to promote healthy lifestyle would be more cost-effective [30, 31]. However, within this context, there is a need to identify those people who are genetically at risk, especially those who are young and lean, in whom PRS may identify those who require pharmacological treatment to halt the disease progression. In this light, in the Diabetes Prevention Programme (DPP), among 823 individuals with pre-diabetes who were randomized to the intensive lifestyle intervention (ILS) arm and remained free of diabetes 1 year after enrolment, genetic risk for T2D identified individuals with differential risk of T2D despite achieving ILS goals of 7% weight loss, 150 min/week leisure-time physical activity, and <25% weekly dietary calories from fat, highlighting that achieving weight loss does not completely ameliorate the genetic risk [32].

Precision Monitoring in T2D

The need for self-monitoring and the use of more advanced glycaemic monitoring such as ambulatory CGM can be adjusted according to clinical profile and overall glucose control. Another potential application of precision monitoring is the interpretation of HbA1c in relation to genetic makeup. For example, a multi-ethnic study of 159,940 individuals identified 60 common variants associated with HbA1c. Of note, a common X-linked G202A variant in the glucose 6 phosphate dehydrogenase (G6PD) gene present in 11% of African Americans was associated with approximately 0.81% units lower HbA1c and hence gives rise to falsely low HbA1c in carriers. This highlights the potential need to screen for the G6PD variant when using HbA1c to diagnose diabetes in populations with high prevalence of G6PD deficiency to provide more precision in monitoring glycaemic control using HbA1c [33].

Precision Treatment in T2D

The aforementioned efforts of sub-classifying T2D, in part by delineating underlying pathophysiological defects, lend themselves to precision treatment of T2D. Thus, patients with predisposition to beta-cell defect would benefit from earlier insulin treatment, whilst those with obesity-related diabetes should be targeted for weight-reduction intervention, including very-low-calorie diet, for diabetes remission [34]. In a proof-of-concept study, using C peptide to define insulin sufficiency, Chinese patients with T2D with low C peptide value treated with insulin had the lowest mortality incidence compared with the highest rate in those with high C peptide and treated with insulin, in part due to long disease duration [35]. Similarly, in a prospective cohort of Chinese patients with young-onset T2D, 8% of patients had latent autoimmune diabetes in adult (LADA) with positive anti-GAD antibodies. Among the insulin-treated patients, patients with LADA had 1.7% reduction in HbA1c compared with 0.8% in the non-LADA patients. Importantly, these patients with LADA had threefold increased risk of end-stage kidney disease than their peers with classical T1D presentation, raising the possibility that delayed diagnosis and treatment in patients with LADA might have contributed to these prognostic differences [36]. In a similar vein, the use of Homeostatic Model for Assessment of insulin resistance and beta cell function (HOMA-IR and HOMA-Beta) derived from fasting plasma glucose and C peptide have also been shown to predict incident diabetes in high risk individuals and, insulin requirement in patients with diabetes [37]. These observational studies have provided the support to develop strategies of matching treatment to underlying pathophysiology. However, randomized clinical trials are needed to incorporate such algorithm-guided treatment to examine long-term clinical outcome.

The need to tailor treatment to clinical characteristics was also highlighted by earlier clinical trials on intensive glucose control. Clinical trials such as the Action to Control Cardiovascular Risk in Diabetes (ACCORD) have highlighted that intensive glucose control (targeting a HbA1c of below 6.0%) in specific patient populations with T2D may be hazardous and was associated with increased mortality among patients randomized to the intensive-therapy group [38]. Some of these patients with severe hypoglycaemia, often unmasked by intensive treatment or failure to adjust treatment, exhibited a "frail" phenotype with multiple morbidities notably chronic kidney disease (CKD) disease with some of them at increased risk of premature death due to multiple causes including cancer [39, 40]. Findings from these studies, together with results from other trials of intensive glucose lowering, have highlighted the need for individualizing treatment targets and led to the recommendation of proposing treatment algorithms for T2D taking into consideration patient profile and co-morbidities [41, 42]. Interestingly, in a subsequent GWAS utilizing the ACCORD cohort, 2 loci, rs9299870 near O6-Methylguanine-DNA Methyltransferase (MGMT) and rs57922 near LINC01333, were found to be associated with increased risk of cardiovascular mortality among participants in the intensive glucose-lowering arm, but not in participants in the standard arm [43]. The modulatory effect of a GRS composed of these two SNPs on association between glycaemic control and cardiovascular mortality was confirmed in an independent cohort from the Joslin clinic [43], highlighting the potential to use biomarkers to identify subjects who may have altered risk-benefit ratio from intensive glucose control.

Another application of precision treatment in T2D is the use of biomarkers or other information to guide treatment selection, including strategies utilizing pharmacogenomics. For example, clinical risk factors including low and high BMI, earlier age at onset, elevated triglyceride and low HDL concentration were found to be associated with increased risk of glycaemic progression and need for insulin in different populations with T2D [44, 45]. Several genetic variants have also been identified to be associated with sulphonylurea and metformin response and may be used to guide treatment dosing [46–49]. In two cohorts of Chinese patients with T2D in Hong Kong, PRS including genetic variants associated with T2D or metformin response were found to show association with glycaemic progression and need for insulin therapy [45].

Precision Prognostics in T2D

There is marked inter-individual variation in the risk of susceptibility to different diabetes complications as well as other emerging comorbidities such as dementia and cancers. Several risk scores or algorithms have been developed to predict risk of cardiovascular and other complications, including the United Kingdom Prospective Diabetes Study (UKPDS) risk engine [50] and the Risk Equations for Complications Of type 2 Diabetes (RECODe) [51]. Several validation studies have suggested that the UKPDS risk engine tend to overestimate risk for CAD in contemporary cohorts [52, 53], thus highlighting the need for additional algorithms and population-specific adaptions.

Using data from the Multi-Ethnic Study of Atherosclerosis (MESA) cohort and the Jackson Heart Study, the Risk Equations for Complications of Type 2 Diabetes (RECODe) provided improved risk stratification compared to the UKPDS outcome model 2 [54]. A series of risk equations have also been developed to predict risk of diabetes complications in Asians with T2D [55].

In Hong Kong, as part of a quality improvement program, the Hong Kong Diabetes Register (HKDR) was set up in 1995 where nurses performed periodic assessment of risk factors and complications (blood, urine, eye and feet), guided by a protocol. This systematic data collection was used to stratify risk, empower self-management, identify care gaps and facilitate shared decision-making. Leveraging the unique healthcare system with a territory-wide electronic medical record system, we were able to develop a series of risk equations with different combinations of risk factors to predict multiple complications including stroke, CAD, heart failure, end-stage kidney disease and all-cause death with 70–90% specificity and sensitivity [56]. This risk stratification program was subsequently incorporated into the web-based Joint Asia Diabetes Evaluation (JADE) portal complete with care protocol, risk engine, personalized reporting system with data visualization including treatment targets and trends supplemented by individualized decision support for implementation in real-world setting [55].

Very few studies have evaluated the utility of incorporating such risk algorithms in clinical practice. In a retrospective analysis comparing diabetes management in three different settings, including routine care in public hospital setting, care in public hospital incorporating the JADE system with nurse-led group education and a community-based nurse-led university diabetes centre utilizing the JADE system with individualized nurse explanation and annual phone reminder for engagement, this data-driven personalized diabetes management, augmented by information and communications technology (ICT), was associated with reduced clinical events and mortality in Chinese patients with T2D [57]. In a broad range of clinical settings in Asia, the implementation of the JADE Program combining the use of data and algorithms delivered by a doctor-nurse team had also been shown to be effective in reducing multiple risk factors, empowering self-management and reducing default [58, 59].

In addition to risk stratification using clinical risk scores, recent advances from genetic studies are also making use of genome-wide PRS (gwPRS) as potential tools for risk stratification in clinical practice [60]. Researchers had used different PRS constructed based on genetic variants for CAD or lipid traits to stratify cardiovascular risk in individuals with T2D [61, 62]. Large international genetic consortia have also identified a large number of genetic variants associated with renal function traits, with potential applications in the stratification of diabetic kidney disease [63, 64]. A strategy that incorporates these different genetic markers for prediction and management of T2D across the course of the disease is illustrated in Fig. 5.2 [29].

In addition to use of genetic variants and PRS for risk stratification, other studies have investigated other "omics" associated with diabetes complications. For example, epigenetic markers such as cytosine methylation markers have been found to improve prediction of renal function decline in diabetic kidney disease [65, 66]. Other epigenetic markers such as circulating microRNA (miRNA) are also showing promise as potential tools for risk stratification for diabetes complications [67] (Fig. 5.3).

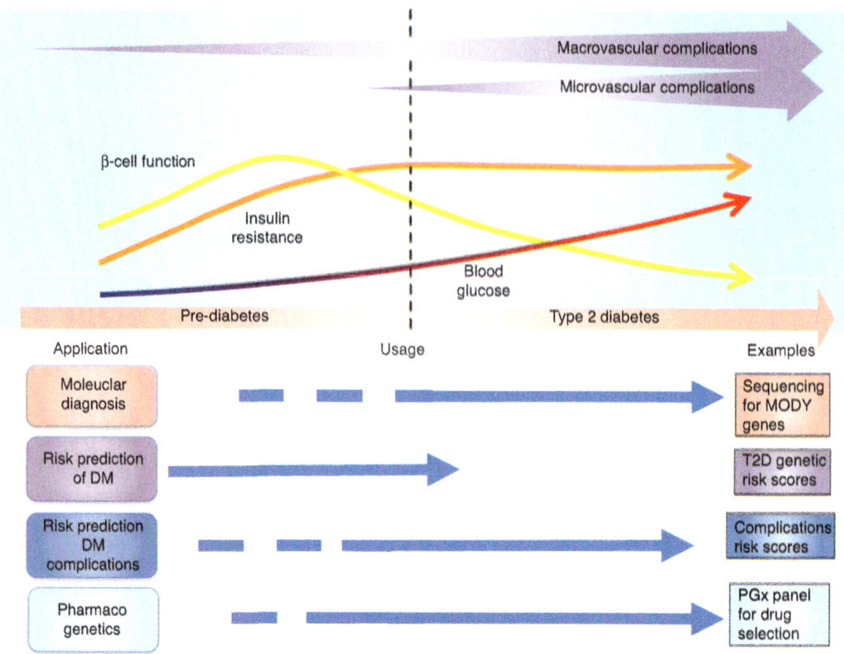

Fig. 5.3 A schematic diagram highlighting potential applications of precision medicine at different stages of type 2 diabetes. (Reproduced with permission from Xie, et al. [29])

Another example of a biomarker-based strategy for risk stratification is the use of CKD risk scores based on proteomic measurement of 273 urinary peptides (CKD273-classifier), which has been shown to predict microalbuminuria during follow-up [68]. In a recent multicentre, prospective, observational study with embedded randomized controlled trial (PRIORITY), patients with T2D and normal urinary albumin excretion were recruited from 15 European centres and stratified for CKD risk using the CKD273-classifier. Patients identified as high risk for CKD were randomized in 1:1 ratio to receive spironolactone or placebo. The study confirmed the utility of the CKD273-classifer in identifying increased risk of progression from normoalbuminuria to microalbuminuria, though spironolactone did not reduce the risk among high-risk subjects randomized to receive spironolactone [69].

Implementation of Precision Medicine for Diabetes

Although much of the discussion so far has centred on the identification of strategies or biomarkers that can facilitate the delivery of precision medicine in diabetes, the identification of such disease-specific biomarkers only represents one of the first steps in the realization of precision medicine. The path to precision medicine, as

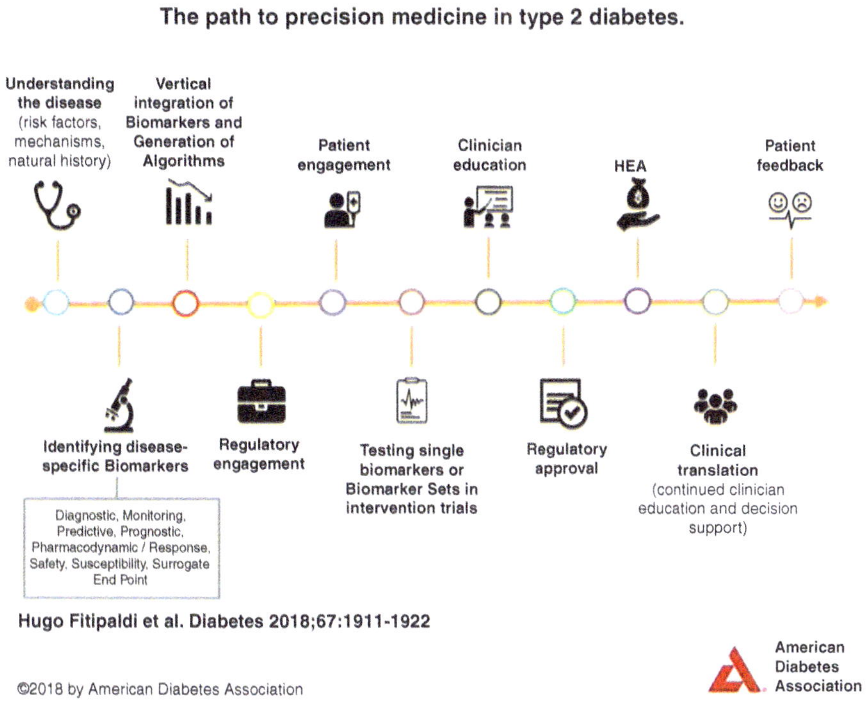

Fig. 5.4 The path towards implementation of precision medicine in diabetes. HEA, health economic assessment. (Reproduced with permission from Fitapaldi, et al. [70])

summarized in a review article [70](Fig. 5.4), requires a concerted effort of integrating the biomarkers and other relevant data into actionable algorithms, engaging approval agencies, empowering clinicians for the appropriate clinical use, generating the evidence of utility in biomarker-driven clinical trials, obtaining regulatory approval, educating users such as patients and high-risk individuals as well as seeking reimbursement from payers, in order for such strategies to be widely adopted by the clinical community (Fig. 5.3). The roadmap described thus highlights the different hurdles and barriers that need to be overcome at different stages of the implementation plan. Among these steps are the need to demonstrate utility of incorporating these strategies compared to traditional approach of diabetes management. Furthermore, both patients and clinicians need to acquire a certain degree of "biomarker" or "genetic literacy" in order to fully utilize these information to make decisions, change behaviours and improve outcomes. Given the complexity of the information being provided, there is also a need to design care models to gather, analyse and communicate this wealth of information relating to risk, or disease subclassification, in order to educate, empower and engage both patients and care providers in accepting these new approaches to diabetes management. Most importantly, these models need to be sustainable with full alignment among patients, providers, payors and policymakers whilst taking into consideration the local setting and cultures.

Whilst the implementation of precision medicine does pose certain challenges as described above, there has been increasing interest and enthusiasm from the diabetes community to incorporate precision medicine into practice. Pilot trials incorporating personalized genetic counselling to motivate diabetes prevention have demonstrated the feasibility to test these hypotheses in clinical settings [71]. In an 8-week randomized clinical trial comparing participants at risk of diabetes given standard lifestyle advice ($N = 190$), lifestyle advice together with genetic risk estimate for T2D ($N = 189$) or lifestyle advice supplemented with phenotypic risk for T2D ($N = 190$) yielded similar outcomes in terms of self-reported diet, self-reported weight, worry and anxiety [72]. In a systematic review including 18 studies reporting on seven different behavioural outcomes, including smoking cessation, diet and physical activity, the meta-analysis revealed no significant effects of communicating DNA-based risk estimates on these health-related behaviours [73]. Future studies would need to explore how best to utilize risk information to enhance preventive strategies. With regard to other biomarkers for risk stratification, most have not been evaluated formally in clinical trial settings. Several clinical trials incorporating biomarkers for diabetes complications are ongoing or have recently been completed which may provide further guidance toward future implementation of precision medicine in diabetes [69]. For example, we have recently completed a randomized clinical trial to examine the utility of implementation of genetic testing for variants related to the risk of diabetes complications [74]. Another trial is currently underway to explore the utility of bio-genetic testing for the management of young-onset diabetes [75]. Against this background, given the genetic and phenotypic heterogeneity underlying the risks for diabetes and its complications, the needs of technologies including devices and medications to alter such risks as well as the cognitive-psychological-social factors that determine behavioural changes, a multicomponent strategy focusing on access to care, provider-patient relationships, data sharing and personalized decision, supported by a practising environment conducive to this model of care delivery, is essential in order to create impact of precision medicine [76].

Conclusions

In this chapter, we have provided some emerging examples of how precision medicine can be helpful in the management of T1D and T2D and some of the challenges involved. Implementation of precision medicine in diabetes requires a multipronged approach in biomarker discovery, validation, clinician education and patient empowerment, as well as regulatory support and reimbursement. Whilst there are still many unknowns, several large international initiatives are underway to systematically evaluate the evidence to help support implementation of precision medicine in diabetes. By combining our existing knowledge and newer technologies (e.g. biogenetic markers, CGMS, HbA1c, artificial intelligence, etc.), we are now in a much better position to integrate these wealth of data to reclassify diabetes and make better prediction for personalized prevention and treatment strategies. It is anticipated that the next few years will witness exciting developments in the delivery of precision medicine in diabetes, which would go hand in hand with the rapid technological developments in big data analytics, large-scale biomarker profiling and artificial intelligence, to bring diabetes care to the forefront of twenty-first-century genomic medicine and care management.

Acknowledgement RCWM acknowledges support from the Research Grants Council Research Impact Fund (CU R4012-18) and a Croucher Senior Medical Research Fellowship. JCNC acknowledges the support of the Hong Kong Government Health and Medical Research Fund for an implementation study of Precision Medicine to Redefine Insulin Secretion and Monogenic Diabetes in Chinese Patients with Young-onset Diabetes (PRISM).

References

1. Robertson CC, Inshaw JRJ, Onengut-Gumuscu S, Chen WM, Santa Cruz DF, Yang H, et al. Fine-mapping, trans-ancestral and genomic analyses identify causal variants, cells, genes and drug targets for type 1 diabetes. Nat Genet. 2021;53(7):962–71.
2. Mahajan A, Taliun D, Thurner M, Robertson NR, Torres JM, Rayner NW, et al. Fine-mapping type 2 diabetes loci to single-variant resolution using high-density imputation and islet-specific epigenome maps. Nat Genet. 2018;50(11):1505–13.
3. Spracklen CN, Horikoshi M, Kim YJ, Lin K, Bragg F, Moon S, et al. Identification of type 2 diabetes loci in 433,540 east Asian individuals. Nature. 2020;582(7811):240–5.
4. Chung WK, Erion K, Florez JC, Hattersley AT, Hivert MF, Lee CG, et al. Precision medicine in diabetes: a consensus report from the American Diabetes Association (ADA) and the European Association for the Study of diabetes (EASD). Diabetes Care. 2020;43(7):1617–35.
5. Ewald N, Hardt PD. Diagnosis and treatment of diabetes mellitus in chronic pancreatitis. World J Gastroenterol. 2013;19(42):7276–81.
6. Lao TT, Chan BC, Leung WC, Ho LF, Tse KY. Maternal hepatitis B infection and gestational diabetes mellitus. J Hepatol. 2007;47(1):46–50.
7. Ma RC, Kong AP, Chan N, Tong PC, Chan JC. Drug-induced endocrine and metabolic disorders. Drug Saf. 2007;30(3):215–45.
8. Fisher EB, Chan JC, Nan H, Sartorius N, Oldenburg B. Co-occurrence of diabetes and depression: conceptual considerations for an emerging global health challenge. J Affect Disord. 2012;142(Suppl):S56–66.
9. Jones AG, McDonald TJ, Shields BM, Hagopian W, Hattersley AT. Latent autoimmune diabetes of adults (LADA) is likely to represent a mixed population of autoimmune (type 1) and nonautoimmune (type 2) diabetes. Diabetes Care. 2021.
10. Oram RA, Patel K, Hill A, Shields B, McDonald TJ, Jones A, et al. A type 1 diabetes genetic risk score can aid discrimination between type 1 and type 2 diabetes in young adults. Diabetes Care. 2016;39(3):337–44.
11. Bingley PJ, Wherrett DK, Shultz A, Rafkin LE, Atkinson MA, Greenbaum CJ. Type 1 diabetes TrialNet: a multifaceted approach to bringing disease-modifying therapy to clinical use in type 1 diabetes. Diabetes Care. 2018;41(4):653–61.
12. Herold KC, Bundy BN, Long SA, Bluestone JA, DiMeglio LA, Dufort MJ, et al. An anti-CD3 antibody, Teplizumab, in relatives at risk for type 1 diabetes. N Engl J Med. 2019;381(7):603–13.

13. Ferrat LA, Vehik K, Sharp SA, Lernmark A, Rewers MJ, She JX, et al. A combined risk score enhances prediction of type 1 diabetes among susceptible children. Nat Med. 2020;26(8):1247–55.
14. McAuley SA, Lee MH, Paldus B, Vogrin S, de Bock MI, Abraham MB, et al. Six months of hybrid closed-loop versus manual insulin delivery with Fingerprick blood glucose monitoring in adults with type 1 diabetes: a randomized controlled trial. Diabetes Care. 2020;43(12):3024–33.
15. Tyler NS, Mosquera-Lopez CM, Wilson LM, Dodier RH, Branigan DL, Gabo VB, et al. An artificial intelligence decision support system for the management of type 1 diabetes. Nat Metab. 2020;2(7):612–9.
16. Chaimowitz NS, Ebenezer SJ, Hanson IC, Anderson M, Forbes LR. STAT1 gain of function, type 1 diabetes, and reversal with JAK inhibition. N Engl J Med. 2020;383(15):1494–6.
17. Akil AA, Yassin E, Al-Maraghi A, Aliyev E, Al-Malki K, Fakhro KA. Diagnosis and treatment of type 1 diabetes at the dawn of the personalized medicine era. J Transl Med. 2021;19(1):137.
18. Chen S, Du K, Zou C. Current progress in stem cell therapy for type 1 diabetes mellitus. Stem Cell Res Ther. 2020;11(1):275.
19. Ma RC. Genetics of cardiovascular and renal complications in diabetes. J Diabetes Investig. 2016;7(2):139–54.
20. Ma RC, Cooper ME. Genetics of diabetic kidney disease-from the worst of nightmares to the light of Dawn? J Am Soc Nephrol. 2017;28(2):389–93.
21. Sandholm N, Groop PH. Genetic basis of diabetic kidney disease and other diabetic complications. Curr Opin Genet Dev. 2018;50:17–24.
22. Salem RM, Todd JN, Sandholm N, Cole JB, Chen WM, Andrews D, et al. Genome-wide association study of diabetic kidney disease highlights biology involved in glomerular basement membrane collagen. J Am Soc Nephrol. 2019;30(10):2000–16.
23. Costacou T, Ferrell RE, Orchard TJ. Haptoglobin genotype: a determinant of cardiovascular complication risk in type 1 diabetes. Diabetes. 2008;57(6):1702–6.
24. Redondo MJ, Hagopian WA, Oram R, Steck AK, Vehik K, Weedon M, et al. The clinical consequences of heterogeneity within and between different diabetes types. Diabetologia. 2020;63(10):2040–8.
25. Ahlqvist E, Tuomi T, Groop L. Clusters provide a better holistic view of type 2 diabetes than simple clinical features. Lancet Diabetes Endocrinol. 2019;7(9):668–9.
26. Udler MS, Kim J, von Grotthuss M, Bonas-Guarch S, Cole JB, Chiou J, et al. Type 2 diabetes genetic loci informed by multi-trait associations point to disease mechanisms and subtypes: a soft clustering analysis. PLoS Med. 2018;15(9):e1002654.
27. Shields BM, McDonald TJ, Ellard S, Campbell MJ, Hyde C, Hattersley AT. The development and validation of a clinical prediction model to determine the probability of MODY in patients with young-onset diabetes. Diabetologia. 2012;55(5):1265–72.
28. Zhu D, Gan S, Liu Y, Ma J, Dong X, Song W, et al. Dorzagliatin monotherapy in Chinese patients with type 2 diabetes: a dose-ranging, randomised, double-blind, placebo-controlled, phase 2 study. The lancet Diabetes & endocrinology. 2018;6:627–36.
29. Xie F, Chan JC, Ma RC. Precision medicine in diabetes prevention, classification and management. J Diabetes Investig. 2018.
30. Langenberg C, Sharp SJ, Franks PW, Scott RA, Deloukas P, Forouhi NG, et al. Gene-lifestyle interaction and type 2 diabetes: the EPIC InterAct Case-cohort study. PLoS Med. 2014;11(5):e1001647.
31. Chan JCN, Lim LL, Wareham NJ, Shaw JE, Orchard TJ, Zhang P, et al. The lancet commission on diabetes: using data to transform diabetes care and patient lives. Lancet. 2021;396(10267):2019–82.
32. Raghavan S, Jablonski K, Delahanty LM, Maruthur NM, Leong A, Franks PW, et al. Interaction of diabetes genetic risk and successful lifestyle modification in the diabetes prevention Programme. Diabetes Obes Metab. 2021;23(4):1030–40.

33. Wheeler E, Leong A, Liu CT, Hivert MF, Strawbridge RJ, Podmore C, et al. Impact of common genetic determinants of hemoglobin A1c on type 2 diabetes risk and diagnosis in ancestrally diverse populations: a transethnic genome-wide meta-analysis. PLoS Med. 2017;14(9):e1002383.
34. Lean ME, Leslie WS, Barnes AC, Brosnahan N, Thom G, McCombie L, et al. Primary care-led weight management for remission of type 2 diabetes (DiRECT): an open-label, cluster-randomised trial. Lancet. 2018;391(10120):541–51.
35. Ko GT, So WY, Tong PC, Chan WB, Yang X, Ma RC, et al. Effect of interactions between C peptide levels and insulin treatment on clinical outcomes among patients with type 2 diabetes mellitus. CMAJ. 2009;180(9):919–26.
36. Luk AOY, Lau ESH, Lim C, Kong APS, Chow E, Ma RCW, et al. Diabetes-related complications and mortality in patients with young-onset latent autoimmune diabetes: a 14-year analysis of the prospective Hong Kong diabetes register. Diabetes Care. 2019;42(6):1042–50.
37. Fan B, Wu H, Shi M, Yang A, Lau ESH, Tam CHT, et al. associations of the homa2-%b and homa2-ir with progression to diabetes and glycaemic deterioration in young and middle-aged chinese. Diabetes/metabolism research and reviews. 2022:e3525.
38. Gerstein HC, Miller ME, Byington RP, Goff DC, Jr., Bigger JT, Action to Control Cardiovascular Risk in Diabetes Study G, et al. Effects of intensive glucose lowering in type 2 diabetes. New England J Med. 2008;358(24):2545–59.
39. Kong AP, Yang X, Luk A, Ma RC, So WY, Ozaki R, et al. Severe hypoglycemia identifies vulnerable patients with type 2 diabetes at risk for premature death and all-site cancer: the Hong Kong diabetes registry. Diabetes Care. 2014;37(4):1024–31.
40. Kong AP, Yang X, Luk A, Cheung KK, Ma RC, So WY, et al. Hypoglycaemia, chronic kidney disease and death in type 2 diabetes: the Hong Kong diabetes registry. BMC Endocr Disord. 2014;14:48.
41. Pozzilli P, Leslie RD, Chan J, De Fronzo R, Monnier L, Raz I, et al. The A1C and ABCD of glycaemia management in type 2 diabetes: a physician's personalized approach. Diabetes Metab Res Rev. 2010;26(4):239–44.
42. Inzucchi SE, Bergenstal RM, Buse JB, Diamant M, Ferrannini E, Nauck M, et al. Management of hyperglycaemia in type 2 diabetes: a patient-centered approach. Position statement of the American Diabetes Association (ADA) and the European Association for the Study of diabetes (EASD). Diabetologia. 2012;55(6):1577–96.
43. Shah HS, Gao H, Morieri ML, Skupien J, Marvel S, Pare G, et al. Genetic predictors of cardiovascular mortality during intensive glycemic control in type 2 diabetes: findings from the ACCORD clinical trial. Diabetes Care. 2016;39(11):1915–24.
44. Zhou K, Donnelly LA, Morris AD, Franks PW, Jennison C, Palmer CN, et al. Clinical and genetic determinants of progression of type 2 diabetes: a DIRECT study. Diabetes Care. 2014;37(3):718–24.
45. Jiang G, Luk AO, Tam CHT, Lau ES, Ozaki R, Chow EYK, et al. Obesity, clinical, and genetic predictors for glycemic progression in Chinese patients with type 2 diabetes: a cohort study using the Hong Kong diabetes register and Hong Kong diabetes biobank. PLoS Med. 2020;17(7):e1003209.
46. Zhou K, Donnelly L, Burch L, Tavendale R, Doney AS, Leese G, et al. Loss-of-function CYP2C9 variants improve therapeutic response to sulfonylureas in type 2 diabetes: a go-DARTS study. Clin Pharmacol Ther. 2010;87(1):52–6.
47. Zhou K, Bellenguez C, Spencer CC, GoDarts, Group UDPS, Wellcome Trust Case Control C, et al. Common variants near ATM are associated with glycemic response to metformin in type 2 diabetes. Nat Genet. 2011;43(2):117–20.
48. Zhou K, Yee SW, Seiser EL, van Leeuwen N, Tavendale R, Bennett AJ, et al. Variation in the glucose transporter gene SLC2A2 is associated with glycemic response to metformin. Nat Genet. 2016;48(9):1055–9.

49. Wang K, Yang A, Shi M, Tam CCH, Lau ESH, Fan B, et al. CYP2C19 Loss-of-function polymorphisms are associated with reduced risk of sulfonylurea treatment failure in chinese patients with type 2 diabetes. Clinical pharmacology and therapeutics. 2021.
50. Stevens RJ, Coleman RL, Adler AI, Stratton IM, Matthews DR, Holman RR. Risk factors for myocardial infarction case fatality and stroke case fatality in type 2 diabetes: UKPDS 66. Diabetes Care. 2004;27(1):201–7.
51. Basu S, Sussman JB, Berkowitz SA, Hayward RA, Yudkin JS. Development and validation of risk equations for complications of type 2 diabetes (RECODe) using individual participant data from randomised trials. Lancet Diabetes Endocrinol. 2017;5(10):788–98.
52. Bannister CA, Poole CD, Jenkins-Jones S, Morgan CL, Elwyn G, Spasic I, et al. External validation of the UKPDS risk engine in incident type 2 diabetes: a need for new type 2 diabetes-specific risk equations. Diabetes Care. 2014;37(2):537–45.
53. Yang X, So WY, Kong AP, Ma RC, Ko GT, Ho CS, et al. Development and validation of a total coronary heart disease risk score in type 2 diabetes mellitus. Am J Cardiol. 2008;101(5):596–601.
54. Basu S, Sussman JB, Berkowitz SA, Hayward RA, Bertoni AG, Correa A, et al. Validation of risk equations for complications of type 2 diabetes (RECODe) using individual participant data from diverse longitudinal cohorts in the U.S. Diabetes Care. 2018;41(3):586–95.
55. Chan JCN, Lim LL, Luk AOY, Ozaki R, Kong APS, Ma RCW, et al. From Hong Kong diabetes register to JADE program to RAMP-DM for data-driven actions. Diabetes Care. 2019;42(11):2022–31.
56. Chan JC, So W, Ma RC, Tong PC, Wong R, Yang X. The complexity of vascular and non-vascular complications of diabetes: the Hong Kong diabetes registry. Curr Cardiovasc Risk Rep. 2011;5(3):230–9.
57. Lim LL, Lau ESH, Ozaki R, Chung H, Fu AWC, Chan W, et al. Association of technologically assisted integrated care with clinical outcomes in type 2 diabetes in Hong Kong using the prospective JADE program: a retrospective cohort analysis. PLoS Med. 2020;17(10):e1003367.
58. Tutino GE, Yang WY, Li X, Li WH, Zhang YY, Guo XH, et al. A multicentre demonstration project to evaluate the effectiveness and acceptability of the web-based joint Asia diabetes evaluation (JADE) programme with or without nurse support in Chinese patients with type 2 diabetes. Diabet Med. 2017;34(3):440–50.
59. Lim LL, Lau ESH, Fu AWC, Ray S, Hung YJ, Tan ATB, et al. Effects of a technology-assisted integrated diabetes care program on Cardiometabolic risk factors among patients with type 2 diabetes in the Asia-Pacific region: the JADE program randomized clinical trial. JAMA Netw Open. 2021;4(4):e217557.
60. Khera AV, Chaffin M, Aragam KG, Haas ME, Roselli C, Choi SH, et al. Genome-wide polygenic scores for common diseases identify individuals with risk equivalent to monogenic mutations. Nat Genet. 2018;50(9):1219–24.
61. Morieri ML, Gao H, Pigeyre M, Shah HS, Sjaarda J, Mendonca C, et al. Genetic tools for coronary risk assessment in type 2 diabetes: a cohort study from the ACCORD clinical trial. Diabetes Care. 2018;41(11):2404–13.
62. Tam CHT, Lim CKP, Luk AOY, Ng ACW, Lee HM, Jiang G, et al. Development of genome-wide polygenic risk scores for lipid traits and clinical applications for dyslipidemia, subclinical atherosclerosis, and diabetes cardiovascular complications among east Asians. Genome Med. 2021;13(1):29.
63. Wuttke M, Li Y, Li M, Sieber KB, Feitosa MF, Gorski M, et al. A catalog of genetic loci associated with kidney function from analyses of a million individuals. Nat Genet. 2019;51(6):957–72.
64. Stanzick KJ, Li Y, Schlosser P, Gorski M, Wuttke M, Thomas LF, et al. Discovery and prioritization of variants and genes for kidney function in >1.2 million individuals. Nat Commun. 2021;12(1):4350.
65. Qiu C, Hanson RL, Fufaa G, Kobes S, Gluck C, Huang J, et al. Cytosine methylation predicts renal function decline in American Indians. Kidney Int. 2018;93(6):1417–31.

66. Gluck C, Qiu C, Han SY, Palmer M, Park J, Ko YA, et al. Kidney cytosine methylation changes improve renal function decline estimation in patients with diabetic kidney disease. Nat Commun. 2019;10(1):2461.
67. Fan B, Luk AOY, Chan JCN, Ma RCW. MicroRNA and diabetic complications: a clinical perspective. Antioxid Redox Signal. 2018;29(11):1041–63.
68. Lindhardt M, Persson F, Zurbig P, Stalmach A, Mischak H, de Zeeuw D, et al. Urinary proteomics predict onset of microalbuminuria in normoalbuminuric type 2 diabetic patients, a sub-study of the DIRECT-protect 2 study. Nephrol Dial Transplant. 2017;32(11):1866–73.
69. Tofte N, Lindhardt M, Adamova K, Bakker SJL, Beige J, Beulens JWJ, et al. Early detection of diabetic kidney disease by urinary proteomics and subsequent intervention with spironolactone to delay progression (PRIORITY): a prospective observational study and embedded randomised placebo-controlled trial. Lancet Diabetes Endocrinol. 2020;8(4):301–12.
70. Fitipaldi H, McCarthy MI, Florez JC, Franks PW. A global overview of precision medicine in type 2 diabetes. Diabetes. 2018;67(10):1911–22.
71. Grant RW, O'Brien KE, Waxler JL, Vassy JL, Delahanty LM, Bissett LG, et al. Personalized genetic risk counseling to motivate diabetes prevention: a randomized trial. Diabetes Care. 2013;36(1):13–9.
72. Godino JG, van Sluijs EM, Marteau TM, Sutton S, Sharp SJ, Griffin SJ. Lifestyle advice combined with personalized estimates of genetic or phenotypic risk of type 2 diabetes, and objectively measured physical activity: a randomized controlled trial. PLoS Med. 2016;13(11):e1002185.
73. Hollands GJ, French DP, Griffin SJ, Prevost AT, Sutton S, King S, et al. The impact of communicating genetic risks of disease on risk-reducing health behaviour: systematic review with meta-analysis. BMJ (Clinical Res Ed). 2016;352:i1102.
74. Ma RC, Xie F, Lim CJ, Lau SH, Luk AO, Ozaki R, et al. Genetic testing and counseling to reduce diabetic complications (NCT02364323). Available from: https://clinicaltrials.gov/ct2/show/NCT02364323?term=ma%2C+ronald&draw=2&rank=1. Last accessed 14 Aug, 2021.
75. Chan JC. Precision medicine in chinese patients with young onset diabetes (NCT04049149). Available from: https://clinicaltrials.gov/ct2/show/NCT04049149?term=chan%2C+juliana&cond=diabetes+AND+prism&draw=2&rank=1. Last accessed 14 Aug, 2021.
76. Lim LL, Lau ESH, Kong APS, Davies MJ, Levitt NS, Eliasson B, et al. Aspects of multicomponent integrated care promote sustained improvement in surrogate clinical outcomes: a systematic review and meta-analysis. Diabetes Care. 2018;41(6):1312–20.

Chapter 6
Precision Genetics for Monogenic Diabetes

Andrea O. Y. Luk and Lee-Ling Lim

Introduction

Monogenic diabetes arises from mutation in a single gene and accounts for roughly 1–3% of people with young-onset diabetes [1, 2]. The mode of inheritance may be autosomal dominant or recessive, although some mutations may occur de novo. People with monogenic diabetes generally present at a young age (below 30 years) and report a strong family history of diabetes [3]. They are typically lean without signs of insulin resistance and are not insulin-dependent. Because of the similarity in clinical presentation, monogenic diabetes may be incorrectly diagnosed as type 1 diabetes or type 2 diabetes. Confirmation of monogenic diabetes requires molecular genetic testing. To date, around 40 monogenic diabetes genes have been identified, the majority of which regulate pancreatic beta-cell function. The most common monogenic diabetes form is maturity-onset diabetes of the young (MODY), and the most commonly implicated genes are glucokinase (*GCK*), hepatocyte nuclear factor 1-alpha (*HNF1A*), hepatocyte nuclear factor 4-alpha (*HNF4A*), and hepatocyte nuclear factor 1-beta (*HNF1B*).

A. O. Y. Luk (✉)
Department of Medicine and Therapeutics, The Chinese University of Hong Kong, Hong Kong, SAR, China

Hong Kong Institute of Diabetes and Obesity, The Chinese University of Hong Kong, Hong Kong, SAR, China
e-mail: andrealuk@cuhk.edu.hk

L.-L. Lim
Hong Kong Institute of Diabetes and Obesity, The Chinese University of Hong Kong, Hong Kong, SAR, China

Department of Medicine, University of Malaya, Kuala Lumpur, Malaysia

R. Basu (ed.), *Precision Medicine in Diabetes*,
https://doi.org/10.1007/978-3-030-98927-9_6

Epidemiology of Monogenic Diabetes

The majority of population-based studies on the prevalence of monogenic diabetes have been conducted in Europe and North America. In most of these studies, only the common MODY forms were considered. The prevalence of MODY varies between studies depending on the criteria used for case finding. From a large Germany and Austria clinical database of over 40,000 youth aged below 20 years with diabetes, 0.8% were classified to have MODY by their physicians [4]. The Norwegian Childhood Diabetes Registry, which accrued 2756 children aged below 15 years, detected monogenic diabetes in 1.1% through genetic screening of individuals without autoimmune antibodies [2]. In a Swedish cohort of 3933 people aged 1–18 years with recently diagnosed diabetes, the minimal prevalence of MODY was 1.2% [5]. The US SEARCH for Diabetes in Youth Study consecutively sequenced 586 diabetic youth who were negative for autoimmune antibodies and had preserved beta-cell function based on detectable fasted C-peptide level for mutations in the three common genes reported prevalence of 8% of the tested sample or 1.2% of the whole diabetes youth population [6]. In a UK-based study, 3.6% of 1365 people with diabetes diagnosed at age below 30 years had monogenic diabetes including both common MODY forms and rare mutations [1]. As these studies mainly reported disease prevalence among young people with diabetes, the prevalence across the full age spectrum of diabetes population is not known.

Classification of Monogenic Diabetes

There is no consensus for classification or nomenclature of monogenic diabetes. It is generally recognized that monogenic diabetes may present as neonatal diabetes (NDM) (diabetes presenting before the age of 6 months), MODY, monogenic diabetes with multisystem syndromes, mitochondrial diabetes, or monogenic diabetes associated with severe insulin resistance or with lipodystrophy [7].

Earlier literatures assigned MODY subtypes according to the order by which the disease-causing mutation was discovered. For example, diabetes due to mutation in the *HNF4A* has been referred to as MODY1, diabetes related to *GCK* mutation as MODY2, etc. This nomenclature scheme is problematic because of the increasing number of genes being incriminated. An alternative classification scheme combining the implicated gene and clinical presentation has been proposed. Under this classification, *HNF4A*-MODY will replace MODY1, *GCK*-MODY will replace MODY2, and so forth. Table 6.1 lists the common monogenic diabetes types based on implicated genes and clinical manifestation.

Table 6.1 Four common subtypes of maturity-onset diabetes of the young (MODY) [9, 28, 32, 37, 38, 49, 52, 57, 60]

Genetic defect	Function on beta-cell	Inheritance	Clinical features	Extra pancreatic features	Treatment	Implications on pregnancy
GCK	Glucose sensor	Autosomal dominant	Incidental diagnosis via screening of asymptomatic individuals Mild fasting hyperglycemia OGTT: Increment <3.0 mmol/L Slow deterioration in beta-cell function with age (comparable to the general population) Very low prevalence of microvascular and macrovascular complications (comparable to the general population)	Nil	**First line:** Diet and exercise Glucose-lowering drugs: Not indicated, unless there is coexisting type 1 or type 2 diabetes, obesity, or pregnancy	Fetal genotype and serial fetal growth guide treatment decisions If both the mother and offspring have *GCK* mutations: Insulin is not required due to an increased risk of low birth weight If the mother has *GCK* mutations and the offspring is unaffected: To initiate insulin if fetal abdominal circumference >75th centile
HNF1A	Transcription factor	Autosomal dominant	Progressive deterioration in beta-cell function Glycosuria due to a low renal glucose threshold Enhanced sensitivity to sulfonylureas Normal body weight Normal lipid levels	Nil	**First line:** Low-dose sulfonylureas or meglitinides **Second line:** Insulin, GLP1-RA, DPP-4 inhibitors	Neonatal hyperinsulinemia, hypoglycemia, and macrosomia: Rare Maternal glycemia determines fetal outcomes Two options with shared decision-making: (a). Stop sulfonylurea and transition to insulin therapy before pregnancy (b). Continue sulfonylurea during early pregnancy, and transition to insulin therapy in the second trimester (only for mothers with optimal glycemic control before pregnancy)

(continued)

Table 6.1 (continued)

Genetic defect	Function on beta-cell	Inheritance	Clinical features	Extra pancreatic features	Treatment	Implications on pregnancy
HNF4A	Transcription factor	Autosomal dominant	Similar to that seen in *HNF1A*-MODY Sequencing for *HNF4A* mutations is indicated if *HNF1A* mutations are absent	Nil	**First line:** Low-dose sulfonylureas **Second line:** Insulin, GLP1-RA	Neonatal hyperinsulinemia, hypoglycemia, and macrosomia: More common than *HNF1A*-MODY Fetal genotype determines fetal outcomes Same treatment approaches as in *HNF1A*-MODY
HNF1B	Transcription factor	Autosomal dominant	Catabolic symptoms: 47% Ketoacidosis: Rare HbA1c ≥13% (119 mmol/Mol) BMI <25 kg/m^2: 80% 43% had ≥4 coexistent cardiovascular risk factors Decreased insulin sensitivity compared with *HNF1A*-MODY	Pancreatic exocrine dysfunction Multi-organ developmental abnormalities (e.g., kidney, genitourinary tract, liver)	**First line:** Sulfonylureas or meglitinides 49% required insulin therapy at diagnosis	If both the mother and offspring have *HNF1B*-MODY: Birth weight is increased If the mother is unaffected and the offspring has *HNF1B* mutations: Low birth weight is common Insulin therapy is a conservative approach

Footnotes: BMI, body mass index; DPP-4, dipeptidyl peptidase-4; *GCK*, glucokinase; GLP1-RA, glucagon-like peptide-1 receptor analogues; *HNF1A*, hepatocyte nuclear factor 1-alpha; *HNF1B*, hepatocyte nuclear factor 1-beta; *HNF4A*, hepatocyte nuclear factor 4-alpha; OGTT, 75-gram oral glucose tolerance test

Diagnosis of Monogenic Diabetes

Correct identification of monogenic diabetes is a prime example of precision medicine as molecular confirmation of this condition will affect medical therapy, direct investigations for possible extra-pancreatic features, and prompt screening in other family members. Depending on the incriminated monogenic diabetes gene, response to glucose-lowering drugs varies, and prognosis with respect to the risks of vascular complications differs. For example, *GCK* mutation, which is linked to a shift in the glucose-sensing threshold of pancreatic beta-cell resulting in mild fasting hyperglycemia, is associated with extremely low risks of vascular complications from diabetes and does not require pharmacological treatment [8, 9]. In contrast, people with mutations in *HNF1A* and *HNF4A* have significant post-meal glucose excursions which are sensitive to the action of sulfonylureas [10, 11]. Unlike people with mutations in *GCK*, those with *HNF1A*, *HNF4A*, and *HNF1B* mutations are susceptible to kidney and retinal complications at an early age, and close monitoring and preventive measures instituted in a timely manner can minimize irreversible end-organ damage.

Diagnosis of monogenic diabetes requires molecular testing using either Sanger sequencing or next-generation sequencing (NGS). Sequencing is the process of determining the order of nucleotides in a gene fragment. The Sanger method sequences one gene at a time, whereas NGS is a high-throughput method and is able to uncover variants in a larger pool of genes simultaneously. Sanger sequencing remains the most frequently used method in clinical practice for identifying common MODY mutations in people with specific phenotypes. With narrowing in the cost differential between Sanger sequencing and NGS, there is gradual trend toward using NGS to screen for genetic variants. In a study of 82 individuals with suspected MODY or neonatal diabetes in whom mutations could not be identified using traditional methods, 17% were found to harbor mutations within the less common monogenic diabetes genes using NGS [12]. In another study in which people with evidence of endogenous insulin secretion and negative islet autoantibodies were sequenced using NGS, mutations in rare genes contributed to about half of all cases of monogenic diabetes [1]. Many facilities have developed targeted NGS gene panels for monogenic diabetes. However, one should be cognizant of the possibility of revealing variants of uncertain clinical significance or those that have little information available in the medical literature. Determining whether these variants are disease-causing poses major challenges even among experts. Recently, the American College of Medical Genetics and Genomics and Association for Molecular Pathology have standardized the procedures for assigning pathogenicity to genetic variants [13]. The Clinical Genome Resource funded by the National Human Genome Research Institute is an expanding knowledge base that is accruing genetic and clinical information from researchers and clinicians from across the globe with the overarching aim to develop consensus methods for interpreting genetic variants in the clinical context [14]. In the case of finding variants associated with extra-pancreatic manifestations, inappropriate interpretation may lead to unnecessary investigations and anxiety for both the affected individual and their family members.

Challenges with Diagnosing Monogenic Diabetes

It was estimated that over 80% of cases of MODY were not detected in clinical practice highlighting the need for better case finding [6, 15]. From the Young Diabetes in Oxford study which actively recruited people from community and hospital-based clinics, 10% of those previously labelled type 1 diabetes and 15% of those diagnosed to have type 2 diabetes up to the age of 45 years had mutation in MODY genes [16]. The low diagnostic rate is multifactorial. Firstly, genetic testing is expensive and not widely available. In areas that do not have a well-developed genetic service, samples will need to be sent to other cities or countries for sequencing. Secondly, as it is not feasible to test everyone with diabetes, the selection of individuals to undergo genetic testing is at the discretion of the physicians. However, the current recommendations are very restrictive leaving many people undiagnosed. The awareness of this condition is also low among general physicians and even among endocrinologists. Thirdly, Sanger sequencing may miss detecting rare monogenic diabetes forms because only the few common genes are tested.

Early guidelines recommend MODY testing for people with age of diabetes diagnosis <25 years, who have known parental history of diabetes, and who are non-insulin dependent. Additionally, low body mass index (BMI) has been frequently identified as one of the discriminatory features for MODY. However, such criteria are neither sensitive nor specific.

Young-onset type 2 diabetes is becoming increasingly common as a result of a rising prevalence of childhood obesity [17, 18]. Exposed to the same obesogenic environment, people with monogenic diabetes are equally as likely to acquire the metabolic syndrome as the general population. In the Young Diabetes in Oxford study, metabolic syndrome was present in a quarter of those with newly confirmed MODY [16]. Among 47 people aged <20 years with screen-detected MODY, acanthosis nigricans was found in 40% and dyslipidemia in 60% [6]. Hence, an obese phenotype and indicators of insulin resistance do not rule out the possibility of MODY.

Positive family history of diabetes is prevalent in type 2 diabetes. Up to 60% of young people with type 2 diabetes report having at least one affected family member [19]. It is noteworthy that with the growing preference for smaller sized families, pedigree analysis as a tool to identify inheritance patterns may become less reliable because the number of family members available to study is few. In this connection, only half of the individuals with MODY detected through population screening reported a transgenerational history of diabetes [6, 16].

Risk Calculator and Screening Algorithm for MODY

Given poor discriminative value of traditional criteria, several research groups have developed risk equations or screening algorithms to improve pre-test probability for genetic testing. Using data from 1191 patients with confirmed MODY and type 1 and type 2 diabetes, investigators from Exeter, UK, constructed risk calculators that demonstrated good performance in differentiating individuals with MODY from the other two diabetes types [20]. Usability of the risk calculator was enhanced by incorporation of simple clinical variables including age of diagnosis, present age, gender, parental history, BMI, HbA1c, and use of insulin or oral glucose-lowering drugs. Of note, the risk calculator has not been validated in non-White ethnic groups.

Biomarkers can also help identify people who are more likely to have monogenic diabetes. These biomarkers include C-peptide, islet autoimmune antibodies, high-sensitivity C-reactive protein (hsCRP), and 1,5-anhydroglucitol [21–24].

C-peptide is a protein that is co-secreted with insulin in equimolar quantities and may serve as a surrogate of insulin secretion. C-peptide levels are undetectable in people with absolute insulin deficiency and therefore can be used to differentiate between type 1 and non-type 1 diabetes [21]. It should be pointed out that endogenous insulin secretion may persist for several years or during honeymoon period in people with type 1 diabetes. Duration of diabetes should be considered when interpreting C-peptide levels.

Anti-islet autoimmune markers include anti-glutamate decarboxylase (GAD), tyrosine phosphatase-related islet antigen-2 (IA-2A), zinc transporter 8 (ZnT8A), and (pro)insulin (IAA) autoantibodies. In general, the presence of anti-islet autoantibodies indicates type 1 diabetes. However, about 10–20% of White people with type 1 diabetes and close to 40% of their non-White counterparts do not harbor anti-islet autoantibodies [5, 25]. Overtime, autoantibody titers decline and seroconversion may occur. As such, absence of antibodies does not fully exclude type 1 diabetes especially for non-White populations.

A study conducted in the UK tested the diagnostic value of a screening pathway consisting of biomarkers in 1365 people with diabetes onset <30 years and an enrolment age <50 years [1]. In this algorithm, molecular genetic testing was performed for individuals with evidence of endogenous insulin secretion based on non-use of insulin therapy or detectable urine C-peptide to creatinine ratio, and negative anti-islet autoantibodies. Using this pathway, monogenic diabetes will be uncovered in one of every five people sequenced, improving the efficiency and cost-effectiveness of testing. In another study consisting of 3933 people aged 1–18 years with newly diagnosed diabetes, 88% were positive for at least one of four anti-islet autoantibodies. MODY was detected in 15% of people who were autoantibody negative and in none of those with positive autoantibodies who likely had type 1 diabetes. As expected, people with MODY had less severe hyperglycemia and were less likely to present with osmotic symptoms or diabetic ketoacidosis. Narrowing the case selection to those with negative autoantibody and either an HbA1c level <7.5% at diagnosis or having a parental history of diabetes increased MODY detection rate to 33% and captured over 90% of all MODY cases.

It should be highlighted that these risk calculators or algorithms may not be generalizable to non-White ethnic groups. Firstly, the distribution of diabetes types among youth or young adults with diabetes differs by ethnicity. For example, in Chinese people, type 2 diabetes contributes to over half of youth (aged <20 years) with diabetes, whereas type 1 diabetes is the predominant diabetes type in White people [17]. Screening methods that differentiate between type 2 diabetes and monogenic diabetes may be more relevant in non-White populations. Secondly, there are huge variations in BMI distribution between ethnic groups. As such, the usual correlation between BMI and diabetes types may not apply equally. Thirdly, the types and frequencies of monogenic diabetes gene mutation may be dissimilar between people of different ethnicities. Differences in genetic makeup will also influence clinical expression of these variants. In a study of predominantly White people, mutations in common MODY genes were detected in 51% of people with age of diabetes onset below 25 years, with at least one affected parent and not insulin treated [15]. In a Chinese diabetes cohort, however, only 10% of individuals fulfilling similar clinical criteria were found to have mutations, leaving the majority undefined [26].

Common Subtypes of MODY: Clinical Phenotypes, Management, and Implications on Pregnancy

GCK-*MODY*

People with *GCK*-MODY have mild fasting hyperglycemia with a slow deterioration of beta-cell function over time. Glucose homeostasis is tightly regulated at a higher set point with the HbA1c levels range between 5.8 and 7.6% (40–60 mmol/mol) and a fasting plasma glucose level of 5.4–8.3 mmol/L (97–149 mg/dL) (Table 6.1) [27, 28]. They are usually non-obese and have normal blood pressure and lipid levels [29, 30].

A cross-sectional study in the UK evaluated the prevalence and severity of diabetes-related complications in 99 individuals with *GCK*-MODY (median age 48.6 years; median HbA1c 6.9% [52 mmol/mol]), 91 non-mutation carriers without diabetes (median age 52.2 years; median HbA1c 5.8% [40 mmol/mol]), and 83 patients with young-onset type 2 diabetes (median age 54.7 years; median HbA1c 7.8% [62 mmol/mol]) [9]. Despite prolonged exposure to mild fasting hyperglycemia from birth, long-term complications are uncommon in patients with *GCK*-MODY. Compared with non-mutation carriers without diabetes, people with *GCK*-MODY reported a similar prevalence of microvascular complications (defined as either persistent albuminuria or preproliferative and advanced stages of retinopathy; 1% versus 3%) and macrovascular complications (4% versus 11%) [9]. The corresponding prevalence was lower than people with young-onset type 2 diabetes (1% versus 36% for microvascular complications and 4% versus 30% for macrovascular complications) [9]. Although people with *GCK*-MODY had a higher prevalence of non-proliferative retinopathy than non-mutation carriers (30% versus 14%), 81% of them were mild in severity with fewer than five microaneurysms [9]. Given its low yield, annual screening for retinopathy is currently not recommended for *GCK*-MODY [28, 31].

Although adequate glycemic control is required to prevent complications in other types of diabetes, people with *GCK*-MODY do not usually require glucose-lowering drugs [31, 32] in the absence of coexisting type 1 or type 2 diabetes, obesity, or pregnancy [28]. The Exeter group reported that 13.5% and 7.5% of people with *GCK*-MODY were treated with a low dose of oral glucose-lowering drugs (5 mg glibenclamide and 660 mg metformin daily) and insulin therapy (0.1–0.8 units/kg/day), respectively, prior to genetic testing [32]. HbA1c levels were not significantly different in those with and without treatment (median HbA1c 6.5% [48 mmol/mol] versus 6.4% [46 mmol/mol]) [32]. Of note, after genetic testing, HbA1c levels remained unchanged post-cessation of treatment, indicating that glucose-lowering treatment is generally not required in *GCK*-MODY [32].

The prevalence of MODY in women with gestational diabetes mellitus ranges between 0.1% and 6.0% [28, 33]. To differentiate *GCK*-MODY from gestational diabetes mellitus, genetic testing can be performed in women with a fasting glucose level ≥5.5 mmol/L (99 mg/dL) and BMI <25 kg/m^2 [34]. Compared with *HNF1A*-MODY, *GCK*-MODY is more difficult to control with higher glycemic excursions and higher rate of miscarriage (33.3% versus 14.0%), especially during the first trimester of pregnancy [33]. Given the risk of miscarriage associated with invasive fetal genotyping, serial monitoring of fetal growth is a pragmatic approach to guide insulin use in pregnant women with *GCK*-MODY [31, 33, 35]. If the offspring inherits the maternal GCK mutation, the offspring's glucose setpoint is increased with normal fetal growth, and thus, insulin therapy is not required during pregnancy [28, 31]. Injudicious use of insulin therapy in such a case has been reported to reduce endogenous maternal insulin secretion with increased risk of small for gestational age [35, 36]. If the offspring is unaffected, in utero exposure to maternal hyperglycemia increases fetal insulin secretion leading to macrosomia, defined as fetal abdominal circumference >75th centile (Table 6.1). Insulin therapy is therefore recommended with labor induction at 38 weeks in these pregnant women with *GCK*-MODY [28, 31].

HNF1A-*MODY*

Compared with GCK-MODY, people with *HNF1A*-MODY have progressive beta-cell dysfunction with marked symptomatic hyperglycemia. Similar to that seen in type 2 diabetes, people with *HNF1A*-MODY tend to develop microvascular and macrovascular complications that are strongly related to glycemic control (Table 6.1)

[37, 38]. In a UK cohort, a lower proportion of people with *HNF1A*-MODY reported any degree of retinopathy than age-, BMI- and diabetes duration-matched patients with type 1 diabetes (13.5% versus 50.0%) [39]. Compared with non-mutation carriers, individuals with *HNF1A*-MODY had 1.9 and 2.6 times increased risk of all-cause and cardiovascular deaths, respectively, after adjusting for sex and smoking status [40]. Hence, annual screening for diabetes-related complications is recommended [31].

First-line treatment for people with *HNF1A*-MODY is low-dose sulfonylureas, which act via potassium-sensitive ATP channels to increase insulin secretion [39]. Given its increased sensitivity to sulfonylureas with a risk of hypoglycemia, sulfonylureas should be initiated at a low dose and slowly titrated to target with dose reduction or discontinuation of concurrent insulin therapy [38]. Despite treatment with sulfonylureas, glycemic control continues to deteriorate after 3 to 25 years due to progressive beta-cell dysfunction [37]. In an observational study in which 21 people with either *HNF1A*- or *HNF4A*-MODY switched from metformin and/or insulin therapy to diet alone or sulfonylurea alone. At 2 years, about 60% achieved target glycemic control of HbA1c ≤7.5% (58 mmol/mol). The major predictors for response to sulfonylureas included short diabetes duration, low pre-treatment HbA1c, and low BMI, highlighting the importance of early diagnosis [41]. Nateglinide has also been shown to reduce postprandial glucose levels with a lower risk of hypoglycemia compared with glyburide [42].

Apart from insulin therapy, glucagon-like peptide-1 receptor analogues (GLP-1 RA) and dipeptidyl peptidase-4 (DPP-4) inhibitors have been investigated as potential adjuvant therapies in *HNF1A*-MODY [43–45]. In a 6-week randomized, double-blinded, crossover trial involving 16 individuals with *HNF1A*-MODY (mean age 39 years, HbA1c 6.4% (46 mmol/mol) and BMI 24.9 kg/m^2), both liraglutide (1.8 mg weekly) and glimepiride (1.0–4.0 mg daily) reduced fasting plasma glucose without significant between-group differences [44]. Compared with liraglutide, glimepiride was associated with a 10 times increased risk of mild hypoglycemia [44]. In another 36-week randomized, double-blinded, crossover trial involving 19 people with *HNF1A*-MODY (mean age 43 years, HbA1c 7.4% (57 mmol/mol) and BMI 24.8 kg/m^2), the addition of linagliptin to glimepiride improved glycemic variability, insulin sensitivity, and HbA1c by 0.5% without increasing the risk of hypoglycemia [46]. By contrast, the use of sodium-glucose co-transporter-2 (SGLT2) inhibitors in *HNF1A*-MODY is cautioned against due to reports of severe volume depletion and diabetic ketoacidosis [31, 47, 48].

Majority of pregnancies affected by *HNF1A*-MODY are not associated with an increased risk of fetal hyperinsulinemia, hypoglycemia, and macrosomia [49]. Maternal glycemia determines fetal outcomes, but there is limited data on the best treatment approach during pregnancy. Although sulfonylureas (especially glyburide as it has been extensively studied in pregnancy) are a reasonable treatment for *HNF1A*-MODY during pregnancy, recent reports about transplacental transfer of glyburide [50] with 2–3 times increased risk of neonatal hypoglycemia and macrosomia have raised safety concerns [51]. In this light, there are two potential treatment approaches, namely, [1] stop glyburide and transition to insulin therapy preconception, or [2] continue glyburide until late first trimester and complete transition to insulin therapy by 26 weeks gestation [50]. The latter is suggested only for women with glyburide-treated *HNF1A*-MODY who have attained optimal glycemic control preconception [50].

HNF4A-*MODY*

Given *HNF1A*-MODY and *HNF4A*-MODY have similar phenotypes, sequencing for *HNF4A* mutations should be performed when *HNF1A* mutations are absent [52]. Likewise, annual screening for diabetes-related complications is recommended. People with *HNF4A*-MODY may present with transient neonatal hyperinsulinemia and hypoglycemia, followed by diabetes during adolescence or early adulthood [37, 53].

Similar to *HNF1A*-MODY, first-line treatment for *HNF4A*-MODY is sulfonylureas (Table 6.1) [52, 54]. However, most will require insulin therapy due to more rapid deterioration of beta-cell function [37, 38]. Substantial glycemic improvement with the use of GLP-1 RA has been reported in a father-son pair with *HNF4A*-MODY who have failed either sulfonylureas or basal-bolus insulin therapy [55].

Nearly half of the offspring of pregnant women with *HNF4A*-MODY experience fetal hyperinsulinemia, transient hypoglycemia, and macrosomia [49, 56]. In contrast to *HNF1A*-MODY, the fetal genotype is the key determinant of fetal outcomes in pregnancies with *HNF4A*-MODY [57]. Compared with non-mutation carriers, offspring with *HNF4A* mutations had a median increase in birthweight by 790 grams and a higher incidence of macrosomia (56.0% versus 13.0%) [49]. Treatment approaches are the same as previously described for pregnancies with *HNF1A*-MODY [57].

HNF1B-*MODY*

Hepatocyte nuclear factor 1-beta is a transcription factor expressed in embryonic development of multiple organs [57]. In a European registry, 40% of individuals with *HNF1B*-MODY reported extra-pancreatic features [58] including developmental kidney disease (e.g., renal cystic disease, renal hypoplasia), chronic kidney disease/end-stage kidney disease, liver dysfunction (e.g., unexplained transaminitis, neonatal cholestasis), genital tract malformations (e.g., rudimentary uterus, cryptorchidism), hyperuricemia, and early-onset gout [59, 60]. Screening for these abnormalities at diagnosis is warranted.

Although first-line treatment for *HNF1B*-MODY can be either sulfonylureas or meglitinides (repaglinide), people with *HNF1B*-MODY have decreased insulin sensitivity than those with *HNF1A*-MODY [61]. In a multicenter retrospective cohort study involving 201 individuals with *HNF1B*-MODY, 49% of them were treated with insulin at diagnosis, which increased to 79% after 12 years of follow-up likely due to progressive deterioration of beta-cell and kidney functions [60]. The median total insulin dose was 0.55 units/kg/day (interquartile range [IQR] 0.39–0.70) with a median HbA1c level of 7.3% (56 mmol/mol) (IQR 6.7–8.4% [50–68 mmol/mol]) [60, 61]. Similar to mutations in other HNF-transcription factors, *HNF1B*-MODY is commonly associated with cardiovascular risk factors and diabetes-related complications (Table 6.1) [60, 61].

Given its very low prevalence, evidence about the intrauterine effects of treatment in pregnant women with *HNF1B*-MODY has been limited. In a UK study involving 21 *HNF1B* mutation carriers, among offspring with *HNF1B*-MODY born to unaffected mothers, their birthweights were significantly reduced (median 2.4 kg [IQR 1.8–33]), of whom 69% were small for gestational age [62]. This is due to reduced fetal insulin secretion, leading to a decrease in insulin-mediated fetal growth. By contrast, when both mother and offspring had *HNF1B*-MODY, there was an increase in birthweight (median 3.8 kg [IQR 3.3–4.6]) [62]. Despite *HNF1B* mutations, pancreatic beta-cells of the offspring remain to be glucose-sensitive, and thus, fetal insulin secretion is augmented in the presence of maternal hyperglycemia, leading to an increase in fetal growth.

KCNJ11-*NDM and* ABCC8-*NDM*

Individuals with neonatal diabetes usually present in the first 6 months of age. It affects 1 in 90,000–160,000 live births [63]. The *KCNJ11* and *ABCC8* genes encode for Kir6.2 (inner subunit) and SUR1 (outer subunit) of the ATP-sensitive potassium (K_{ATP}) channel, respectively [64]. Mutations in *KCNJ11* and *ABCC8* account for 40% of cases of NDM with a marked reduction in pancreatic beta-cell insulin section [63]. The median age of diagnosis in people with *KCNJ11* or *ABCC8* mutations was 9.6 weeks (IQR 6.1–18.3 weeks) [65, 66].

Neonatal diabetes should be suspected in infants with acute hyperglycemia, typically with blood glucose levels persistently above 14 mmol/L (252 mg/dL) for more than 7 days. Although neonatal diabetes is commonly diagnosed in the early neonatal period, it can still manifest up to 12 months of age with failure to thrive [67]. The frequency of diabetic ketoacidosis at diagnosis ranges between 30% and 75% [65, 66]. Given that K_{ATP} channels are found in the brain, people with *KCNJ11* mutations may experience sleep disturbances and attention deficit hyperactivity disorder, and even DEND syndrome which is a triad of developmental delays, seizures, and neonatal diabetes [68, 69].

People with *KCNJ11* or *ABCC8* mutations will usually require insulin therapy during acute hyperglycemia. For the majority of them, treatment can be subsequently converted to high-dose sulfonylureas (typically 0.5–1.0 mg/kg/day of glyburide) [63]. A Monogenic Diabetes Registry reported a delay in having genetic diagnosis of neonatal diabetes after clinical diagnosis by a median of 10.4 weeks

(IQR 1.6–58.2) [70]. Given the potential for adverse neurocognitive effects, early initiation of sulfonylureas should be considered even before genetic testing.

INS-*NDM*

Mutations in the insulin gene (*INS*) are the second most common cause of neonatal diabetes [71]. These mutations lead to protein misfolding with increased endoplasmic reticulum stress and, subsequently, pancreatic beta-cell death [72]. Individuals with *INS* mutations have similar presentations to that in those with early-onset type 1 diabetes, and 30% of them may present with diabetic ketoacidosis [63]. The majority of cases are diagnosed in the first 6 months of age with a median age of 10 weeks (IQR 6.1–17.4) [63]. Insulin therapy is recommended in these people [63].

Conclusion

A diagnosis of diabetes can adversely influence an individual's life. Although monogenic diabetes is relatively uncommon accounting for less than 5% of diabetes in young people, early and accurate detection allows us to project clinical course, steer the choice of glucose- lowering drugs, and guide screening of at-risk family members. Timely recognition of MODY also influences antenatal care as maternal-offspring genotype concordance or discordance can affect pregnancy outcomes. Given the low diagnostic rate, there is a need to improve the scope and the efficiency to test. This may be achieved by providing education for physicians and/or systematic screening guided by validated screening algorithms.

References

1. Shields BM, Shepherd M, Hudson M, McDonald TJ, Coldough K, Peters J, Knight B, Hyde C, Ellard S, Pearson ER, Hattersley AT, on behalf of the UNITED study team. Population-based assessment of a biomarker-based screening pathway to aid diagnosis of monogenic diabetes in young-onset patients. Diabetes Care. 2017;40:1017–25.
2. Irgens HU, Molnes J, Johansson BB, Ringdal M, Skrivarhaug T, Undlien DE, Sovik O, Joner G, Molven A, Njolstad PR. Prevalence of monogenic diabetes in the population-based Norwegian childhood diabetes registry. Diabetologia. 2013;56:1512–219.
3. Tattersall RB, Fajans SS, Arbor A. Prevalence of diabetes and glucose intolerance in 199 offspring of thirty-seven conjugal diabetic parents. Diabetes. 1975;24:452–62.
4. Schober E, Rami B, Grabert M, Thon A, Kapellen T, Reinehr T, Holl RW. Phenotypical aspects of maturity-onset diabetes of the young (MODY diabetes) in comparison with type 2 diabetes mellitus (T2DM) in children and adolescents: experience from a large multicentre database. Diabet Med. 2009;26:466–73.

5. Carlsson A, Shepherd M, Ellard S, Weedon M, Lernmark A, Forsander G, Colclough K, Brahimi Q, Valtonen-Andre C, Ivarsson SA, Larsson HE, Samuelsson U, Ortqvist E, Groop L, Ludvigsson J, Marcus C, Hattersley AT. Absence of islet autoantibodies and modestly raised glucose values at diabetes diagnosis should lead to testing for MODY: lessons from a 5-year pediatric Swedish national cohort study. Diabetes Care. 2020;43:82–9.
6. Pihoker C, Gilliam LK, Ellard S, Dabelea D, Davis C, Dolan LM, Greenbaum CJ, Imperatore G, Lawrence JM, Marcovina SM, Mayer-Davis E, Rodriguez BL, Steck AK, Williams DE, Hattersley AT. Prevalence, characteristics and clinical diagnosis of maturity onset diabetes of the young due to mutations in HNF1A, HNF4A and glucokinase: results from the SEARCH for diabetes in youth. J Clin Endocrinol Metab. 2013;98:4055–62.
7. Riddle MC, Philipson LH, Rich SS, Carlsson A, Franks PW, Greeley SA, Nolan JJ, Pearson ER, Zeitler PS, Hattersley AT. Monogenic diabetes: from genetic insights to population-based precision in care. Reflections from a diabetes care editors' expert forum. Diabetes Care. 2020;43:3117–28.
8. Froguel P, Zouali H, Vionnet N, et al. Familial hyperglycemia due to mutations in glucokinase. Definition of a subtype of diabetes mellitus. N Engl J Med. 1993;328:697–702.
9. Steele AM, Shields BM, Wensley KJ, Colclough K, Ellard S, Hattersley AT. Prevalence of vascular complications among patients with glucokinase mutations and prolonged, mild hyperglycemia. JAMA. 2014;311:279–86.
10. Yamagata K, Oda N, Kaisaki PJ, et al. Mutations in the hepatocyte nuclear factor-1α gene in maturity-onset diabetes of the young (MODY3). Nature. 1996;384:455–8.
11. Yamagata K, Furuta H, Oda N, et al. Mutations in the hepatocyte nuclear factor-4α gene in maturity-onset diabetes of the young (MODY1). Nature. 1996;384:458–60.
12. Ellard S, Allen HL, De Franco E, Flanagan SE, Hysenaj G, Colclough K, Houghton JA, Shepherd M, Hattersley AT, Weedon MN, Caswell R. Improved genetic testing for monogenic diabetes using targeted next-generation sequencing. Diabetologia. 2013;56:1958–63.
13. Richards S, Aziz N, Bale S, et al. ACMG laboratory quality assurance committee. Standards and guidelines for the interpretation of sequence variants: a joint consensus recommendation of the American College of Medical Genetics and Genomics and the Association for Molecular Pathology. Genet Med. 2015;17:405–24.
14. Clinical Genome Resource. https://www.clinicalgenome.org/. Access date: 4 March 2021.
15. Shields BM, Hicks S, Shepherd MH, Colclough K, Hattersley AT, Ellard S. Maturity-onset diabetes of the young (MODY): how many cases are we missing? Diabetologia. 2010;53:2504–8.
16. Thanabalasingham G, Pal A, Selwood MP, Dudley C, Fisher K, Bingley PJ, Ellard S, Aj F, McCarthy MI, Owen KR. Systematic assessment of etiology in adults with a clinical diagnosis of young-onset type 2 diabetes is a successful strategy for identifying maturity-onset diabetes of the young. Diabetes Care. 2012;35:1206–12.
17. Luk A, Ke C, Lau ES, Wu H, Goggins W, Ma RC, Chow E, Kong A, So WY, Chan JC. Secular trends in incidence of type 1 and type 2 diabetes in Hong Kong: a retrospective cohort study. PLoS Med. 2020.
18. Magliano DJ, Sacre JW, Harding JL, Gregg EW, Zimmet PZ, Shaw JE. Young-onset type 2 diabetes mellitus – implications for morbidity and mortality. Nature Rev. 2019.
19. Chan JC, Lau ES, Luk AO, Cheung KK, Kong AP, Yu LW, Choi KC, Chow FC, Ozaki R, Brown N, Yang X, Bennett PH, Ma RC, So WY. Premature mortality and comorbidities in young-onset diabetes: a 7-year prospective analysis. Am J Med. 2014;127:616–24.
20. Shields BM, McDonald TJ, Ellard S, Campbell MJ, Hyde C, Hattersley AT. The development and validation of a clinical prediction model to determine the probability of MODY in patients with young-onset diabetes. Diabetologia. 2012;55:1265–72.
21. Besser RE, Shepherd MH, McDonald TJ, et al. Urinary C-peptide creatinine ratio is a practical outpatient tool for identifying hepatocyte nuclear factor 1-alpha/hepatocyte nuclear factor 4-alpha maturity-onset diabetes of the young from long-duration type 1 diabetes. Diabetes Care. 2011;34:286–91.

22. McDonald TJ, Colclough K, Brown R, et al. Islet autoantibodies can discriminate maturity-onset diabetes of the young (MODY) from type 1 diabetes. Diabet Med. 2011;28:1028–33.
23. Owen KR, Thanabalasingham G, James TJ, Karpe F, Farmer AJ, McCarthy MI, Gloyn AL. Assessment of high-sensitivity C-reactive protein levels as diagnostic discriminator of maturity-onset diabetes of the young due to HNF1A mutations. Diabetes Care. 2010;33:1919–24.
24. Pal A, Farmer AJ, Dudley C, Selwood MP, Barrow BA, Klyne R, Grew JP, McCarthy MI, Gloyn AL, Owen KR. Evaluation of serum 1,5anhydroglucitol levels as a clinical test to differentiate subtypes of diabetes. Diabetes Care. 2010;33:252–7.
25. Tuomi T, Zimmet P, Rowley MJ, Min HK, Vichayanrat A, Lee HK, Rhee BD, Vannasaeng S, Humphrey AR, Mackay IR. Differing frequency of autoantibodies to glutamic acid decarboxylase among Koreans, Thais, and Australians with diabetes mellitus. Clin Immumol Immunopathol. 1995;74:202–6.
26. Xu JY, Dan QH, Chan V, Wat NM, Tam S, Tiu SC, Lee KF, Siu SC, Tsang MW, Fung LM, Chan KW, Lam KS. Genetic and clinical characteristics of maturity-onset diabetes of the young in Chinese patients. Eur J Hum Genet. 2005;13:422–7.
27. Steele AM, Wensley KJ, Ellard S, Murphy R, Shepherd M, Colclough K, et al. Use of HbA1c in the identification of patients with hyperglycaemia caused by a glucokinase mutation: observational case control studies. PLoS One. 2013;8(6):e65326.
28. Chakera AJ, Steele AM, Gloyn AL, Shepherd MH, Shields B, Ellard S, et al. Recognition and management of individuals with hyperglycemia because of a heterozygous glucokinase mutation. Diabetes Care. 2015;38(7):1383–92.
29. Page RC, Hattersley AT, Levy JC, Barrow B, Patel P, Lo D, et al. Clinical characteristics of subjects with a missense mutation in glucokinase. Diabet Med. 1995;12(3):209–17.
30. Velho G, Blanché H, Vaxillaire M, Bellanné-Chantelot C, Pardini VC, Timsit J, et al. Identification of 14 new glucokinase mutations and description of the clinical profile of 42 MODY-2 families. Diabetologia. 1997;40(2):217–24.
31. Broome DT, Pantalone KM, Kashyap SR, Philipson LH. Approach to the patient with MODY-monogenic diabetes. J Clin Endocrinol Metab. 2021;106(1):237–50.
32. Stride A, Shields B, Gill-Carey O, Chakera AJ, Colclough K, Ellard S, et al. Cross-sectional and longitudinal studies suggest pharmacological treatment used in patients with glucokinase mutations does not alter glycaemia. Diabetologia. 2014;57(1):54–6.
33. Bacon S, Schmid J, McCarthy A, Edwards J, Fleming A, Kinsley B, et al. The clinical management of hyperglycemia in pregnancy complicated by maturity-onset diabetes of the young. Am J Obstet Gynecol. 2015;213(2):236.e1–7.
34. Chakera AJ, Spyer G, Vincent N, Ellard S, Hattersley AT, Dunne FP. The 0.1% of the population with glucokinase monogenic diabetes can be recognized by clinical characteristics in pregnancy: the Atlantic diabetes in pregnancy cohort. Diabetes Care. 2014;37(5):1230–6.
35. Spyer G, Hattersley AT, Sykes JE, Sturley RH, MacLeod KM. Influence of maternal and fetal glucokinase mutations in gestational diabetes. Am J Obstet Gynecol. 2001;185(1):240–1.
36. Spyer G, Macleod KM, Shepherd M, Ellard S, Hattersley AT. Pregnancy outcome in patients with raised blood glucose due to a heterozygous glucokinase gene mutation. Diabet Med. 2009;26(1):14–8.
37. Fajans SS, Bell GI. MODY: history, genetics, pathophysiology, and clinical decision making. Diabetes Care. 2011;34(8):1878–84.
38. Hattersley AT, Patel KA. Precision diabetes: learning from monogenic diabetes. Diabetologia. 2017;60(5):769–77.
39. Bacon S, Kyithar MP, Rizvi SR, Donnelly E, McCarthy A, Burke M, et al. Successful maintenance on sulphonylurea therapy and low diabetes complication rates in a HNF1A-MODY cohort. Diabet Med. 2016;33(7):976–84.
40. Steele AM, Shields BM, Shepherd M, Ellard S, Hattersley AT, Pearson ER. Increased all-cause and cardiovascular mortality in monogenic diabetes as a result of mutations in the HNF1A gene. Diabet Med. 2010;27(2):157–61.

41. Shepherd MH, Shields BM, Hudson M, Pearson ER, Hyde C, Ellard S, Hattersley AT, Patel KA, for the UNITED study. A UK nationwide prospective study of treatment change in MODY: genetic subtype and clinical characteristics predict optimal glycaemic control after discontinuing insulin and metformin. Diabetologia. 2018;61:2520–7.
42. Tuomi T, Honkanen EH, Isomaa B, Sarelin L, Groop LC. Improved prandial glucose control with lower risk of hypoglycemia with nateglinide than with glibenclamide in patients with maturity-onset diabetes of the young type 3. Diabetes Care. 2006;29(2):189–94.
43. Docena MK, Faiman C, Stanley CM, Pantalone KM. Mody-3: novel HNF1A mutation and the utility of glucagon-like peptide (GLP)-1 receptor agonist therapy. Endocr Pract. 2014;20(2):107–11.
44. Østoft SH, Bagger JI, Hansen T, Pedersen O, Faber J, Holst JJ, et al. Glucose-lowering effects and low risk of hypoglycemia in patients with maturity-onset diabetes of the young when treated with a GLP-1 receptor agonist: a double-blind, randomized, crossover trial. Diabetes Care. 2014;37(7):1797–805.
45. Fantasia KL, Steenkamp DW. Optimal glycemic control in a patient with HNF1A MODY with GLP-1 RA monotherapy: implications for future therapy. J Endocr Soc. 2019;3(12):2286–9.
46. Christensen AS, Hædersdal S, Støy J, Storgaard H, Kampmann U, Forman JL, et al. Efficacy and safety of glimepiride with or without Linagliptin treatment in patients with HNF1A diabetes (maturity-onset diabetes of the young type 3): a randomized, double-blinded, placebo-controlled, crossover trial (GLIMLINA). Diabetes Care. 2020;43(9):2025–33.
47. Pruhova S, Dusatkova P, Neumann D, Hollay E, Cinek O, Lebl J, et al. Two cases of diabetic ketoacidosis in HNF1A-MODY linked to severe dehydration: is it time to change the diagnostic criteria for MODY? Diabetes Care. 2013;36(9):2573–4.
48. Hohendorff J, Szopa M, Skupien J, Kapusta M, Zapala B, Platek T, et al. A single dose of dapagliflozin, an SGLT-2 inhibitor, induces higher glycosuria in GCK- and HNF1A-MODY than in type 2 diabetes mellitus. Endocrine. 2017;57(2):272–9.
49. Pearson ER, Boj SF, Steele AM, Barrett T, Stals K, Shield JP, et al. Macrosomia and hyperinsulinaemic hypoglycaemia in patients with heterozygous mutations in the HNF4A gene. PLoS Med. 2007;4(4):e118.
50. Shepherd M, Brook AJ, Chakera AJ, Hattersley AT. Management of sulfonylurea-treated monogenic diabetes in pregnancy: implications of placental glibenclamide transfer. Diabet Med. 2017;34(10):1332–9.
51. Poolsup N, Suksomboon N, Amin M. Efficacy and safety of oral antidiabetic drugs in comparison to insulin in treating gestational diabetes mellitus: a meta-analysis. PLoS One. 2014;9(10):e109985.
52. Pearson ER, Pruhova S, Tack CJ, Johansen A, Castleden HA, Lumb PJ, et al. Molecular genetics and phenotypic characteristics of MODY caused by hepatocyte nuclear factor 4alpha mutations in a large European collection. Diabetologia. 2005;48(5):878–85.
53. Bacon S, Kyithar MP, Condron EM, Vizzard N, Burke M, Byrne MM. Prolonged episodes of hypoglycaemia in HNF4A-MODY mutation carriers with IGT. Evidence of persistent hyperinsulinism into early adulthood. Acta Diabetol. 2016;53(6):965–72.
54. Pearson ER, Starkey BJ, Powell RJ, Gribble FM, Clark PM, Hattersley AT. Genetic cause of hyperglycaemia and response to treatment in diabetes. Lancet. 2003;362(9392):1275–81.
55. Broome DT, Tekin Z, Pantalone KM, Mehta AE. Novel use of GLP-1 receptor agonist therapy in HNF4A-MODY. Diabetes Care. 2020;43(6):e65.
56. Colclough K, Bellanne-Chantelot C, Saint-Martin C, Flanagan SE, Ellard S. Mutations in the genes encoding the transcription factors hepatocyte nuclear factor 1 alpha and 4 alpha in maturity-onset diabetes of the young and hyperinsulinemic hypoglycemia. Hum Mutat. 2013;34(5):669–885.
57. Dickens LT, Naylor RN. Clinical Management of Women with monogenic diabetes during pregnancy. Curr Diab Rep. 2018;18(3):12.

58. Warncke K, Kummer S, Raile K, Grulich-Henn J, Woelfle J, Steichen E, et al. Frequency and characteristics of MODY 1 (HNF4A mutation) and MODY 5 (HNF1B mutation): analysis from the DPV database. J Clin Endocrinol Metab. 2019;104(3):845–55.
59. Clissold RL, Hamilton AJ, Hattersley AT, Ellard S, Bingham C. HNF1B-associated renal and extra-renal disease-an expanding clinical spectrum. Nat Rev Nephrol. 2015;11(2):102–12.
60. Dubois-Laforgue D, Cornu E, Saint-Martin C, Coste J, Bellanné-Chantelot C, Timsit J. Diabetes, associated clinical Spectrum, long-term prognosis, and genotype/phenotype correlations in 201 adult patients with hepatocyte nuclear factor 1B (HNF1B) molecular defects. Diabetes Care. 2017;40(11):1436–43.
61. Pearson ER, Badman MK, Lockwood CR, Clark PM, Ellard S, Bingham C, et al. Contrasting diabetes phenotypes associated with hepatocyte nuclear factor-1alpha and -1beta mutations. Diabetes Care. 2004;27(5):1102–7.
62. Edghill EL, Bingham C, Slingerland AS, Minton JA, Noordam C, Ellard S, et al. Hepatocyte nuclear factor-1 beta mutations cause neonatal diabetes and intrauterine growth retardation: support for a critical role of HNF-1beta in human pancreatic development. Diabet Med. 2006;23(12):1301–6.
63. Lemelman MB, Letourneau L, Greeley SAW. Neonatal diabetes mellitus: an update on diagnosis and management. Clin Perinatol. 2018;45(1):41–59.
64. Pipatpolkai T, Usher S, Stansfeld PJ, Ashcroft FM. New insights into K(ATP) channel gene mutations and neonatal diabetes mellitus. Nat Rev Endocrinol. 2020;16(7):378–93.
65. Rafiq M, Flanagan SE, Patch AM, Shields BM, Ellard S, Hattersley AT. Effective treatment with oral sulfonylureas in patients with diabetes due to sulfonylurea receptor 1 (SUR1) mutations. Diabetes Care. 2008;31(2):204–9.
66. Gloyn AL, Pearson ER, Antcliff JF, Proks P, Bruining GJ, Slingerland AS, et al. Activating mutations in the gene encoding the ATP-sensitive potassium-channel subunit Kir6.2 and permanent neonatal diabetes. N Engl J Med. 2004;350(18):1838–49.
67. Rubio-Cabezas O, Ellard S. Diabetes mellitus in neonates and infants: genetic heterogeneity, clinical approach to diagnosis, and therapeutic options. Horm Res Paediatr. 2013;80(3):137–46.
68. Carmody D, Pastore AN, Landmeier KA, Letourneau LR, Martin R, Hwang JL, et al. Patients with KCNJ11-related diabetes frequently have neuropsychological impairments compared with sibling controls. Diabet Med. 2016;33(10):1380–6.
69. Landmeier KA, Lanning M, Carmody D, Greeley SAW, Msall ME. ADHD, learning difficulties and sleep disturbances associated with KCNJ11-related neonatal diabetes. Pediatr Diabetes. 2017;18(7):518–23.
70. Carmody D, Bell CD, Hwang JL, Dickens JT, Sima DI, Felipe DL, et al. Sulfonylurea treatment before genetic testing in neonatal diabetes: pros and cons. J Clin Endocrinol Metab. 2014;99(12):E2709–R2714.
71. Edghill EL, Flanagan SE, Patch AM, Boustred C, Parrish A, Shields B, et al. Insulin mutation screening in 1,044 patients with diabetes: mutations in the INS gene are a common cause of neonatal diabetes but a rare cause of diabetes diagnosed in childhood or adulthood. Diabetes. 2008;57(4):1034–42.
72. Park SY, Ye H, Steiner DF, Bell GI. Mutant proinsulin proteins associated with neonatal diabetes are retained in the endoplasmic reticulum and not efficiently secreted. Biochem Biophys Res Commun. 2010;391(3):1449–54.

Chapter 7
Diabetic Kidney Disease: Identification, Prevention, and Treatment

M. Luiza Caramori and Peter Rossing

Abbreviations

ACR	Albumin-to-creatinine ratio
CKD	Chronic kidney disease
CVD	Cardiovascular disease
DKD	Diabetic kidney disease
ESKD	End-stage kidney disease
eGFR	Estimated glomerular filtration rate
GBM	Glomerular basement membrane
GFR	Glomerular filtration rate
KDIGO	Kidney Disease: Improving Global Outcomes
RAS	Renin-angiotensin system
T1D	Type 1 diabetes
T2D	Type 2 diabetes

M. L. Caramori (✉)
Division of Diabetes, Endocrinology and Metabolism, Department of Medicine, Division of Pediatric Nephrology, Department of Pediatrics, University of Minnesota, Minneapolis, MN, USA
e-mail: caram001@umn.edu

P. Rossing
Steno Diabetes Center Copenhagen, Herlev, Denmark

Department of Clinical Medicine, University of Copenhagen, Copenhagen, Denmark

R. Basu (ed.), *Precision Medicine in Diabetes*,
https://doi.org/10.1007/978-3-030-98927-9_7

Introduction and Epidemiology

Diabetes and its complications are a very extensive public health problem, and about 10% of the world's population has diabetes [1]. Diabetes is associated with increased mortality and morbidity, and it is the most common cause of end-stage kidney disease (ESKD) in the USA and other developed countries [1], being responsible for more than 47% of the new ESKD cases in the USA. This is in large part due to type 2 diabetes (T2D) as most patients with diabetes have T2D rather than type 1 diabetes (T1D). However, the proportion of individuals starting kidney replacement therapy due to diabetes varies significantly, ranging from 13% in China to 66% in Singapore [1]. The likelihood of a patient with diabetes developing chronic kidney disease (CKD) is about 50% for patients with T1D and 30% for those with T2D. Although data from NHANES have shown an overall stable prevalence of CKD among patients with T2D (about 28.4% in 1988–1994 and 26.2% in 2009–2014), there was an increase in the proportion of patients with T2D with reduced GFR and a decline in the prevalence of albuminuria over time [2]. Importantly, patients with T2D and CKD are at a higher risk for cardiovascular morbidity and mortality than those without CKD [3, 4]. The 10-year standardized cardiovascular mortality increased from 3.4% in patients without diabetes or CKD to 6.7% among those with diabetes and no CKD and to 19.6% (a 3x increase compared to diabetes only) among those with both diabetes and CKD [4]. These patients often require multiple therapies aimed at prevention of progressive CKD and its associated comorbidities and mortality, which adds to their burden. Underserved/under-represented populations are disproportionately affected by both T2D and CKD. ESKD is devastating to the individual and their families and of enormous financial and social consequences. Rare in the past, in the more recent decades, we have observed a vast increase in the frequency of T2D in children and adolescents. These individuals have a high prevalence of hypertension and albuminuria [5], and ESKD and death are particularly common among underrepresented/underserved youth [6–8].

Pathophysiology

Diabetic nephropathy is a chronic condition that develops over many years, and it is characterized by a gradual increase in urinary albumin excretion, blood pressure levels and cardiovascular risk, declining glomerular filtration rate (GFR), and eventual ESKD. Over the past two decades, studies indicate the presence of another phenotype, one that does not follow the classical natural history of disease. Thus, reduced GFR in the presence of normal urinary albumin levels has been reported in 25 to 50% of patients with T1D [9, 10] and 45–57% of those with T2D [11–13]. The clinical syndrome is associated with characteristic histopathological features [14–16] and also with other conditions such as hypertensive renal disease, and obesity-related glomerulopathy. Kidney biopsy studies in patients with T2D indicate that IgA nephropathy, acute tubular necrosis, and others may also be present in these patients [17–19]. Their frequency is related to the frequency of these conditions in the background population as well as to reasons for a kidney biopsy indication, which often include atypical course [17–19]. Other causes of reduced GFR or albuminuria should be considered if proteinuria in patients with T1D for <5 years, in the presence of active urinary sediment, and if other systemic diseases that can cause renal dysfunction are present.

Screening, Diagnosis and Stages, and Monitoring

CKD in diabetes is diagnosed by the presence of abnormal kidney function, namely, estimated glomerular filtration rate (eGFR) and albuminuria [20]. The pathogenic mechanisms associated with these findings may be distinct.

Screening

Multiple guidelines recommend annual CKD screening of patients with diabetes, starting about 5 years after T1D diagnosis and at diagnosis in patients with T2D. Screening tests should include both albuminuria measurements and estimates of GFR.

Albuminuria

First-morning-void urinary albumin-to-creatinine ratio (ACR) measurement is the test of choice. It is less cumbersome than timed urine collections and has lower day-to-day variability compared to other methods [21]. If the results are abnormal, this needs confirmation by collecting another urine sample, ideally within 1–3 months. At least two out of three measurements should be abnormal before a diagnosis of albuminuria is made. Acute illnesses, acute hyperglycemia, exercise, and upright posture can transiently increase albuminuria.

GFR

GFR is usually estimated using equations that include patient's age, sex, race, and serum creatinine. Many laboratories currently calculate the eGFR using the serum creatinine CKD-EPI equation [22] (https://www.mdcalc.com/ckd-epi-equations-glomerular-filtration-rate-gfr), with race being now optional on this equation. Importantly, serum creatinine should be measured by an accredited and standardized assay (isotope dilution mass spectrometry reference method (IDMS)-traceable).

Diagnosis and Stages

CKD is diagnosed when two eGFRs (at least 3 months apart) are <60 mL/min/1.73 m^2 and/or two out of three ACR measurements are $\geq$30 mg/g [20]. CKD staging considers both eGFR and albuminuria values (Fig. 7.1). This heat map serves as an indicator of risk of progression to ESKD and is also a good indicator of cardiovascular morbidity and mortality [20].

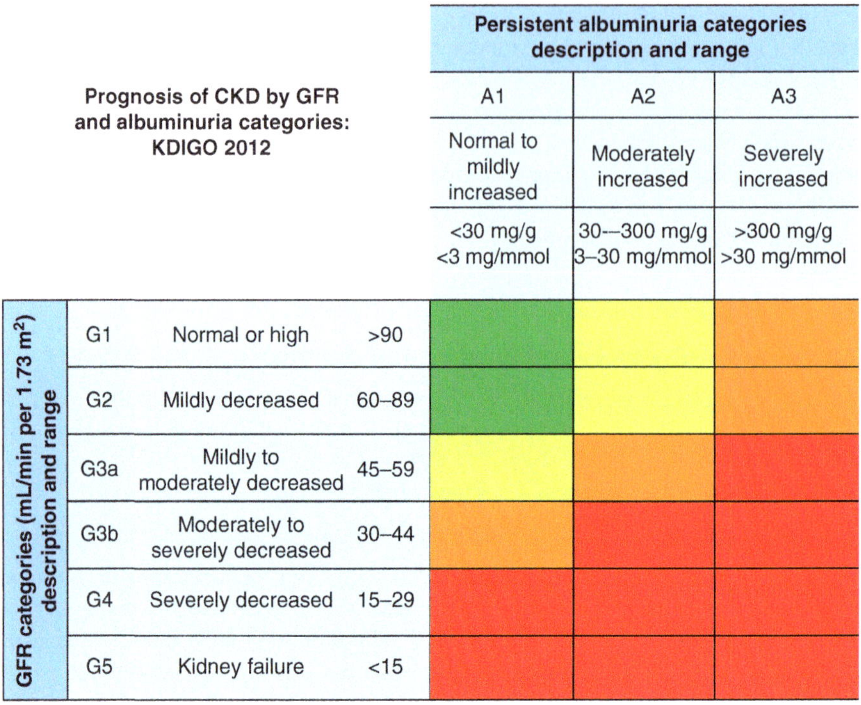

Prognosis of CKD by GFR and albuminuria categories: KDIGO 2012			Persistent albuminuria categories description and range		
			A1	A2	A3
			Normal to mildly increased	Moderately increased	Severely increased
			<30 mg/g <3 mg/mmol	30--300 mg/g 3–30 mg/mmol	>300 mg/g >30 mg/mmol
GFR categories (mL/min per 1.73 m²) description and range: G1	Normal or high	>90			
G2	Mildly decreased	60–89			
G3a	Mildly to moderately decreased	45–59			
G3b	Moderately to severely decreased	30–44			
G4	Severely decreased	15–29			
G5	Kidney failure	<15			

Fig. 7.1 Prognosis of chronic kidney disease by estimated glomerular filtration rate and albuminuria. (Source: Reprinted by permission from KDIGO – Kidney Disease: Improving Outcomes [158])

Monitoring Kidney Disease

Once urinary albumin excretion is abnormal, ACR should be measured every 3 months and eGFR every 3–6 months, depending on the CKD stage.

Structural Kidney Lesions in Diabetes

DKD manifests as a constellation of structural changes considered unique to this disease [15, 23–25]. In patients with T1D, glomerular lesions can be demonstrated after diabetes has been present for about 5 years, while in T2D, they can be present at diagnosis, probably reflecting delayed T2D diagnosis. The severity of these lesions is related to diabetes duration, glycemic control, and genetic factors and correlates with functional abnormalities (albuminuria and decreased GFR). Renal hypertrophy is the earliest renal structural change in T1D. Thickening of the glomerular basement membrane (GBM), mesangial expansion, and arteriolar hyalinosis follow. Kimmelstiel-Wilson nodules or nodular mesangial expansion is observed in 40–50% of patients with proteinuria. Tubular atrophy and interstitial fibrosis, common to most chronic renal disorders, can be present at later stages. Foot processes (podocyte) changes can be observed by electron microscopy, and the severity of these abnormalities has been associated with kidney function [26].

Relationships Between Kidney Structure and Function

There are strong relationships between kidney structure and function in T1D [15, 27, 28]. Mesangial fractional volume is inversely correlated with GFR and directly correlated with albuminuria [15, 28] and blood pressure [28, 29]. GBM width is a strong independent predictor of progression to clinically advanced kidney disease among normoalbuminuric patients with T1D [30]. Global glomerular sclerosis [30, 31] and interstitial expansion [25, 30] are additional independent predictors of GFR loss in these patients. Although increases in podocyte foot process width also correlate with albuminuria increases in T1D [32–34], our longitudinal studies indicate that podocyte parameters did not predict progression in patients with T1D who had no clinical manifestations of CKD at time of their research kidney biopsies [35].

Risk Factors

Multiple factors are associated with CKD in diabetes, and diabetes duration is one of the strongest risk factors for diabetic nephropathy, particularly in T1D. Factors that influence the development of kidney disease may not be the same as those influencing its progression.

Blood Glucose

Data from multiple observational and intervention studies in both T1D and T2D support indicate that hyperglycemia is an important risk factor for the development and progression of diabetic nephropathy [36]. Greater variability in HbA_{1c} is independently associated with albuminuria and diabetic nephropathy [37–39], and variability in blood glucose by continuous glucose monitoring (CGM) has also been associated with complications.

Blood Pressure

Elevated blood pressure levels are among the most important risk factors for the development and progression of diabetic kidney disease. Variability in systolic and diastolic blood pressure independently predicts the development of albuminuria in T1D [37, 38]. Changes in blood pressure may be subtle, sometimes manifesting only as reduced nocturnal diastolic blood pressure dipping [40]. Hypertension is present in about 40% of newly diagnosed patients with T2D [41].

Additional risk factors include lipids [42–45],smoking [46], insulin resistance [47, 48], uric acid levels [49], metabolic syndrome [50], ethnicity [51–55], and genetic and epigenetic factors [56–62]. Many of the risk factors for kidney disease in diabetes overlap with cardiovascular risk factors [63].

Albuminuria and GFR

Albuminuria and eGFR levels are associated with CKD development and progression [46, 64]. Baseline albuminuria strongly predicts ESKD [65]. Higher levels of normoalbuminuria [66] and lower eGFR [67] predict a faster decline in eGFR. Conversely, a short-term reduction in albuminuria with intervention suggests reduced progression of kidney and cardiovascular complications [68, 69].

Comorbidities and Associated Complications

Patients with diabetic nephropathy often have other microvascular complications. Significant retinopathy is almost always present in individuals with T1D and albuminuria [70]. This relationship is less strong among patients with T2D [71]. Peripheral neuropathy is also more common in diabetic nephropathy and associated with both albuminuria and declining GFR [72]. Autonomic neuropathy, diagnosed by loss of nocturnal blood pressure dipping, is frequently present [73, 74], and it predicts decline in kidney function [75].

Albuminuria and reduced GFR contribute independently and synergistically to the increased cardiovascular risk and are associated with increased morbidity and mortality [4, 76–79]. While individuals with T1D and normoalbuminuria do not have a higher risk of premature death [80, 81], those with moderately elevated albuminuria have a two- to threefold higher risk, those with severely increased albuminuria have a ninefold higher risk, and those with ESKD have an 18-fold increased risk of premature death versus the non-diabetic population [80]. CVD is 1.2-fold more common in patients with diabetes and moderately increased albuminuria [82] and tenfold higher in those with severely increased albuminuria compared with those with normoalbuminuria [83].

Similarly, in T2D, CVD risk is increased two- to fourfold with moderately increased albuminuria [84, 85] and ninefold in severely increased albuminuria [86]. Once serum creatinine is outside the normal range, cardiovascular risk increases exponentially [87].

Prevention and Treatment

The Kidney Disease Improving Global Outcomes (KDIGO) guideline on management of diabetes in CKD emphasizes a holistic approach for the management of cardiorenal risk factors, including lifestyle modification (diet, exercise, and cessation of smoking); glucose, blood pressure, and lipid control; use of agents blocking the renin-angiotensin-aldosterone system; and use of SGLT2 inhibitors in patients with T2D (Fig. 7.2) [88]. This is supported by data from the Steno 2 trial, where patients with T2D randomized to intensive lifestyle intervention (weight loss,

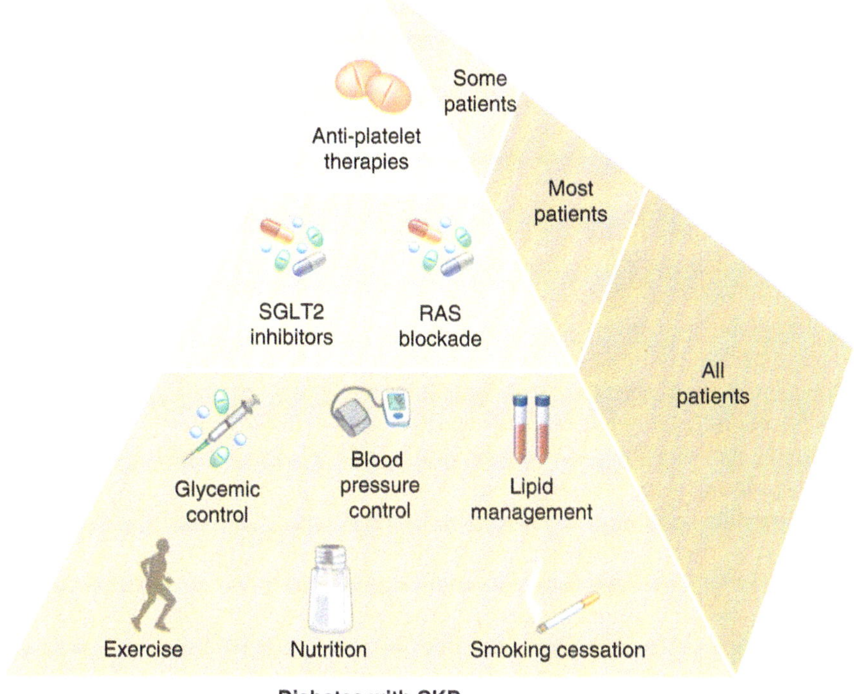

Fig. 7.2 Management of risk factors for kidney and heart disease. (Source: Reprinted by permission from KDIGO – Kidney Disease: Improving Outcomes [20])

glucose and blood pressure control with RAS blockers, aspirin, and lipid-lowering agents) had lower CKD rates [89].

The risk of developing diabetic nephropathy is significantly reduced by achievement and maintenance of good blood glucose and blood pressure control. Moreover, multiple strategies are now available to reduce the rate of CKD progression slow in diabetes.

Lifestyle and dietary modifications: Dietary modifications target sodium, protein, lipid content, and caloric content. Dietary sodium restriction reduces albuminuria [90] and potentiates ARB treatment effects [91] when added to RAS blockade. Reduction of sodium intake to <2 g of sodium per day is recommended for patients with diabetic nephropathy [88]. Low-protein diet (0.8 g protein/kg body weight/day) improves GFR but not albuminuria in patients with diabetes on all stages of nephropathy [92] and reduced mortality and progression to ESKD among proteinuric patients with T1D [93]. However, a higher protein intake (1.0–1.2 g protein/kg body weight/day) is recommended for patients in peritoneal dialysis [88]. The eGFR and albuminuria impact of low-carbohydrate, Mediterranean, and low-fat diets seem to be similar [94]. Bariatric surgery was also associated with reduced albuminuria among adults with T2D [95] and adolescents with or without T2D [96]. While there have been no good trials of smoking cessation, smoking increases the likelihood of CKD, and smoking cessation should be encouraged.

Glycemic Control

The Diabetes Control and Complications Trial (DCCT) indicate that patients randomized to intensive control had a 39% relative risk reduction for development of moderately elevated albuminuria (or microalbuminuria) and a 54% risk reduction for development of macroalbuminuria or proteinuria [97]. Mean achieved HbA_{1c} was 7.0% and 9.1%, respectively. Importantly, there was no HbA_{1c} threshold below which risk was not reduced [98]. Additionally, the Epidemiology of Diabetes and Its Complications (EDIC) follow-up of the DCCT cohort described a significant reduction in the risk of having eGFR <60 mL/min/1.73 m^2 [98] and ESKD [99] among individuals who were previously randomized to the intensive arm. Glycemic variability and time in range (time in glycemic target) in patients with T1D may also be important for the development of renal complications [100, 101].

The UKPDS also demonstrated a significant benefit of improved glycemic control on the risk of developing elevated urinary albumin levels [102]. Like the T1D data [98], no threshold of HbA_{1c} and risk was observed [103]. In the ADVANCE study, patients randomized to intensive therapy (HbA1c 6.5% versus 7.3%) had a 9% relative risk reduction of moderately elevated albuminuria, a 30% reduction in the development of severely increased albuminuria, and a 65% reduction in ESKD over 5 years [104, 105]. These findings were corroborated by the ACCORD study [106]; progression of albuminuria was reduced and regression increased. However, patients with CKD randomized to the intensive glucose management arm had a significantly greater risk of cardiovascular and all-cause mortality [107], supporting the recommendation of individualized HbA1c targets.

Organ Protection

SGLT2 Inhibitor

In the recent years, the concept of organ protection in diabetes has evolved, and currently specific classes of glucose-lowering agents are recommended for kidney and/or cardiovascular protection. Although there are differences in the beneficial effects and safety profile among the various FDA-approved sodium-glucose cotransporter-2 (SGLT2) inhibitors, these agents (empagliflozin, canagliflozin, and dapagliflozin) have shown to reduce major adverse cardiovascular events, rates of hospitalization for heart failure, and renal protection [108, 109]. CREDENCE, the first SGLT2 inhibitor study dedicated to T2D patients with CKD, showed a major benefit on renal outcomes, heart failure, and major adverse cardiovascular events [110]. The primary outcome was a composite of ESKD, doubling of the serum creatinine, or death from renal or cardiovascular causes. The study was stopped early as canagliflozin showed a benefit effect with 30% reduction in the rates of the primary outcome. These data were confirmed and extended by the DAPA-CKD study including individuals with CKD with or without diabetes [111]. Small studies in T1D show an increased risk of diabetic ketoacidosis, particularly among ambulatory insulin pimp users. There are no studies in diabetic nephropathy in T1D. In patients with T2D with CKD, SGLT2 inhibitors are recommended, independent of HbA1c, for organ protection [88, 112, 113] (Fig. 7.3).

GLP1-RA

Cardiovascular benefits in individuals with T2D and pre-existing atherosclerotic CVD have also been demonstrated for some (liraglutide, semaglutide, and dulaglutide) but not all glucagon-like peptide 1 receptor agonists (GLP1-RA) [112, 113]. Benefit on CVD outcomes was also demonstrated in CKD populations, and thus GLP1-RA are recommended for patients with T2D and CKD when metformin and SGLT2 inhibition cannot control glucose levels [88, 114](Fig. 7.3).

RAS Inhibition

Intensive control of blood pressure drastically improves the prognosis in diabetic nephropathy. RAS inhibitors do not prevent albuminuria in normotensive individuals with T1D [115–117]. There is also no evidence that control of hypertension in T1D with normoalbuminuria prevents kidney disease progression; however, this seems highly likely. Once albuminuria is present, RAS inhibition is clearly indicated and associated with decreased likelihood of progression and increased likelihood of regression to normoalbuminuria levels [118]. RAS inhibitors should be offered to all individuals with T1D and albuminuria, regardless of blood pressure.

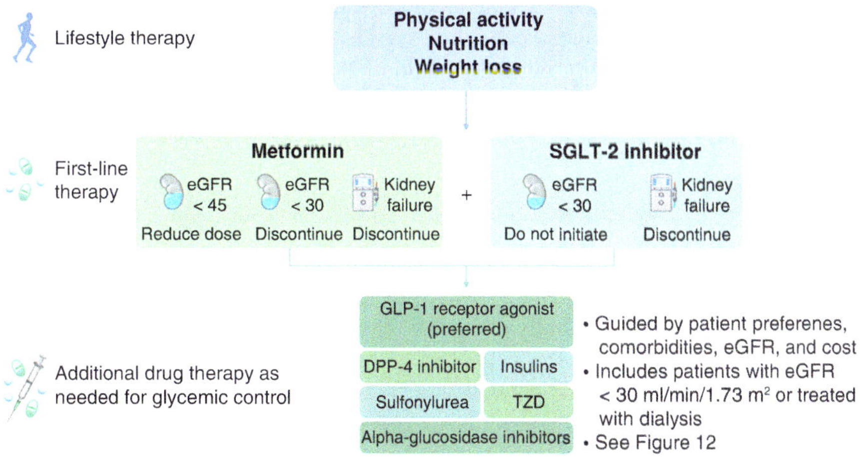

Fig. 7.3 Treatment algorithm for selecting antihyperglycemic drugs for patients with type 2 diabetes and chronic kidney disease, in addition to lifestyle therapy. (Source: Reprinted by permission from KDIGO – Kidney Disease: Improving Outcomes [20])

An often-overlooked concept is the importance of titrating these agents up to the maximum recommended or tolerated dose, to obtain maximal antiproteinuric effect. Studies indicate that the rate of GFR decline can be reduced from 10–12 mL/min/year to <5 mL/min/year if blood pressure levels are controlled [119]. Often multiple blood pressure-lowering agents are needed in patients with CKD stage 3 and beyond.

Data in patients with T2D also indicates that control of hypertension reduces the risk of increased albuminuria [120–123]. Inhibition of the renin-angiotensin system may be of particular benefit [124–126], but lowering blood pressure is the key. Most guidelines suggest a blood pressure target of 130/80 mmHg in patients with T2D. Systolic blood pressure levels below 120–130 mmHg were associated with increased mortality and ESKD in patients with T2D [127]. In T2D, RAS inhibition is clearly indicated in the presence of albuminuria [119, 121]. In more advanced CKD, RAS inhibition with angiotensin receptor blockers (ARB) reduces kidney disease progression, ESKD, or death [128, 129]. With worsening of CKD, hyperkalemia is a common problem [130], and general measures to lower potassium levels, such as dietary changes, diuretics, and use of potassium binders, should be considered [88]. Introduction of a RAS inhibitor often leads to an acute decline in GFR, which then stabilizes. Individuals with the greatest initial fall in GFR have the slowest subsequent decline in kidney function [131]. Dual blockade of the RAS is not recommended [132–137].

Mineralocorticoid Receptor Antagonists (MRA)
Short-term studies indicate that spironolactone or eplerenone reduces albuminuria by about 30% in patients with CKD [138]. However, a longer-term study (3-year intervention) including high-risk patients with T2D did not show a benefit of spironolactone on the progression of kidney disease [139]. A novel nonsteroidal MRA, finerenone conferred an 18%reduction in progression to kidney failure, decrease of eGFR ≥40%, or kidney death among patients with T2D and CKD [140]. In a separated RCT, finerenone reduced the risk of cardiovascular death or nonfatal cardiovascular events (myocardial infarction, stroke, or heart failure hospitalization) by 13% [141]. MRA are associated with an increased risk of hyperkalemia, and potassium levels should be carefully monitored and managed in these patients.

Other Agents
Atrasentan, an endothelin receptor A antagonist, showed kidney but no major adverse cardiovascular events benefit, with a tendency to increased heart failure [142].

Additional Agents Modifying Cardiovascular Risk and Their Potential Impact in the Kidneys
Lipid-lowering therapy is recommended to reduce the risk for CVD in patients with CKD. There is also some evidence that lipid-lowering agents may be potentially beneficial to the kidney [143].

Aspirin is indicated in patients with established CVD and should be considered for prevention in high-risk patients. Patients with diabetes and CKD not only have a higher risk of atrial fibrillation but also higher morbidity and mortality associated with atrial fibrillation complications [144], and anticoagulation is often recommended. Direct oral anticoagulants are usually preferred due to their reduced risk for bleeding, equivalent or superior thrombosis prevention, and possible reduction in progression of CKD [145].

Monitoring

In progressive CKD from stage 3 onward, bone chemistry, full blood count, and iron stores should be assessed 3–6 monthly.

- Glucose control: Red blood cell and protein turnover are abnormal in CKD, making the interpretation of HbA_{1c}, glycated albumin, and fructosamine results difficult, especially when eGFR is <30 mL/min/1.73m^2. Self-monitoring of blood glucose and use of continuous glucose monitoring (CGM) systems are indicated, particularly if treatment can cause hypoglycemia [88].
- Medication dosage: Metformin should be used with caution in patients with eGFR <45 mL/min/1.73 m^2 and discontinued when eGFR reaches 30 mL/min/1.73 m^2 [146]. The dose of some but not all DPP-4 inhibitors and GLP-1 RA may need to be reduced as kidney function declines. SGLT2 inhibitors become less effective as GFR falls but should not be discontinued as they continue to confer cardiovascular protection. Sulfonylurea (glibenclamide, gliclazide, and tolbutamide) dose needs to be reduced in CKD. Meglitinides have minimal renal excretion and can be used in CKD. Thiazolidinediones (rosiglitazone and pioglitazone) are predominantly metabolized in the liver, but fluid retention may limit their use in patients with advanced CKD and ESKD. It is important to consider that insulin is also excreted by the kidney, and dose reduction may be indicated once eGFR reaches 50 mL/min/1.73m^2.

Pregnancy in Women with Diabetes and Chronic Kidney Disease

Pregnancy outcomes are poorer in patients with DKD [147]. Both T1D and T2D patients with CKD have an even greater risk of hypertension, preeclampsia, abnormal fetal growth, and preterm delivery than patients with diabetes and no CKD [148, 149]. These patients are also at increased risk of retinopathy progression. Pre-pregnancy counseling and pregnancy planning can potentially improve outcomes. Glucose and blood pressure control should be optimized, glucose-lowering therapies need to be revised and may require modification, and RAS inhibitors should be discontinued and substituted by therapies which are safe in pregnancy. Statins are also contraindicated in pregnancy.

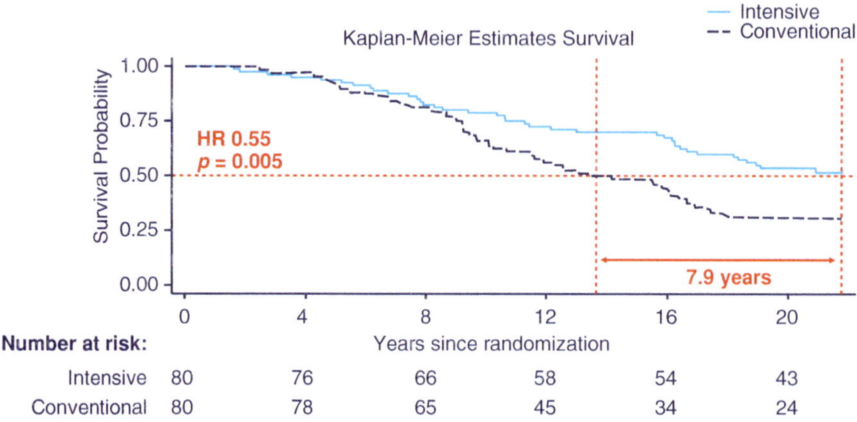

Fig. 7.4 Long-term effects of 8 years of intensive multifactorial intervention targeting lifestyle and heart and kidney risk factors compared to standard of care

Organization of Care

Structured care of patients with T2D and CKD delivered by specialists working in close collaboration and using clear protocols with specific treatment goals and targets reduces the rates of albuminuria [150, 151] and severe retinopathy and provides greater kidney and cardiovascular benefits than routine care [88, 152–157]. The 8-year structured intensive multifactorial intervention described above (Steno-2 study) extended patients' median survival for almost 8 years [154] (Fig. 7.4).

References

1. United States Renal Data System. 2020 USRDS Annual Data Report: Epidemiology of Kidney Disease in the United States. In: National Institutes of Health NIoDaDaKD, editor. Bethesda, MD; 2020.
2. Afkarian M, Zelnick LR, Hall YN, Heagerty PJ, Tuttle K, Weiss NS, et al. Clinical manifestations of kidney Disease among US adults with diabetes, 1988–2014. JAMA. 2016;316(6):602–10.
4. Afkarian M, Sachs MC, Kestenbaum B, Hirsch IB, Tuttle KR, Himmelfarb J, et al. Kidney disease and increased mortality risk in type 2 diabetes. Journal of the American Society of Nephrology : JASN. 2013;24(2):302–8.
3. Fox CS, Matsushita K, Woodward M, Bilo HJ, Chalmers J, Heerspink HJ, et al. Associations of kidney disease measures with mortality and end-stage renal disease in individuals with and without diabetes: a meta-analysis. Lancet. 2012;380(9854):1662–73.
5. Group TS. Rapid rise in hypertension and nephropathy in youth with type 2 diabetes: the TODAY clinical trial. Diabetes Care. 2013;36(6):1735–41.
6. Dyck RF, Jiang Y, Osgood ND. The long-term risks of end stage renal disease and mortality among first nations and non-first nations people with youth-onset diabetes. Can J Diabetes. 2014;38(4):237–43.

7. Dart AB, Sellers EA, Martens PJ, Rigatto C, Brownell MD, Dean HJ. High burden of kidney disease in youth-onset type 2 diabetes. Diabetes Care. 2012;35(6):1265–71.
8. Chan JC, Lau ES, Luk AO, Cheung KK, Kong AP, Yu LW, et al. Premature mortality and comorbidities in young-onset diabetes: a 7-year prospective analysis. Am J Med. 2014;127(7):616–24.
9. Molitch ME, Steffes M, Sun W, Rutledge B, Cleary P, de Boer IH, et al. Development and progression of renal insufficiency with and without albuminuria in adults with type 1 diabetes in the diabetes control and complications trial and the epidemiology of diabetes interventions and complications study. Diabetes Care. 2010;33(7):1536–43.
10. Krolewski AS, Niewczas MA, Skupien J, Gohda T, Smiles A, Eckfeldt JH, et al. Early progressive renal decline precedes the onset of microalbuminuria and its progression to macroalbuminuria. Diabetes Care. 2014;37(1):226–34.
11. Vistisen D, Andersen GS, Hulman A, Persson F, Rossing P, Jorgensen ME. Progressive decline in estimated glomerular filtration rate in patients with diabetes after moderate loss in kidney function-even without albuminuria. Diabetes Care. 2019;42(10):1886–94.
12. Retnakaran R, Cull CA, Thorne KI, Adler AI, Holman RR, Group US. Risk factors for renal dysfunction in type 2 diabetes: U.K. prospective diabetes study 74. Diabetes. 2006;55(6):1832–9.
13. Thomas MC, Macisaac RJ, Jerums G, Weekes A, Moran J, Shaw JE, et al. Nonalbuminuric renal impairment in type 2 diabetic patients and in the general population (national evaluation of the frequency of renal impairment cO-existing with NIDDM [NEFRON] 11). Diabetes Care. 2009;32(8):1497–502.
14. Caramori ML, Fioretto P, Mauer M. Low glomerular filtration rate in normoalbuminuric type 1 diabetic patients: an indicator of more advanced glomerular lesions. Diabetes. 2003;52(4):1036–40.
15. Caramori ML, Kim Y, Huang C, Fish AJ, Rich SS, Miller ME, et al. Cellular basis of diabetic nephropathy: 1. Study design and renal structural-functional relationships in patients with long-standing type 1 diabetes. Diabetes. 2002;51(2):506–13.
16. Mauer M, Caramori ML, Fioretto P, Najafian B. Glomerular structural-functional relationship models of diabetic nephropathy are robust in type 1 diabetic patients. Nephrol Dial Transplant. 2015;30(6):918–23.
17. Mazzucco G, Bertani T, Fortunato M, Bernardi M, Leutner M, Boldorini R, et al. Different patterns of renal damage in type 2 diabetes mellitus: a multicentric study on 393 biopsies. American Journal of Kidney Diseases: The Official Journal of the National Kidney Foundation. 2002;39(4):713–20.
18. Chong YB, Keng TC, Tan LP, Ng KP, Kong WY, Wong CM, et al. Clinical predictors of non-diabetic renal disease and role of renal biopsy in diabetic patients with renal involvement: a single Centre review. Ren Fail. 2012;34(3):323–8.
19. Sharma SG, Bomback AS, Radhakrishnan J, Herlitz LC, Stokes MB, Markowitz GS, et al. The modern spectrum of renal biopsy findings in patients with diabetes. Clinical Journal of the American Society of Nephrology: CJASN. 2013;8(10):1718–24.
20. Kidney Disease: Improving Global Outcomes Diabetes Work G. KDIGO 2020 Clinical Practice Guideline for Diabetes Management in Chronic Kidney Disease. Kidney Inter. 2020;98(4S):S1–115.
21. Gansevoort RT, Brinkman J, Bakker SJ, De Jong PE, de Zeeuw D. Evaluation of measures of urinary albumin excretion. Am J Epidemiol. 2006;164(8):725–7.
22. Levey AS, Stevens LA, Schmid CH, Zhang YL, Castro AF 3rd, Feldman HI, et al. A new equation to estimate glomerular filtration rate. Ann Intern Med. 2009;150(9):604–12.
23. Mauer SM. Structural-functional correlations of diabetic nephropathy. Kidney Int. 1994;45(2):612–22.
24. Mauer SM, Steffes MW, Brown DM. The kidney in diabetes. Am J Med. 1981;70(3):603–12.
25. Lane PH, Steffes MW, Fioretto P, Mauer SM. Renal interstitial expansion in insulin-dependent diabetes mellitus. Kidney Int. 1993;43(3):661–7.

26. Toyoda M, Najafian B, Kim Y, Caramori ML, Mauer M. Podocyte detachment and reduced glomerular capillary endothelial fenestration in human type 1 diabetic nephropathy. Diabetes. 2007;56(8):2155–60.
27. Ellis EN, Steffes MW, Goetz FC, Sutherland DE, Mauer SM. Glomerular filtration surface in type I diabetes mellitus. Kidney Int. 1986;29(4):889–94.
28. Mauer SM, Steffes MW, Ellis EN, Sutherland DE, Brown DM, Goetz FC. Structural-functional relationships in diabetic nephropathy. J Clin Invest. 1984;74(4):1143–55.
29. Mauer SM, Sutherland DE, Steffes MW. Relationship of systemic blood pressure to nephropathology in insulin-dependent diabetes mellitus. Kidney Int. 1992;41(4):736–40.
30. Caramori ML, Parks A, Mauer M. Renal lesions predict progression of diabetic nephropathy in type 1 diabetes. Journal of the American Society of Nephrology: JASN. 2013;24(7):1175–81.
31. Harris RD, Steffes MW, Bilous RW, Sutherland DE, Mauer SM. Global glomerular sclerosis and glomerular arteriolar hyalinosis in insulin dependent diabetes. Kidney Int. 1991;40(1):107–14.
32. Ellis EN, Steffes MW, Chavers B, Mauer SM. Observations of glomerular epithelial cell structure in patients with type I diabetes mellitus. Kidney Int. 1987;32(5):736–41.
33. Bjorn SF, Bangstad HJ, Hanssen KF, Nyberg G, Walker JD, Viberti GC, et al. Glomerular epithelial foot processes and filtration slits in IDDM patients. Diabetologia. 1995;38(10):1197–204.
34. Pagtalunan ME, Miller PL, Jumping-Eagle S, Nelson RG, Myers BD, Rennke HG, et al. Podocyte loss and progressive glomerular injury in type II diabetes. J Clin Invest. 1997;99(2):342–8.
35. Harindhanavudhi T, Parks A, Mauer M, Caramori ML. Podocyte structural parameters do not predict progression to diabetic nephropathy in normoalbuminuric type 1 diabetic patients. Am J Nephrol. 2015;41(4–5):277–83.
36. Nordwall M, Abrahamsson M, Dhir M, Fredrikson M, Ludvigsson J, Arnqvist HJ. Impact of HbA1c, followed from onset of type 1 diabetes, on the development of severe retinopathy and nephropathy: the VISS study (vascular diabetic complications in Southeast Sweden). Diabetes Care. 2015;38(2):308–15.
37. Kilpatrick ES, Rigby AS, Atkin SL. A1C variability and the risk of microvascular complications in type 1 diabetes: data from the diabetes control and complications trial. Diabetes Care. 2008;31(11):2198–202.
38. Rotbain Curovic V, Theilade S, Winther SA, Tofte N, Tarnow L, Jorsal A, et al. Visit-to-visit variability of clinical risk markers in relation to long-term complications in type 1 diabetes. Diabet Med. 2021;38(5):e14459.
39. Hsu CC, Chang HY, Huang MC, Hwang SJ, Yang YC, Lee YS, et al. HbA1c variability is associated with microalbuminuria development in type 2 diabetes: a 7-year prospective cohort study. Diabetologia. 2012;55(12):3163–72.
40. Dost A, Klinkert C, Kapellen T, Lemmer A, Naeke A, Grabert M, et al. Arterial hypertension determined by ambulatory blood pressure profiles: contribution to microalbuminuria risk in a multicenter investigation in 2,105 children and adolescents with type 1 diabetes. Diabetes Care. 2008;31(4):720–5.
41. Hypertension in Diabetes Study (HDS): I. Prevalence of hypertension in newly presenting type 2 diabetic patients and the association with risk factors for cardiovascular and diabetic complications. J Hypertens. 1993;11(3):309–17.
42. Daousi C, Bain SC, Barnett AH, Gill GV. Hypertriglyceridaemia is associated with an increased likelihood of albuminuria in extreme duration (>50 years) type 1 diabetes. Diabet Med. 2008;25(10):1234–6.
43. Thomas MC, Rosengard-Barlund M, Mills V, Ronnback M, Thomas S, Forsblom C, et al. Serum lipids and the progression of nephropathy in type 1 diabetes. Diabetes Care. 2006;29(2):317–22.
44. Tolonen N, Forsblom C, Thorn L, Waden J, Rosengard-Barlund M, Saraheimo M, et al. Relationship between lipid profiles and kidney function in patients with type 1 diabetes. Diabetologia. 2008;51(1):12–20.

45. Tofte N, Suvitaival T, Ahonen L, Winther SA, Theilade S, Frimodt-Moller M, et al. Lipidomic analysis reveals sphingomyelin and phosphatidylcholine species associated with renal impairment and all-cause mortality in type 1 diabetes. Sci Rep. 2019;9(1):16398.
46. Rossing P, Hougaard P, Parving HH. Risk factors for development of incipient and overt diabetic nephropathy in type 1 diabetic patients: a 10-year prospective observational study. Diabetes Care. 2002;25(5):859–64.
47. Bjornstad P, Snell-Bergeon JK, Rewers M, Jalal D, Chonchol MB, Johnson RJ, et al. Early diabetic nephropathy: a complication of reduced insulin sensitivity in type 1 diabetes. Diabetes Care. 2013;36(11):3678–83.
48. Hsu CC, Chang HY, Huang MC, Hwang SJ, Yang YC, Tai TY, et al. Association between insulin resistance and development of microalbuminuria in type 2 diabetes: a prospective cohort study. Diabetes Care. 2011;34(4):982–7.
49. Hovind P, Rossing P, Tarnow L, Johnson RJ, Parving HH. Serum uric acid as a predictor for development of diabetic nephropathy in type 1 diabetes: an inception cohort study. Diabetes. 2009;58(7):1668–71.
50. Thorn LM, Forsblom C, Waden J, Saraheimo M, Tolonen N, Hietala K, et al. Metabolic syndrome as a risk factor for cardiovascular disease, mortality, and progression of diabetic nephropathy in type 1 diabetes. Diabetes Care. 2009;32(5):950–2.
51. Allawi J, Rao PV, Gilbert R, Scott G, Jarrett RJ, Keen H, et al. Microalbuminuria in non-insulin-dependent diabetes: its prevalence in Indian compared with Europid patients. Br Med J (Clin Res Ed). 1988;296(6620):462–4.
52. Sinha SK, Shaheen M, Rajavashisth TB, Pan D, Norris KC, Nicholas SB. Association of race/ethnicity, inflammation, and albuminuria in patients with diabetes and early chronic kidney disease. Diabetes Care. 2014;37(4):1060–8.
53. Nelson RG, Knowler WC, Pettitt DJ, Hanson RL, Bennett PH. Incidence and determinants of elevated urinary albumin excretion in Pima Indians with NIDDM. Diabetes Care. 1995;18(2):182–7.
54. Joshy G, Dunn P, Fisher M, Lawrenson R. Ethnic differences in the natural progression of nephropathy among diabetes patients in New Zealand: hospital admission rate for renal complications, and incidence of end-stage renal disease and renal death. Diabetologia. 2009;52(8):1474–8.
55. Collins VR, Dowse GK, Finch CF, Zimmet PZ, Linnane AW. Prevalence and risk factors for micro- and macroalbuminuria in diabetic subjects and entire population of Nauru. Diabetes. 1989;38(12):1602–10.
56. Sandholm N, Van Zuydam N, Ahlqvist E, Juliusdottir T, Deshmukh HA, Rayner NW, et al. The genetic landscape of renal complications in type 1 diabetes. Journal of the American Society of Nephrology: JASN. 2017;28(2):557–74.
57. van Zuydam NR, Ahlqvist E, Sandholm N, Deshmukh H, Rayner NW, Abdalla M, et al. A genome-wide association study of diabetic kidney Disease in subjects with type 2 diabetes. Diabetes. 2018;67(7):1414–27.
58. Seaquist ER, Goetz FC, Rich S, Barbosa J. Familial clustering of diabetic kidney disease. Evidence for genetic susceptibility to diabetic nephropathy [see comments]. N Engl J Med. 1989;320(18):1161–5.
59. Fagerudd JA, Pettersson-Fernholm KJ, Gronhagen-Riska C, Groop PH. The impact of a family history of type II (non-insulin-dependent) diabetes mellitus on the risk of diabetic nephropathy in patients with type I (insulin-dependent) diabetes mellitus. Diabetologia. 1999;42(5):519–26.
60. Thorn LM, Forsblom C, Fagerudd J, Pettersson-Fernholm K, Kilpikari R, Groop PH, et al. Clustering of risk factors in parents of patients with type 1 diabetes and nephropathy. Diabetes Care. 2007;30(5):1162–7.
61. Wuttke M, Li Y, Li M, Sieber KB, Feitosa MF, Gorski M, et al. A catalog of genetic loci associated with kidney function from analyses of a million individuals. Nat Genet. 2019;51(6):957–72.

62. Keating ST, van Diepen JA, Riksen NP, El-Osta A. Epigenetics in diabetic nephropathy, immunity and metabolism. Diabetologia. 2018;61(1):6–20.
63. Pilemann-Lyberg S, Hansen TW, Tofte N, Winther SA, Theilade S, Ahluwalia TS, et al. Uric acid is an independent risk factor for decline in kidney function, cardiovascular events, and mortality in patients with type 1 diabetes. Diabetes Care. 2019;42(6):1088–94.
64. Murussi M, Campagnolo N, Beck MO, Gross JL, Silveiro SP. High-normal levels of albuminuria predict the development of micro- and macroalbuminuria and increased mortality in Brazilian type 2 diabetic patients: an 8-year follow-up study. Diabet Med. 2007;24(10):1136–42.
65. de Zeeuw D, Ramjit D, Zhang Z, Ribeiro AB, Kurokawa K, Lash JP, et al. Renal risk and renoprotection among ethnic groups with type 2 diabetic nephropathy: a post hoc analysis of RENAAL. Kidney Int. 2006;69(9):1675–82.
66. Babazono T, Nyumura I, Toya K, Hayashi T, Ohta M, Suzuki K, et al. Higher levels of urinary albumin excretion within the normal range predict faster decline in glomerular filtration rate in diabetic patients. Diabetes Care. 2009;32(8):1518–20.
67. Zoppini G, Targher G, Chonchol M, Ortalda V, Negri C, Stoico V, et al. Predictors of estimated GFR decline in patients with type 2 diabetes and preserved kidney function. Clinical Journal of the American Society of Nephrology: CJASN. 2012;7(3):401–8.
68. Rossing P, Hommel E, Smidt UM, Parving HH. Reduction in albuminuria predicts a beneficial effect on diminishing the progression of human diabetic nephropathy during antihypertensive treatment. Diabetologia. 1994;37(5):511–6.
69. Heerspink HJL, Greene T, Tighiouart H, Gansevoort RT, Coresh J, Simon AL, et al. Change in albuminuria as a surrogate endpoint for progression of kidney disease: a meta-analysis of treatment effects in randomised clinical trials. Lancet Diabetes Endocrinol. 2019;7(2):128–39.
70. Kramer CK, Retnakaran R. Concordance of retinopathy and nephropathy over time in type 1 diabetes: an analysis of data from the diabetes control and complications trial. Diabet Med. 2013;30(11):1333–41.
71. Penno G, Solini A, Zoppini G, Orsi E, Zerbini G, Trevisan R, et al. Rate and determinants of association between advanced retinopathy and chronic kidney disease in patients with type 2 diabetes: the renal insufficiency and cardiovascular events (RIACE) Italian multicenter study. Diabetes Care. 2012;35(11):2317–23.
72. Margolis DJ, Hofstad O, Feldman HI. Association between renal failure and foot ulcer or lower-extremity amputation in patients with diabetes. Diabetes Care. 2008;31(7):1331–6.
73. Ko SH, Park SA, Cho JH, Song KH, Yoon KH, Cha BY, et al. Progression of cardiovascular autonomic dysfunction in patients with type 2 diabetes: a 7-year follow-up study. Diabetes Care. 2008;31(9):1832–6.
74. Nielsen FS, Hansen HP, Jacobsen P, Rossing P, Smidt UM, Christensen NJ, et al. Increased sympathetic activity during sleep and nocturnal hypertension in type 2 diabetic patients with diabetic nephropathy. Diabet Med. 1999;16(7):555–62.
75. Tahrani AA, Dubb K, Raymond NT, Begum S, Altaf QA, Sadiqi H, et al. Cardiac autonomic neuropathy predicts renal function decline in patients with type 2 diabetes: a cohort study. Diabetologia. 2014;57(6):1249–56.
76. Amin AP, Whaley-Connell AT, Li S, Chen SC, McCullough PA, Kosiborod MN, et al. The synergistic relationship between estimated GFR and microalbuminuria in predicting long-term progression to ESRD or death in patients with diabetes: results from the kidney early evaluation program (KEEP). American Journal of Kidney Diseases: The Official Journal of the National Kidney Foundation. 2013;61(4 Suppl 2):S12–23.
77. McCullough PA, Jurkovitz CT, Pergola PE, McGill JB, Brown WW, Collins AJ, et al. Independent components of chronic kidney disease as a cardiovascular risk state: results from the kidney early evaluation program (KEEP). Arch Intern Med. 2007;167(11):1122–9.
78. So WY, Kong AP, Ma RC, Ozaki R, Szeto CC, Chan NN, et al. Glomerular filtration rate, cardiorenal end points, and all-cause mortality in type 2 diabetic patients. Diabetes Care. 2006;29(9):2046–52.

79. Bruno G, Merletti F, Bargero G, Novelli G, Melis D, Soddu A, et al. Estimated glomerular filtration rate, albuminuria and mortality in type 2 diabetes: the Casale Monferrato study. Diabetologia. 2007;50(5):941–8.
80. Groop PH, Thomas MC, Moran JL, Waden J, Thorn LM, Makinen VP, et al. The presence and severity of chronic kidney disease predicts all-cause mortality in type 1 diabetes. Diabetes. 2009;58(7):1651–8.
81. Orchard TJ, Secrest AM, Miller RG, Costacou T. In the absence of renal disease, 20 year mortality risk in type 1 diabetes is comparable to that of the general population: a report from the Pittsburgh epidemiology of diabetes complications study. Diabetologia. 2010;53(11):2312–9.
82. Deckert T, Yokoyama H, Mathiesen E, Ronn B, Jensen T, Feldt-Rasmussen B, et al. Cohort study of predictive value of urinary albumin excretion for atherosclerotic vascular disease in patients with insulin dependent diabetes. BMJ. 1996;312(7035):871–4.
83. Tuomilehto J, Borch-Johnsen K, Molarius A, Forsen T, Rastenyte D, Sarti C, et al. Incidence of cardiovascular disease in type 1 (insulin-dependent) diabetic subjects with and without diabetic nephropathy in Finland. Diabetologia. 1998;41(7):784–90.
84. Targher G, Marra F, Marchesini G. Increased risk of cardiovascular disease in non-alcoholic fatty liver disease: causal effect or epiphenomenon? Diabetologia. 2008;51(11):1947–53.
85. Dinneen SF, Gerstein HC. The association of microalbuminuria and mortality in non-insulin-dependent diabetes mellitus. A systematic overview of the literature. Arch Intern Med. 1997;157(13):1413–8.
86. Fuller JH, Stevens LK, Wang SL. Risk factors for cardiovascular mortality and morbidity: the WHO Mutinational study of vascular disease in diabetes. Diabetologia. 2001;44(Suppl 2):S54–64.
87. Adler AI, Stevens RJ, Manley SE, Bilous RW, Cull CA, Holman RR. Development and progression of nephropathy in type 2 diabetes: the United Kingdom prospective diabetes study (UKPDS 64). Kidney Int. 2003;63(1):225–32.
88. de Boer IH, Caramori ML, Chan JCN, Heerspink HJL, Hurst C, Khunti K, et al. Executive summary of the 2020 KDIGO diabetes management in CKD guideline: evidence-based advances in monitoring and treatment. Kidney Int. 2020;98(4):839–48.
89. Forouhi NG, Koulman A, Sharp SJ, Imamura F, Kroger J, Schulze MB, et al. Differences in the prospective association between individual plasma phospholipid saturated fatty acids and incident type 2 diabetes: the EPIC-InterAct case-cohort study. Lancet Diabetes Endocrinol. 2014;2(10):810–8.
90. Kwakernaak AJ, Krikken JA, Binnenmars SH, Visser FW, Hemmelder MH, Woittiez AJ, et al. Effects of sodium restriction and hydrochlorothiazide on RAAS blockade efficacy in diabetic nephropathy: a randomised clinical trial. Lancet Diabetes Endocrinol. 2014;2(5):385–95.
91. Lambers Heerspink HJ, Holtkamp FA, Parving HH, Navis GJ, Lewis JB, Ritz E, et al. Moderation of dietary sodium potentiates the renal and cardiovascular protective effects of angiotensin receptor blockers. Kidney Int. 2012;82(3):330–7.
92. Nezu U, Kamiyama H, Kondo Y, Sakuma M, Morimoto T, Ueda S. Effect of low-protein diet on kidney function in diabetic nephropathy: meta-analysis of randomised controlled trials. BMJ Open. 2013;3(5).
93. Hansen HP, Tauber-Lassen E, Jensen BR, Parving HH. Effect of dietary protein restriction on prognosis in patients with diabetic nephropathy. Kidney Int. 2002;62(1):220–8.
94. Tirosh A, Golan R, Harman-Boehm I, Henkin Y, Schwarzfuchs D, Rudich A, et al. Renal function following three distinct weight loss dietary strategies during 2 years of a randomized controlled trial. Diabetes Care. 2013;36(8):2225–32.
95. Jackson S, le Roux CW, Docherty NG. Bariatric surgery and microvascular complications of type 2 diabetes mellitus. Curr Atheroscler Rep. 2014;16(11):453.
96. Bjornstad P, Nehus E, Jenkins T, Mitsnefes M, Moxey-Mims M, Dixon JB, et al. Five-year kidney outcomes of bariatric surgery differ in severely obese adolescents and adults with and without type 2 diabetes. Kidney Int. 2020;97(5):995–1005.

97. The effect of intensive treatment of diabetes on the development and progression of long-term complications in insulin-dependent diabetes mellitus. The Diabetes Control and Complications Trial Research Group. N Engl J Med. 1993;329(14):977–86.
98. The absence of a glycemic threshold for the development of long-term complications: the perspective of the Diabetes Control and Complications Trial. Diabetes. 1996;45(10):1289–98.
99. Group DER, de Boer IH, Sun W, Cleary PA, Lachin JM, Molitch ME, et al. Intensive diabetes therapy and glomerular filtration rate in type 1 diabetes. N Engl J Med. 2011;365(25):2366–76.
100. Beck RW, Bergenstal RM, Riddlesworth TD, Kollman C, Li Z, Brown AS, et al. Validation of time in range as an outcome measure for diabetes clinical trials. Diabetes Care. 2019;42(3):400–5.
101. Ranjan AG, Rosenlund SV, Hansen TW, Rossing P, Andersen S, Norgaard K. Improved time in range over 1 year is associated with reduced albuminuria in individuals with sensor-augmented insulin pump-treated type 1 diabetes. Diabetes Care. 2020;43(11):2882–5.
102. Intensive blood-glucose control with sulphonylureas or insulin compared with conventional treatment and risk of complications in patients with type 2 diabetes (UKPDS 33). UK Prospective Diabetes Study (UKPDS) Group [published erratum appears in Lancet 1999 Aug 14;354(9178):602] [see comments]. Lancet. 1998;352(9131):837–53.
103. Stratton IM, Adler AI, Neil HA, Matthews DR, Manley SE, Cull CA, et al. Association of glycaemia with macrovascular and microvascular complications of type 2 diabetes (UKPDS 35): prospective observational study. BMJ. 2000;321(7258):405–12.
104. Group AC, Patel A, MacMahon S, Chalmers J, Neal B, Billot L, et al. Intensive blood glucose control and vascular outcomes in patients with type 2 diabetes. N Engl J Med. 2008;358(24):2560–72.
105. Perkovic V, Heerspink HL, Chalmers J, Woodward M, Jun M, Li Q, et al. Intensive glucose control improves kidney outcomes in patients with type 2 diabetes. Kidney Int. 2013;83(3):517–23.
106. Ismail-Beigi F, Craven T, Banerji MA, Basile J, Calles J, Cohen RM, et al. Effect of intensive treatment of hyperglycaemia on microvascular outcomes in type 2 diabetes: an analysis of the ACCORD randomised trial. Lancet. 2010;376(9739):419–30.
107. Papademetriou V, Lovato L, Doumas M, Nylen E, Mottl A, Cohen RM, et al. Chronic kidney disease and intensive glycemic control increase cardiovascular risk in patients with type 2 diabetes. Kidney Int. 2015;87(3):649–59.
108. Zinman B, Wanner C, Lachin JM, Fitchett D, Bluhmki E, Hantel S, et al. Empagliflozin, cardiovascular outcomes, and mortality in type 2 diabetes. N Engl J Med. 2015;373(22):2117–28.
109. Wanner C, Inzucchi SE, Lachin JM, Fitchett D, von Eynatten M, Mattheus M, et al. Empagliflozin and progression of kidney Disease in type 2 diabetes. N Engl J Med. 2016;375(4):323–34.
110. Perkovic V, Jardine MJ, Neal B, Bompoint S, Heerspink HJL, Charytan DM, et al. Canagliflozin and renal outcomes in type 2 diabetes and nephropathy. N Engl J Med. 2019;380(24):2295–306.
111. Heerspink HJL, Stefansson BV, Correa-Rotter R, Chertow GM, Greene T, Hou FF, et al. Dapagliflozin in patients with chronic kidney Disease. N Engl J Med. 2020;383(15):1436–46.
112. Buse JB, Wexler DJ, Tsapas A, Rossing P, Mingrone G, Mathieu C, et al. 2019 update to: Management of Hyperglycemia in type 2 diabetes, 2018. A consensus report by the American Diabetes Association (ADA) and the European Association for the Study of diabetes (EASD). Diabetes Care. 2020;43(2):487–93.
113. Buse JB, Wexler DJ, Tsapas A, Rossing P, Mingrone G, Mathieu C, et al. Erratum. 2019 Update to: Management of Hyperglycemia in Type 2 Diabetes, 2018. A Consensus Report by the American Diabetes Association (ADA) and the European Association for the Study of Diabetes (EASD). Diabetes Care 2020;43:487–93. Diabetes Care. 2020;43(7):1670.
114. Tuttle KR, Lakshmanan MC, Rayner B, Busch RS, Zimmermann AG, Woodward DB, et al. Dulaglutide versus insulin glargine in patients with type 2 diabetes and moderate-to-severe

chronic kidney disease (AWARD-7): a multicentre, open-label, randomised trial. Lancet Diabetes Endocrinol. 2018;6(8):605–17.

115. Randomised placebo-controlled trial of lisinopril in normotensive patients with insulin-dependent diabetes and normoalbuminuria or microalbuminuria. The EUCLID Study Group. Lancet. 1997;349(9068):1787–92.
116. Bilous R, Chaturvedi N, Sjolie AK, Fuller J, Klein R, Orchard T, et al. Effect of candesartan on microalbuminuria and albumin excretion rate in diabetes: three randomized trials. Ann Intern Med. 2009;151(1):11–20. W3-4.
117. Mauer M, Zinman B, Gardiner R, Suissa S, Sinaiko A, Strand T, et al. Renal and retinal effects of enalapril and losartan in type 1 diabetes. N Engl J Med. 2009;361(1):40–51.
118. Group ACEIiDNT. Should all patients with type 1 diabetes mellitus and microalbuminuria receive angiotensin-converting enzyme inhibitors? A meta-analysis of individual patient data. Ann Intern Med. 2001;134(5):370–9.
119. Parving HH, Lehnert H, Brochner-Mortensen J, Gomis R, Andersen S, Arner P. The effect of irbesartan on the development of diabetic nephropathy in patients with type 2 diabetes. N Engl J Med. 2001;345(12):870–8.
120. Tight blood pressure control and risk of macrovascular and microvascular complications in type 2 diabetes: UKPDS 38. UK Prospective Diabetes Study Group [see comments] [published erratum appears in BMJ 1999 Jan 2;318(7175):29]. BMJ. 1998;317(7160):703–13.
121. Effects of ramipril on cardiovascular and microvascular outcomes in people with diabetes mellitus: results of the HOPE study and MICRO-HOPE substudy. Heart Outcomes Prevention Evaluation Study Investigators. Lancet. 2000;355(9200):253–9.
122. Ruggenenti P, Fassi A, Ilieva AP, Bruno S, Iliev IP, Brusegan V, et al. Preventing microalbuminuria in type 2 diabetes. N Engl J Med. 2004;351(19):1941–51.
123. Patel A, Group AC, MacMahon S, Chalmers J, Neal B, Woodward M, et al. Effects of a fixed combination of perindopril and indapamide on macrovascular and microvascular outcomes in patients with type 2 diabetes mellitus (the ADVANCE trial): a randomised controlled trial. Lancet. 2007;370(9590):829–40.
124. Persson F, Lindhardt M, Rossing P, Parving HH. Prevention of microalbuminuria using early intervention with renin-angiotensin system inhibitors in patients with type 2 diabetes: a systematic review. J Renin Angiotensin Aldosterone Syst. 2016;17(3).
125. Haller H, Ito S, Izzo JL Jr, Januszewicz A, Katayama S, Menne J, et al. Olmesartan for the delay or prevention of microalbuminuria in type 2 diabetes. N Engl J Med. 2011;364(10):907–17.
126. Strippoli GF, Craig M, Schena FP, Craig JC. Antihypertensive agents for primary prevention of diabetic nephropathy. J Am Soc Nephrol: JASN. 2005;16(10):3081–91.
127. Sim JJ, Shi J, Kovesdy CP, Kalantar-Zadeh K, Jacobsen SJ. Impact of achieved blood pressures on mortality risk and end-stage renal disease among a large, diverse hypertension population. J Am Coll Cardiol. 2014;64(6):588–97.
128. Brenner BM, Cooper ME, de Zeeuw D, Keane WF, Mitch WE, Parving HH, et al. Effects of losartan on renal and cardiovascular outcomes in patients with type 2 diabetes and nephropathy. N Engl J Med. 2001;345(12):861–9.
129. Lewis EJ, Hunsicker LG, Clarke WR, Berl T, Pohl MA, Lewis JB, et al. Renoprotective effect of the angiotensin-receptor antagonist irbesartan in patients with nephropathy due to type 2 diabetes. N Engl J Med. 2001;345(12):851–60.
130. Miao Y, Dobre D, Heerspink HJ, Brenner BM, Cooper ME, Parving HH, et al. Increased serum potassium affects renal outcomes: a post hoc analysis of the reduction of endpoints in NIDDM with the angiotensin II antagonist losartan (RENAAL) trial. Diabetologia. 2011;54(1):44–50.
131. Holtkamp FA, de Zeeuw D, Thomas MC, Cooper ME, de Graeff PA, Hillege HJ, et al. An acute fall in estimated glomerular filtration rate during treatment with losartan predicts a slower decrease in long-term renal function. Kidney Int. 2011;80(3):282–7.

132. Mogensen CE, Neldam S, Tikkanen I, Oren S, Viskoper R, Watts RW, et al. Randomised controlled trial of dual blockade of renin-angiotensin system in patients with hypertension, microalbuminuria, and non-insulin dependent diabetes: the candesartan and lisinopril microalbuminuria (CALM) study. BMJ. 2000;321(7274):1440–4.
133. Jacobsen P, Andersen S, Rossing K, Jensen BR, Parving HH. Dual blockade of the renin-angiotensin system versus maximal recommended dose of ACE inhibition in diabetic nephropathy. Kidney Int. 2003;63(5):1874–80.
134. Mann JF, Schmieder RE, McQueen M, Dyal L, Schumacher H, Pogue J, et al. Renal outcomes with telmisartan, ramipril, or both, in people at high vascular risk (the ONTARGET study): a multicentre, randomised, double-blind, controlled trial. Lancet. 2008;372(9638):547–53.
135. Parving HH, Brenner BM, McMurray JJ, de Zeeuw D, Haffner SM, Solomon SD, et al. Cardiorenal end points in a trial of aliskiren for type 2 diabetes. N Engl J Med. 2012;367(23):2204–13.
136. Fried LF, Emanuele N, Zhang JH, Brophy M, Conner TA, Duckworth W, et al. Combined angiotensin inhibition for the treatment of diabetic nephropathy. N Engl J Med. 2013;369(20):1892–903.
137. Ren F, Tang L, Cai Y, Yuan X, Huang W, Luo L, et al. Meta-analysis: the efficacy and safety of combined treatment with ARB and ACEI on diabetic nephropathy. Ren Fail. 2015;37(4):548–61.
138. Currie G, Taylor AH, Fujita T, Ohtsu H, Lindhardt M, Rossing P, et al. Effect of mineralocorticoid receptor antagonists on proteinuria and progression of chronic kidney disease: a systematic review and meta-analysis. BMC Nephrol. 2016;17(1):127.
139. Tofte N, Lindhardt M, Adamova K, Bakker SJL, Beige J, Beulens JWJ, et al. Early detection of diabetic kidney disease by urinary proteomics and subsequent intervention with spironolactone to delay progression (PRIORITY): a prospective observational study and embedded randomised placebo-controlled trial. Lancet Diabetes Endocrinol. 2020;8(4):301–12.
140. Bakris GL, Agarwal R, Anker SD, Pitt B, Ruilope LM, Rossing P, et al. Effect of Finerenone on chronic kidney Disease outcomes in type 2 diabetes. N Engl J Med. 2020;383(23):2219–29.
141. Pitt B, Filippatos G, Agarwal R, Anker SD, Bakris GL, Rossing P, et al. Cardiovascular events with Finerenone in kidney Disease and type 2 diabetes. N Engl J Med. 2021;385(24):2252–63.
142. Heerspink HJL, Parving HH, Andress DL, Bakris G, Correa-Rotter R, Hou FF, et al. Atrasentan and renal events in patients with type 2 diabetes and chronic kidney disease (SONAR): a double-blind, randomised, placebo-controlled trial. Lancet. 2019;393(10184):1937–47.
143. Jun M, Zhu B, Tonelli M, Jardine MJ, Patel A, Neal B, et al. Effects of fibrates in kidney disease: a systematic review and meta-analysis. J Am Coll Cardiol. 2012;60(20):2061–71.
144. Kreutz R, Camm AJ, Rossing P. Concomitant diabetes with atrial fibrillation and anticoagulation management considerations. Eur Heart J Suppl. 2020;22(Suppl O):O78–86.
145. Hernandez AV, Bradley G, Khan M, Fratoni A, Gasparini A, Roman YM, et al. Rivaroxaban vs. warfarin and renal outcomes in non-valvular atrial fibrillation patients with diabetes. Eur Heart J Qual Care Clin Outcomes. 2020;6(4):301–7.
146. Petrie JR, Rossing PR, Campbell IW. Metformin and cardiorenal outcomes in diabetes: a reappraisal. Diabetes Obes Metab. 2020;22(6):904–15.
147. Mathiesen ER. Diabetic nephropathy in pregnancy: new insights from a retrospective cohort study. Diabetologia. 2015;58(4):649–50.
148. Klemetti MM, Laivuori H, Tikkanen M, Nuutila M, Hiilesmaa V, Teramo K. Obstetric and perinatal outcome in type 1 diabetes patients with diabetic nephropathy during 1988-2011. Diabetologia. 2015;58(4):678–86.
149. Damm JA, Asbjornsdottir B, Callesen NF, Mathiesen JM, Ringholm L, Pedersen BW, et al. Diabetic nephropathy and microalbuminuria in pregnant women with type 1 and type 2 diabetes: prevalence, antihypertensive strategy, and pregnancy outcome. Diabetes Care. 2013;36(11):3489–94.

150. Lim LL, Lau ESH, Ozaki R, Chung H, Fu AWC, Chan W, et al. Association of technologically assisted integrated care with clinical outcomes in type 2 diabetes in Hong Kong using the prospective JADE program: a retrospective cohort analysis. PLoS Med. 2020;17(10):e1003367.
151. Tu ST, Chang SJ, Chen JF, Tien KJ, Hsiao JY, Chen HC, et al. Prevention of diabetic nephropathy by tight target control in an asian population with type 2 diabetes mellitus: a 4-year prospective analysis. Arch Intern Med. 2010;170(2):155–61.
152. Gaede P, Lund-Andersen H, Parving HH, Pedersen O. Effect of a multifactorial intervention on mortality in type 2 diabetes. N Engl J Med. 2008;358(6):580–91.
153. Chan JC, So WY, Yeung CY, Ko GT, Lau IT, Tsang MW, et al. Effects of structured versus usual care on renal endpoint in type 2 diabetes: the SURE study: a randomized multicenter translational study. Diabetes Care. 2009;32(6):977–82.
154. Gaede P, Oellgaard J, Carstensen B, Rossing P, Lund-Andersen H, Parving HH, et al. Years of life gained by multifactorial intervention in patients with type 2 diabetes mellitus and microalbuminuria: 21 years follow-up on the Steno-2 randomised trial. Diabetologia. 2016;59(11):2298–307.
155. Gaede P, Oellgaard J, Kruuse C, Rossing P, Parving HH, Pedersen O. Beneficial impact of intensified multifactorial intervention on risk of stroke: outcome of 21 years of follow-up in the randomised Steno-2 study. Diabetologia. 2019;62(9):1575–80.
156. Oellgaard J, Gaede P, Rossing P, Persson F, Parving HH, Pedersen O. Intensified multifactorial intervention in type 2 diabetics with microalbuminuria leads to long-term renal benefits. Kidney Int. 2017;91(4):982–8.
157. Oellgaard J, Gaede P, Rossing P, Rorth R, Kober L, Parving HH, et al. Reduced risk of heart failure with intensified multifactorial intervention in individuals with type 2 diabetes and microalbuminuria: 21 years of follow-up in the randomised Steno-2 study. Diabetologia. 2018;61(8):1724–33.
158. Kidney Disease: Improving Global Outcomes (KDIGO) CKD Work Group. KDIGO clicical practice guideline for the evaluation and management of chronic kidney disease. Kidney Inter Suppl. 2013;3:1–150.

Chapter 8
Precision Medicine for Diabetic Neuropathy

Long Davalos, Amro M. Stino, Dinesh Selvarajah, Stacey A. Sakowski, Solomon Tesfaye, and Eva L. Feldman

Diabetic Peripheral Neuropathy: Clinical Evaluation and Epidemiology

Evolution of Understanding

The entity referred to as diabetic peripheral neuropathy (DPN) was historically considered a single entity tied to glycemic index. Data accumulated over the last several decades has produced a more precise understanding, one grounded in animal models, which paved the way for more targeted therapies. As early as the 1990s, it was first noted by clinicians that many patients with cryptogenic sensory peripheral neuropathy (CSPN) shared phenotypic features with diabetic patients, particularly with regard to obesity and metabolic syndrome (MetS). Robust international epidemiological data followed, confirming that obesity and MetS, even in the absence of frank diabetes, were associated with peripheral neuropathy [1–6]. It is now clear that type 1 diabetic peripheral neuropathy (T1DPN) and type 2 diabetic peripheral neuropathy (T2DPN) are two separate disease entities [7, 8]. In addition, MetS itself is a bona fide cause of peripheral neuropathy and accelerates the development of peripheral neuropathy, particularly in type 2 diabetes (T2D) [3, 9, 10]. Most recently, murine models have emerged, demonstrating a pathophysiologic foundation for

L. Davalos · A. M. Stino · S. A. Sakowski · E. L. Feldman (✉)
Department of Neurology, University of Michigan, Ann Arbor, MI, USA
e-mail: loda@med.umich.edu; amstino@med.umich.edu; staceysa@med.umich.edu; efeldman@med.umich.edu

D. Selvarajah
Department of Oncology and Metabolism, Medical School, University of Sheffield, Sheffield, UK
e-mail: d.selvarajah@sheffield.ac.uk

S. Tesfaye (✉)
Diabetes Research Unit, Sheffield Teaching Hospital, Sheffield, UK
e-mail: solomon.tesfaye@nhs.net

R. Basu (ed.), *Precision Medicine in Diabetes*,
https://doi.org/10.1007/978-3-030-98927-9_8

Table 8.1 Drug trials on peripheral neuropathy associated with T1DM and T2DM from 2010 to 2020

Drug	Disease or pain modifying	Mechanism of action	Diabetes type	Clinical trial outcome for neuropathy	Reference
OnabotulintoxinA (BoNT/A)	Pain	Inhibits neurogenic inflammation from peripheral nociceptive nerve terminals	T2DM	Improved tactile and mechanical pain perception in painful DPN	[139]
Botulin toxin (BTX-A)	Pain	Potent neurotoxin, used in treatment of dystonia, muscle hyperactivity, and glandular hyperactivity. BTX-A may have analgesic properties	T2DM	Intradermal injection of BTX-A significantly improved painful DPN	[140]
Monochromatic infrared energy (MIRE)	Disease	Increases blood circulation	T2DM	No improvement	[141]
L-arginine	Disease	Substrate for nitric oxide synthesis to improve microcirculation	T2DM	No effect DPN	[142]
Minocycline	Disease and pain	Anti-inflammatory and antiapoptotic properties, suppression of microglial activation	T2DM	Improved vibration perception threshold, reduced neuropathic symptoms, and pain disability index	[143]
Benfotiamine	Disease	Modulates advanced glycation end products	T1DM	No effect on peripheral nerve function	[144]

Reproduced with permission from Stino et al. [15]

initial clinical and epidemiologic observations [11–14]. Despite decades of costly and failed clinical trials (Table 8.1), spanning antioxidants, lipid-lowering agents, aldose reductase inhibitors, neurotrophic factors, and GABA analogues, to name a few, we now stand on the cusp of a targeted therapeutic approach to diabetic neuropathy, one that encompasses interventions such as exercise, dietary control, and more targeted and novel drug therapies [15–17]. Advances in DPN pain research have also refined DPN pain management approaches through more focused sensory and imaging phenotyping.

Type 1 Versus Type 2 Diabetic Peripheral Neuropathy: Towards a More Precise Understanding

DPN is most frequently a distal symmetric sensory predominant neuropathy, which is the most common complication of both type 1 diabetes (T1D) and T2D [18–20]. The incidence of T2DPN (6100 per 100,000 person-years) is higher than T1DPN (2800 per 100,000 person-years) [21–23]. However, the prevalence of neuropathy is similar in T2DPN (8–51%) [18–20] and T1DPN (11–50%) [18, 24]. The observed difference in incidence with similar prevalence in both might be related to multiple factors, including the underlying pathophysiology, as well as differences in age and onset of diabetes.

In T1DPN, hyperglycemia is the major contributor to the development of neuropathy. Intensive glycemic control reduces the risk of developing T1DPN by 60%, and the beneficial effects persist for over 16 years [25, 26]. Other smaller studies reached similar conclusions, evidence that improved glycemic control preserves nerve function and/or decreases likelihood of developing DPN [27].

On the other hand, in T2DPN, hyperglycemia does not seem to be the primary mechanism. Large studies have demonstrated little to no effect of glycemic control on T2DPN, indicating that factors independent of glycemic control are critical in the development of neuropathy [28, 29]. In fact, there is growing evidence that the MetS components (central obesity, dyslipidemia, hypertension) accelerate T2DPN progression and might have equal or greater import than glycemic index alone [9].

Such pathophysiologic differences require distinct management approaches targeted to T1DPN and T2DPN. Improving glycemic control should be the main focus in patients with T1DPN, while lifestyle interventions, specifically diet and exercise, coupled with optimal lipid and blood pressure control, are the optimal therapeutic approaches for patients with T2DPN.

Clinical Approach

DPN often presents with acral pain, numbness, tingling, or dysesthesias involving the feet, which often progresses, if unchecked, to involve the distal upper limbs as well. The Toronto consensus criteria laid out an objective and reproducible framework for diagnosing DPN, applicable in both the clinical and research settings, and predicated upon demonstrating (a) neuropathic signs and symptoms and (b) impairment in validated measures of large and/or small fiber function, namely, nerve conduction studies (NCS) and skin biopsy evaluation of intraepidermal nerve fiber density (IENFD), respectively [30]. NCS are quite useful clinically for evaluating the severity of large fiber DPN; however, normal values do not exclude the presence of small fiber neuropathy. Furthermore, NCS are of limited value in DPN research, while IENFD has emerged as the gold standard outcome measure. MetS and diabetes both preferentially target small nerve fibers early in the disease course. Data has also shown that obesity and hypertriglyceridemia, both MetS components, preferentially target small unmyelinated fibers, while hyperglycemia renders more damage to large myelinated fibers [31]. IENFD testing is now considered the gold standard for diagnosing small fiber DPN and involves immunohistochemical staining and quantitation of unmyelinated axons using an antibody against protein end product 9.5 (PGP 9.5), a neuronal biomarker. IENFD testing is also invaluable to DPN therapeutic development, as it allows sensitive detection of nerve healing and regrowth, given the unique regenerative capacity of small fibers [32, 33].

While our chapter focuses on evaluating and testing somatic DPN, it is worth noting that diabetic autonomic neuropathy represents another equally important area of research. Autonomic neuropathy is tested by the autonomic reflex screen, which encompasses quantitative sudomotor axon reflex testing, Valsalva blood pressure analysis, heart rate variation to deep breathing, heart rate variation to Valsalva, and tilt table testing [34].

Metabolic Syndrome, Obesity, and Peripheral Neuropathy

MetS revolves around dyslipidemia (elevated triglycerides and/or reduced high-density lipoproteins (HDLs), central obesity, insulin resistance (diabetes or prediabetes), and hypertension) and afflicts over one-third of adults in the United States [35]. Seven international population-based studies have now firmly identify MetS as a driver of peripheral neuropathy and highlight the intimate association between central obesity and neuropathy [1–6, 36].

Obesity has emerged as the second most influential metabolic risk factor for neuropathy after diabetes, independent of glycemic status. Recent studies in the United States have shown that obese normoglycemic individuals have a higher prevalence of neuropathy compared to lean controls [37]. In fact, waist circumference is associated with the greatest number of neuropathy outcome measures compared to other metabolic factors [1, 2]. Studies conducted in China and Europe have reached similar conclusions, highlighting that obesity is independently associated with neuropathy, regardless of glycemic status [3–6]. Global population-specific differences, however, are worthy of consideration, as a recent study of South Asian Indian patients found that MetS components or waist circumference did not associate with peripheral neuropathy [38]. In addition, hypertriglyceridemia correlates with CSPN, IENFD loss, sural nerve myelinated fiber loss, and the likelihood of lower limb amputation [31, 39–41].

The optimal disease-modifying approach in obese patients with and without diabetes is to target obesity and its downstream effects. Lifestyle interventions such as diet and exercise are inexpensive and accessible strategies to combat obesity and promote nerve restoration, as highlighted in the Look AHEAD trial [42, 43]. However, since poor exercise and dietary compliance are a natural limitation, the role of alternative strategies, such as pharmacotherapy and bariatric surgery, has become a topic of interest in MetS-related neuropathy. Although initial observations suggested that lipid-lowering therapy reduces DPN development risk and lower limb amputation, a recent population-based Danish study showed that statin therapy did not mitigate DPN risk in T2D patients (9% of whom were obese) [44]. Bariatric surgery, however, seems to improve neuropathic outcome measures in patients with obesity and T2D and is the focus of ongoing evaluation in a randomized controlled clinical trial [45, 46]. Even though these interventions have shown promising results, larger studies are needed to evaluate their cost-effectiveness [47, 48].

Prediabetes and Peripheral Neuropathy

Alongside obesity, prediabetes is another MetS component that has been the focus of much epidemiologic research. Different studies have suggested an association between prediabetes and neuropathy, although, conversely, a few reports have questioned this association.

The San Luis Valley study showed a neuropathy prevalence of 25.8% in diabetic patients, 11.2% in those with impaired glucose tolerance (IGT), and 3.9% in the control group [47]. The MONICA/KORA study reported a 13.3% prevalence of painful neuropathy in diabetic individuals, 8.7% in the IGT group, 4.2% in the impaired fasting glucose (IFG) group, and 1.2% in normoglycemic patients [49]. The longitudinal PROMISE study supported these prior findings, showing a prevalence of 49% in prediabetes patients. Furthermore, the progression to glucose intolerance over 3 years predicted a higher risk of peripheral neuropathy and nerve dysfunction, and, compared to normoglycemic subjects, prediabetic patients had higher Michigan Neuropathy Symptom Inventory (MNSI) scores and vibration detection thresholds [50]. Likewise, a cohort of 32 patients with IGT and neuropathic symptoms exhibited abnormalities in the distal skin biopsy of all subjects, indicating that small fiber damage occurs quite frequently in the prediabetic population [42]. All these studies support the role of prediabetes as a cause of neuropathy. In addition, patients with preexisting CSPN seem more likely to have prediabetes. In a cohort of CSPN patients, 56% were found to have IFG, and 36% had IGT, with the IGT group showing primarily small nerve fiber involvement [51].

Despite the evidence linking prediabetes to neuropathy, there are some studies that do not support this association [39, 52]. One recent single-center study showed that there was no difference between prediabetic and normoglycemic patients regarding small fiber structure and function [53]. Likewise, two studies of a population in Olmsted County, Minnesota, showed that prediabetes did not increase neuropathy risk [54, 55]. Nevertheless, these studies did suggest that other features of MetS increased the likelihood of neuropathy. Adding to the complexity of interpreting the findings is that despite adjusting for obesity, some of the studies used NCS (rather than IENFD) as the primary outcome measure.

The conflicting conclusions of these published studies are most likely related to the different criteria used to diagnose prediabetes and neuropathy. It is well-known that a large proportion of prediabetic individuals develop T2D, and there is growing data suggesting that MetS components are independent neuropathy risk factors. Therefore, interventions that prevent prediabetes progression to diabetes, as well as those that treat MetS, should be expected to reduce neuropathy incidence in prediabetic patients.

Pediatric Diabetic Peripheral Neuropathy

In the pediatric population, T1D is the most prevalent diabetes type, accounting for 98% of diabetic cases in children younger than 10 years, and 87% of those aged 10–19 years [56]. The incidence and prevalence of both T1D and T2D in the pediatric population have increased markedly, along with an associated rise in DPN incidence [57–63].

Estimating the real prevalence of pediatric DPN can be challenging due variability in tests and criteria, as well as the high prevalence of asymptomatic neuropathy. In pediatric and youth patients with T1D, neuropathy prevalence ranges from 3 to 62%. The Epidemiology of Diabetes Complications (EDC) study found T1DPN in 3% of patients ≤18 years old using a standardized neurological exam and clinical history as a tool to detect neuropathy. The EURODIAB insulin-dependent diabetes mellitus (IDDM) complications study assessed symptoms, deep tendon reflexes, vibration perception threshold (VPT), and autonomic function and reported T1DPN in 19% of patients aged 15 to 29 [64, 65]. Conversely, a population-based longitudinal Danish study reported a T1DPN prevalence of 62% in patients aged 12 to 27 using VPT [66]. Likewise, a cohort of 73 patients with a mean age of 13.6 years and a T1D duration ≥5 years found neuropathic symptoms in only 4% but abnormal neurological exam, NCS, and VPT in 36%, 57%, and 51% of subjects, respectively [67]. In these studies, the prevalence was higher with older age and longer disease duration. Pediatric DPN prevalence generally appears to be higher in T2D than T1D patients in studies that have compared both groups, with estimates indicating a prevalence of 17–22% for T2D versus 7–12% for T1D [62, 68, 69]. As previously discussed, the wide range in stated prevalence is the result of testing modalities employed to define DPN.

DPN is infrequently reported in pediatric practice, likely due to a lack of voluntary reporting from children and adolescents and the high rates of asymptomatic manifestations. The DPN symptom profile in this population differs from the one in adults and often consists of paresthesias and fewer intense pain experiences [70]. In terms of risk factors, hyperglycemia is the major T1DPN driver, but there is no data supporting this in T2DPN for pediatric patients [71]. Obesity and dyslipidemia have emerged as potential risk factors, suggesting a multifactorial etiology similar to the adult population. This is alarming considering that approximately one-third of children and adolescents in most resource-rich countries are either overweight or obese, which has fuelled the increase in DPN incidence and prevalence [57, 58, 72, 73]. Management should target glycemic control, as well as focus on weight loss, exercise, and nutrition counseling in order to improve obesity and insulin resistance [74]. Diagnosing DPN early and appropriate interventions in children and adolescents are crucial, since it may improve or even reverse subclinical DPN.

Genetic Risk Factors

Genetic risk factors in DPN development are the focus of much study. Despite numerous potential variants of interest, it is still unclear how such variants impact or associate with DPN development. Nevertheless, certain single-nucleotide polymorphisms of interest, which have gained attention in both adult and pediatric patients, include variants affecting the polyol pathway (aldose reductase gene (*AKR1B1*)) [75], cholesterol transport (apolipoprotein E (*APOE*)) [76], mitochondrial uncoupling (*UCP2* and *UCP3*) [77], oxidative stress defense (superoxide dismutase (*SOD2* and *SOD3*)) [78], catalase (*CAT*) [79], and glutathione peroxidase-1 (*GPX1*) [79].

Epigenetics is another area of active research. A recent genome-wide methylation study explored alterations in the sural nerve DNA methylome and transcriptome, demonstrating differentially methylated genes and differentially expressed genes between T2DPN human subjects with the highest and lowest levels of hemoglobin A1c. Differential gene methylation and expression were enriched in pathways critical to the immune system, extracellular matrix, and axon guidance [80].

Diabetic Peripheral Neuropathy: Pathogenesis and Therapeutic Targets

Animal Models

Murine models of DPN now include leptin (*ob/ob*) and leptin receptor (*db/db*) mutant mice, as well as a C57BL/6 J mice fed high-fat diet as a prediabetes model and C57BL/6 J mice fed high-fat diet and administered low-dose streptozotocin as a T2D model [11–14]. Mitochondrial dysfunction, dysregulated substrate uptake, and inflammation underlie peripheral nerve DPN pathology, especially in T2DPN and MetS-associated peripheral neuropathy [81]. Long-chain fatty acids alter mitochondrial size, morphology, and motility, contributing to compromised mitochondrial bioenergetics [82]. Nerve-lipid signaling is impaired in both murine models and human sural nerve, as shown using transcriptomic and lipidomic analyses [83]. Transport and substrate uptake is also dysregulated in the MetS. Long-chain fatty acid overexposure produces long-chain acylcarnitine, a trigger of mitochondrial dysfunction in both neurons and Schwan cells [84]. Furthermore, peroxisome proliferator-activated receptors (PPARs) are highly dysregulated in T2D [85]. In addition, oxidized cholesterol – oxysterol – a byproduct of reactive oxygen species and low-density lipoproteins (LDLs), binds to various neuronal cell membrane receptors, including oxidized LDL receptor 1 (LOX1), toll-like receptor 4 (TLR4), and receptor for advanced glycation end products (RAGE), triggering further downstream pro-inflammatory signaling via IL-6, COX-2, and TNF-α [86–88]. Nuclear transcription factors upregulate NF-κB expression and free fatty acid β-oxidation, further adding to a pro-inflammatory state [89].

Toll-like receptors (TLRs) also play a key role in DPN, particularly TLR 4 in pain and TLR 2 and 4 in disease pathogenesis, neuropathy progression, and metabolic dysfunction, particularly lipopolysaccharide binding protein (LPB) and phosphatidylinositol-4,5-bisphosphate 3-kinase catalytic subunit beta (PIK3CB). In a recent study, TLR 2 and 4 knockout mice placed on a high-fat diet were evaluated alongside wild-type mice on a high-fat diet and wild-type mice on a standard diet. TLR 2 and 4 knockout mice developed neuropathy at a later time point compared to high-fat diet wild-type mice [90]. The study suggested that TLR signaling impacts early sensory neuron injury in DPN and is mediated via immune modulation.

Potential Therapeutic Avenues

As much as our understanding of pathogenesis has shed led on DPN complexity, it has also opened the door to more precise therapies (Fig. 8.1). Dietary reversal from a high-fat diet to a standard diet or to a diet consisting of a higher ratio of mono- or polyunsaturated fatty acids (relative to long-chain saturated fatty acids) prevents peripheral neuropathy development and restores IENFD in murine models [11]. In addition, such dietary changes improve thermal responsiveness and large fiber sensory nerve conduction velocities [91]. Pioglitazone, a PPAR-γ agonist, improves DPN in T2D *db/db* mice [92]. In addition, sodium glucose cotransporter 2 (SGLT2) inhibitors represent another area of therapeutic interest. SGLT2 inhibitors increase renal glucose excretion and lower blood glucose levels and are thought to lessen microvascular complications. A 10-week regimen of empagliflozin, an SGLT2 inhibitor, improved neuropathy in streptozotocin-induced T1D mice, but not in *db/db* T2D mice [93]. There was also a trending improvement of empagliflozin on retinopathy in T1D animals, but no effect on nephropathy and no effect on either retinopathy or nephropathy in T2D mice. The study emphasized two important aspects – first, that T1DPN differs in pathology than T2DPN since empagliflozin exerts differential effects and, second, that tissue-specific treatments for the various macrovascular complications could be necessary. With regard to inflammatory targets, polyunsaturated fatty acids inhibit NF-κB activation and nuclear translocation, while both pioglitazone and acipimox offer additional mechanisms that block the NF-κB pathway [12]. Pioglitazone is a PPAR-γ agonist that alters glucose and lipid metabolism gene expression and increases insulin sensitivity. Acipimox is a niacin

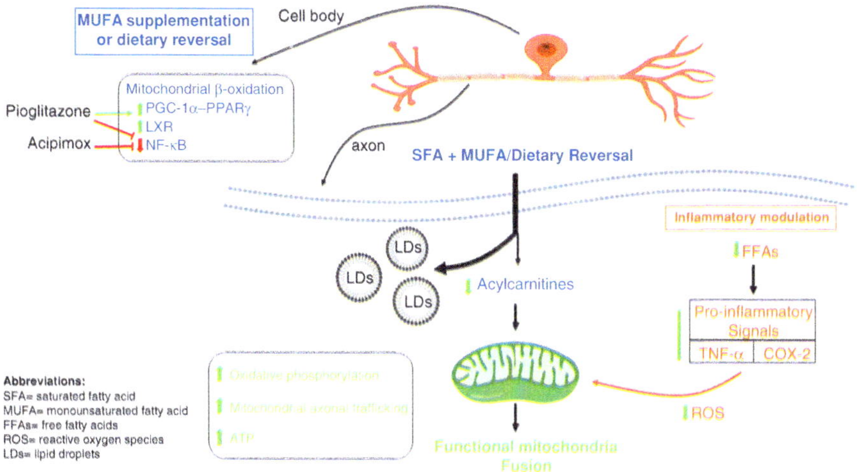

Fig. 8.1 Therapeutic targets identified by dietary intervention and inflammatory pathway studies. Molecular targets were identified in preclinical studies using murine models of dyslipidemia and DPN. Dietary intervention with MUFA supplementation reverses DPN progression potentially through the sequestration of SFAs into LDs in sensory neurons. Dietary reversal from a high-fat diet to a standard diet reduces the level of SFAs in sensory neurons. Subsequent to both dietary intervention paradigms, reduced levels of acylcarnitine improve mitochondrial function and prevent apoptosis. Similarly, stimulation of PGC-1α, PPARγ, and LXR transcription factors by pioglitazone activates FFA β-oxidation, improving mitochondrial function and nerve function. Pioglitazone and acipimox both inhibit NF-κB activation of pro-inflammatory pathways. The reduction in pro-inflammatory TNF-α, IL-6, COX-2, and ROS production prevents downstream mitochondrial dysfunction and sensory neuron apoptosis. (Reproduced with permission from Stino et al. [15])

derivative that inhibits the enzyme triglyceride lipase and reduces fatty acid concentration in the blood. In addition, COX-2 pathway inhibition and *COX-2* gene inactivation as well as heat-shock chaperone protein modulation are other therapies with promising animal model data [94, 95].

Diabetic Peripheral Neuropathy: Pain

Painful Diabetic Peripheral Neuropathy

Painful DPN is highly prevalent in patients with diabetes and often refractory, causing substantial disability and deterioration in quality of life. Much effort has gone into identifying distinguishing risk factors and predispositions between painful and non-painful DPN, including three cross-sectional studies in Britain, Germany/Czech Republic, and Italy, but data was mixed at best [96–100]. The British Pain in Neuropathy Study (PiNS) showed no dependence on BMI, sex, age, or waist-to-hip circumference but did suggest that painful DPN had more profound large and small fiber sensory loss [97]. Patients also tended to be younger and have higher hemoglobin A1c levels.

With regard to managing painful DPN, pharmacotherapy is the treatment mainstay, but the best which can be achieved for a monotherapy is 50% pain relief in only a third of patients [101]. This wide variability in treatment response may in part be due to an underlying heterogeneity in clinical pain phenotypes [102]. This could be one reason several recent randomized clinical trials of painful DPN failed, despite encouraging preclinical and early clinical results [101]. Moreover, most studies use crude summative measures of pain (e.g., numeric rating scales) as primary endpoints. This approach is unlikely to capture the complex and multidimensional nature of pain. The question arises whether it is possible to select more homogenous phenotypic subgroups and/or use an alternative and more salient primary outcome measure, which might increase sensitivity and reveal a positive response in future clinical trials [103]. Currently, there are no biomarkers qualified by the US Food and Drug Administration (FDA) or the European Medicines Agency (EMA) for use in analgesic clinical trials requiring regulatory review [103]. Three types of assessments with established roles in pain research – namely, sensory profile testing, skin biopsy, and brain imaging – could serve as potential candidate biomarkers in analgesic randomized controlled trials.

Sensory Profiling

Quantitative Sensory Profiling

For many years, sensory profiling has been the mainstay for identifying a homogenous subgroup of neuropathic pain patients in clinical pain research. The basis of this approach is that painful symptoms reflect specific pathophysiological mechanisms, which are present to varying degrees in individual patients [102]. Detailed sensory profiling using quantitative sensory testing (QST) can be used to subgroup patients into more homogenous cohorts (pain phenotypes), which could then be targeted with treatments known to act specifically on pathophysiological pathways underlying the phenotypes [104]. QST refers to a battery of standardized, psychophysical tests (e.g., thermal testing, pin prick, pressure algometry, and von Frey filaments) used to assess central and peripheral nervous system sensory function [105]. In DPN, QST has been used for several decades mainly for diagnosing and quantifying the extent of small and large nerve fiber impairment in individuals predominantly with painless DPN. In the context of pain somatosensory phenotyping, a standardized QST protocol was developed by the German Research Network on Neuropathic Pain (DFNS), which includes 12 sensory testing parameters (i.e., cold and warm detection thresholds, paradoxical heat sensations, thermal sensory limen procedure, cold and heat pain thresholds, mechanical detection threshold, mechanical pain threshold, mechanical pain sensitivity, dynamic mechanical allodynia, wind-up ratio, vibration detection threshold, and pressure pain threshold) [106]. The positive and negative results of individual patients are obtained by comparison against a normative QST reference dataset, comprised of age- and sex-stratified healthy individuals [106].

Two Distinct Pain Phenotypes: The Nonirritable and Irritable Nociceptor

Application of the QST technique has shown that there are two distinct subgroups of patients who have particular patterns of sensory symptoms and signs: (1) a predominant differentiation with loss of sensory function (nonirritable nociceptor phenotype) and (2) a relatively preserved small fiber function associated with thermal/mechanical hypersensitivity (irritable nociceptor phenotype) [104]. Using the DFNS protocol, the PiNS reported that the nonirritable nociceptor was the predominant phenotype in painful DPN, while only a minority of patients had the irritable nociceptor phenotype (6.3%) [97]. Nevertheless, a small but significant proportion of patients (15%) did demonstrate signs of sensory gain with dynamic mechanical allodynia, often in combination with hyposensitivity across a range of small and large nerve fiber sensory assessments. The presence of allodynia would suggest that aberrant central processing of sensory inputs has an important role in these patients. Recent studies have demonstrated proof of concept for using sensory profiling to improve clinical trial efficiency by demonstrating that some treatments are more effective in patients with the irritable versus the nonirritable nociceptor phenotype [107–110]. However, most of these studies examined patients with peripheral neuropathy of diverse causes.

Phenotype-Driven Therapeutic Experience in Painful DPN

Examples of studies that focused on painful DPN include an open-label retrospective study using the DFNS protocol, which evaluated key phenotypic differences in sensory profiling associated with response to intravenous lidocaine in patients with severe, intractable painful DPN [111]. Patients with the irritable nociceptor phenotype were more likely to respond to intravenous lidocaine, which inactivates sodium channels, compared to the nonirritable nociceptor phenotype [111]. In fact, dynamic mechanical allodynia and pain summation to repetitive pinprick stimuli were the only evoked "gain-of-function" QST parameters that informed treatment response. The presence of these sensory gain parameters suggests aberrant central processing with hyperexcitable neurons driven by abnormal sodium channel regulation, generating ectopic impulses and amplifying afferent sensory inputs. In another painful DPN study by Campbell et al. of topical clonidine, sensory profiling was performed using the capsaicin challenge test [112]. The post hoc analysis demonstrated a significant reduction in pain in the patient subgroup with increased spontaneous pain following cutaneous capsaicin administration, indicating the presence of functioning and sensitized nociceptors. Bouhassira et al. published post hoc analysis data of treatment response based on sensory profiling using the Neuropathic Pain Symptom Inventory (NPSI) questionnaire from the Combination vs Monotherapy of Pregabalin and Duloxetine in Diabetic Neuropathy (COMBO-DN) study [113]. This study examined the effect of high-dose duloxetine, a serotonin noradrenaline reuptake inhibitor, or pregabalin, a calcium channel blocker, as monotherapy versus combined pregabalin and duloxetine for painful DPN. The investigators showed that adding pregabalin (300 mg) to duloxetine (60 mg) improved the dimensions of "pressing pain" and "evoked pain" more significantly. On the other hand, increasing duloxetine from 60 mg to 120 mg daily improved the dimension "paraesthesia/dysesthesia" to a greater extent.

Sensory Phenotyping to Predict Therapeutic Response

In a randomized, double-blind, placebo-controlled, and phenotype-stratified study of patients with painful DPN, Demant et al. reported that oxcarbazepine was more efficacious for relief of peripheral neuropathic pain in patients with the irritable vs the nonirritable nociceptor phenotype (Fig. 8.2). Based on this and other recent studies, current opinion with regard to neuropathic pain clinical trials recommends a detailed sensory profiling of participants at baseline; and even if there is no significant separation of a drug with placebo, a subgroup analysis can be performed to see if the drug was efficacious in a particular subgroup. If there is a clear signal that this

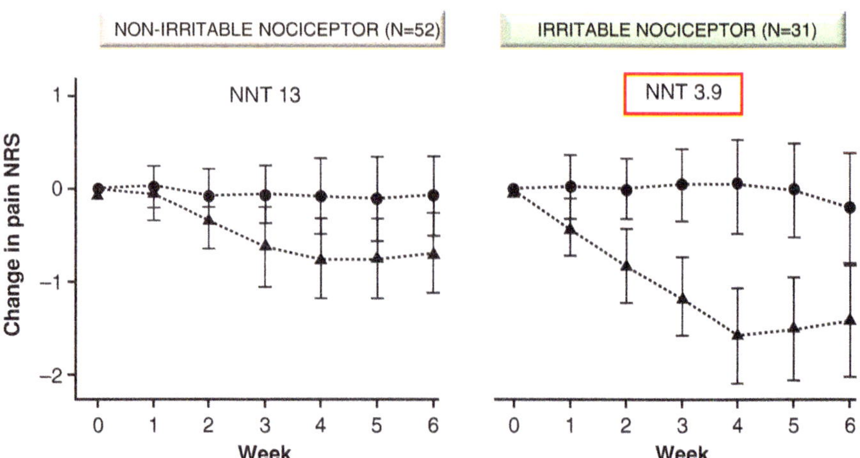

Fig. 8.2 Effect of oxcarbazepine in painful DPN depends on pain phenotype based on detailed quantitative sensory testing. Nonirritable nociceptor phenotype comprise of patients with deafferentiation dominated by sensory loss. Patients with the irritable nociceptor have preserved small fiber function (cold, warm, and pinprick sensation) and contact hypersensitivity (e.g., allodynia). (Adapted from Demant [114])

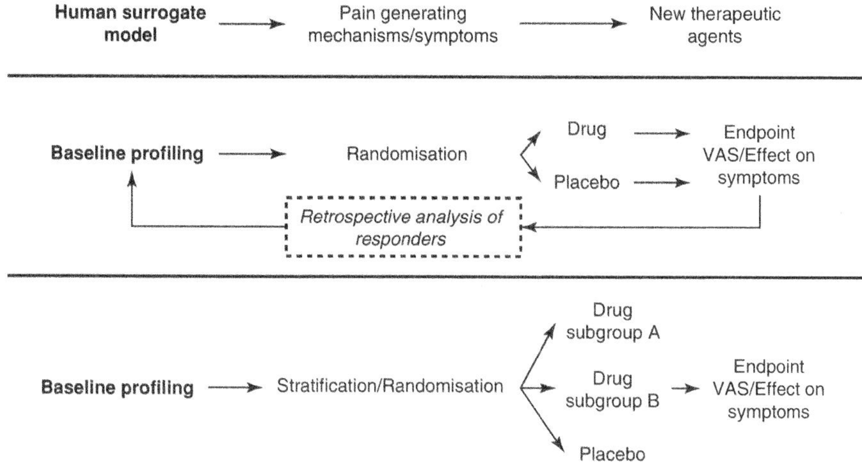

Fig. 8.3 Designing studies to inform personalized pharmacological treatment of neuropathic pain

was the case, a further, adequately powered, phenotype-stratified trial would be designed (Fig. 8.3).

Sensory profiling can also identify subgroups with altered endogenous pain modulation to predict treatment outcomes of drugs and other interventions that affect a given mechanism. In a study of pain modulation in DPN, individuals were assessed using QST for conditioned pain modulation (CPM), a psychophysical paradigm in which central pain inhibition is measured via the phenomenon of "pain inhibiting pain," via the simultaneous administration of a conditioning painful stimulus at a distant body site. The pain in participants with abnormal CPM was more receptive to duloxetine, which is believed to increase descending inhibitory pain pathway activation, than individuals with normal pain modulation, although there was no comparison to placebo in this open-label study [115].

Taken together, these studies support the notion that mechanism-based approaches to pain management may be feasible in painful DPN. However, in an elegant mechanistic study, Haroutounian et al. examined 14 patients with neuropathic pain of mixed etiology [unilateral foot pain from nerve injury ($n = 7$) and distal polyneuropathy ($n = 7$)] to determine the contribution of primary afferent input in maintaining peripheral neuropathic pain [116]. Each patient underwent randomized ultrasound-guided peripheral nerve block with lidocaine versus intravenous lidocaine infusion. They found that peripheral afferent input was critical for maintaining neuropathic pain, but improvement in evoked hypersensitivity was not related to improvements in spontaneous pain intensity. This suggests that further studies are needed to rationalize sensory phenotyping in order to optimize clinical trial outcomes in painful DPN. Moreover, given the rarity of the irritable nociceptor phenotype, as determined by QST, a single assessment modality may be unlikely to help stratify patients, and combining with additional modalities may be necessary (e.g., brain imaging).

Brain Imaging in Painful Diabetic Peripheral Neuropathy

Recent advances in neuroimaging provide us with unique insights into the human central nervous system in chronic pain conditions (Fig. 8.4) [118]. We now have a better understanding how the brain modulates nociceptive inputs to generate the pain experience and how this is disrupted in patients with painful DPN. However, to date, brain imaging serves mainly as a research tool, with minimal direct application in clinical trials for pain or clinical practice. While mechanistic approaches that require carefully evaluating specific responses to guide therapy have significant appeal (e.g., cold, heat, von Frey, etc.), in practice, these are time-consuming and may be difficult to implement in busy clinical practices. Furthermore, these are psychophysical measures which rely on patient responses and may be subjective and biased. Sensory profiling methods also do not capture the complex and multidimensional pain experience, which affects emotional and cognitive processing in addition to sensory processing. For example, chronic pain patients often undergo neuropsychological changes, which include changes in emotion and motivation or changes in cognition [119]. Chronic pain may also arise after the onset of depression, even in patients without a prior history of pain or depression. Collectively, these clinical insights suggest a better strategy for assessing and treating painful DPN, given it is a chronic disease of dynamic process (e.g., evolution of comorbid phenotypes such as anxiety or depression), which is not easily reversed in most patients. It is important to determine specific targets that are relevant to pain across individuals, because modulating activation in these targets may provide evidence that a compound engages a target or attenuates nociceptive processing.

Structural and functional cortical plasticity is a fundamental property of the human central nervous system, which can adjust to nerve injury. However, it can have maladaptive consequences, possibly resulting in chronic pain. Studies using structural magnetic resonance (MR) neuroimaging have demonstrated a clear reduction in both spinal cord cross-sectional area [120] and primary somatosensory cortex (S1) gray matter volume in patients with DPN [121]. These findings are supported by studies in other pain conditions, which have also reported dynamic structural and functional plasticity with profound effects on the brain in patients with neuropathic pain. More recently, it has been demonstrated how brain structural and functional changes are related to painful DPN clinical phenotypes [122]. Patients with the painful insensate phenotype have a more pronounced reduction in S1 cortical thickness and a remapping of S1 sensory processing compared to painful DPN subjects with relatively preserved sensation [122]. Furthermore, the extent to which S1 cortical structure and function is altered is related to the severity of neuropathy and the magnitude of self-reported pain. These data suggest a dynamic plasticity of the brain in DPN driven by the neuropathic process and may ultimately determine an individual's clinical pain phenotypes.

Over the last decade, resting-state functional MR imaging (RS-fMRI) – a quick and simple noninvasive technique – has become an increasingly appealing way to examine spontaneous brain activity in individuals, without relying on external

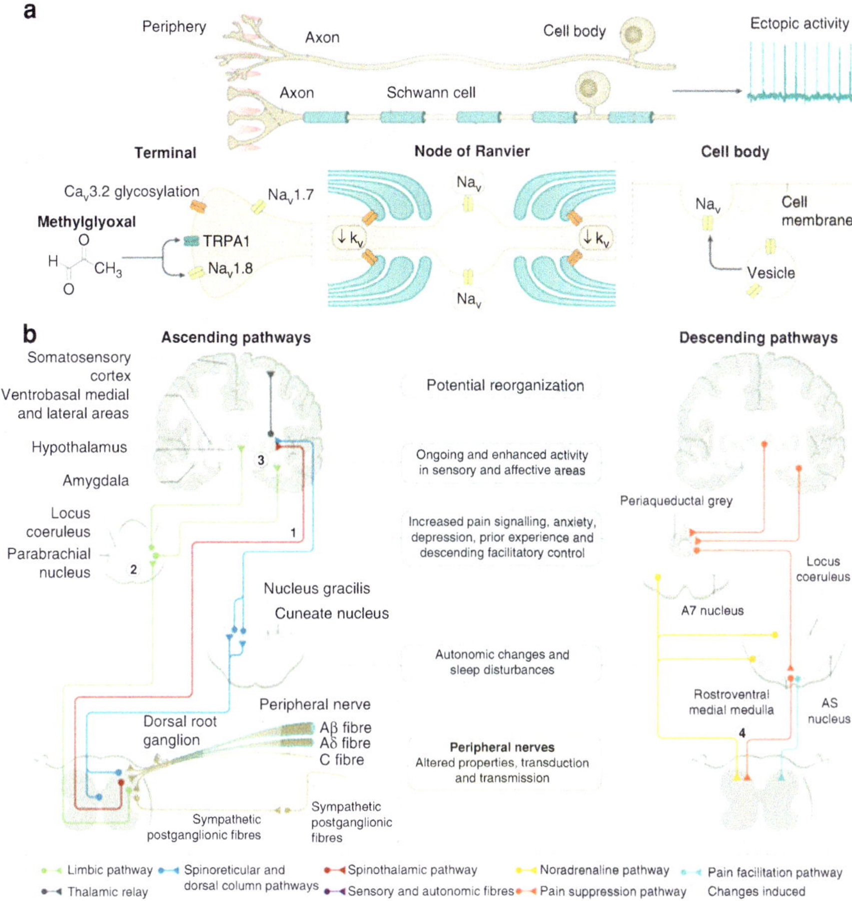

Fig. 8.4 Central and peripheral mechanisms contributing to neuropathic pain in diabetic neuropathy. (**a**) Several alterations to peripheral and central neurons contribute to the pathophysiology of painful diabetic neuropathy. Ion channels at the terminals of nociceptors can undergo glycation through the addition of methylglyoxal to form advanced glycation end products (AGEs), which can contribute to gain of function of these channels and neuronal hyperexcitability. Changes at the perikaryon include increased expression of voltage-gated sodium channels, such as Na$_v$1.8, which can lead to hyperexcitability. In myelinated axons, the expression of shaker-type potassium (K$_v$) channels is reduced, which can also contribute to hyperexcitability. Hyperexcitability of neurons leads to increased stimulus responses and ectopic neuronal activity, leading to excessive nociceptive input to the spinal cord. In the spinal cord, microglia become activated and further enhance excitability within the dorsal horn. (**b**) Several ascending pathways are involved in pain perception and the psychological changes associated with pain, for example, the spinothalamic pathway (1), which is involved in pain perception, and the spinoreticular tract. In addition, ascending pathways that travel via the parabrachial nucleus (2) to the hypothalamus and amygdala (3) are involved in autonomic function, fear, and anxiety. Descending pathways inhibit or facilitate the transmission of nociceptive information at the spinal level (4). Changes induced by peripheral neuropathy are shown in boxes. (Reproduced with permission from Feldman et al. [117])

stimulation tasks. During a typical RS-fMRI examination, the hemodynamic response to spontaneous neuronal activity (blood oxygen level-dependent (BOLD)) signal is acquired while subjects are instructed to simply rest in the MR scanner [123]. The data acquired is used in brain mapping to evaluate regional interactions or functional connectivity, which occur in a resting state. Most studies use a machine learning approach to identify patterns of functional connectivity, which differentiates patients from controls. RS-fMRI experiments in painful DPN have reported greater thalamic-insula functional connectivity and decreased thalamic-somatosensory cortical functional connectivity in patients with the irritable versus nonirritable nociceptor phenotype (Fig. 8.5) [111]. There was a significant positive correlation between thalamic-insula functional connectivities with self-reported pain scores [111]. Conversely, there was a more significant reduction in thalamic-somatosensory cortical functional connectivity in those with more severe neuropathy. This demonstrates how RS-fMRI measures of functional connectivity relate to

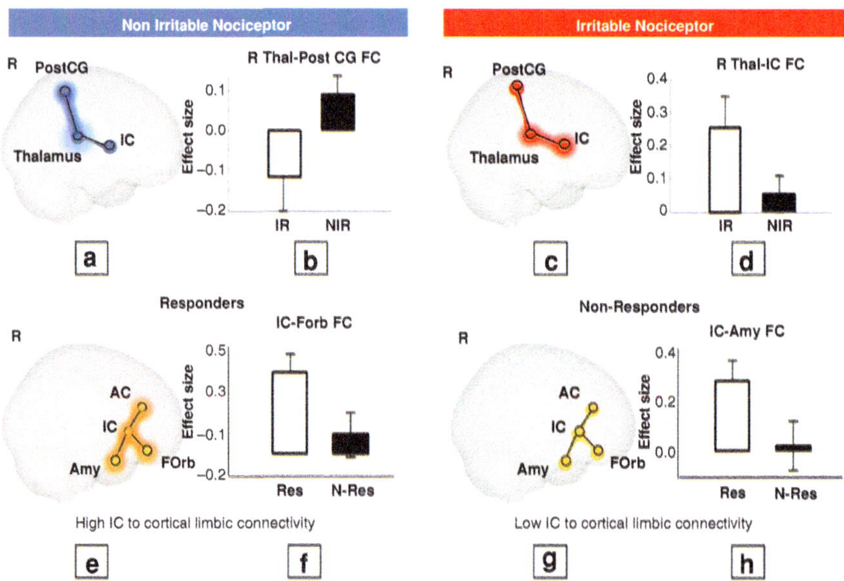

Fig. 8.5 Right view of resting-state functional connectivity in painful diabetic peripheral neuropathy (DPN) patients with the nonirritable nociceptor phenotype (**a**) and irritable nociceptor phenotype (**c**); R, right; IC, insula cortex. Bar charts demonstrating effect size of differences in thalamic-insula (**d**) and thalamic-postcentral (**b**) cortical functional connectivity between study groups. (*IR* irritable nociceptor, *NIR* nonirritable nociceptor. Adapted from Teh et al. Somatosensory network functional connectivity differentiates clinical pain phenotypes in diabetic neuropathy. Diabetologia. 2021;64(6):1412–21). Right view of insula cortical resting-state functional connectivity in responders (**e**) and nonresponders (**g**) to intravenous lidocaine treatment. *IC* insula cortex; *Amy* amygdala; *AC* anterior cingulate gyrus; *FOrb* orbital frontal cortex. Bar charts demonstrating the effect size of differences in resting-state functional connectivity in intravenous lidocaine responders and nonresponders between the insula cortex and the orbital frontal cortex (**f**) and amygdala (**h**) on the right. (Adapted from Wilkinson et al. [111])

both the somatic and non-somatic assessments of painful DPN. In one study, using a machine learning approach to integrate anatomical and functional connectivity data achieved an accuracy of 92% and sensitivity of 90%, indicating good overall performance [111]. Multimodal MR imaging combining structural and RS-fMRI has also been used to predict treatment response in painful DPN. Responders to intravenous lidocaine treatment have significantly greater S1 cortical volume and greater functional connectivity between the insular cortex and corticolimbic system compared to nonresponders (Fig. 8.5) [111]. The insular cortex plays a pivotal role in processing the emotion and cognitive dimensions of the chronic pain experience. The corticolimbic circuits have also long been implicated in reward, decision-making, and fear learning. Hence, these findings suggest that this network may have a role in determining treatment response in painful DPN.

Using advanced multimodal MR neuroimaging, a number of studies have demonstrated alterations in pain processing brain regions, which relate to clinical pain phenotype, treatment response, and behavioral/psychological factors impacted by pain. Taken together, these assessments could serve as a possible central pain signature for painful DPN. The challenge now is to apply this potential pain biomarker at an individual level in order to demonstrate clinical utility. To this end, applying machine learning [124] to leverage brain imaging features from a quick 6-minute RS-fMRI scan to classify individual patients into different clinical pain phenotypes is appealing. Future studies should externally validate and optimize current models in larger patient cohorts to examine if/how such models can be used as biomarkers in clinical trials of pain therapeutics. Although many of the findings described are consistent with neuroimaging studies in other chronic pain conditions, it is difficult to assess convergence of findings across a number of relatively small cohort studies employing different analytical methods to derive complex models involving a large number of distributed brain regions [125]. These are important limitations that are being addressed with (1) a number of large-scale multicenter studies in progress or in preparation (MAPP consortium [126] and placebo imaging consortium [127]) and (2) several consensus statements by key stakeholders, promoting standardized approaches and reporting and transparent/sharable models.

Diabetic Peripheral Neuropathy: Future Directions and Moving Toward Precise Treatments

The gap between pathogenic animal models and human data is large (and growing), and how it all fits together to form a coherent, cumulative understanding of DPN is complex and multifaceted. To promote convergence, human studies should increasingly use results and concepts from animal studies, and vice versa, to constrain and corroborate clinical study findings to move the field toward biomarkers with translational applications. Moreover, despite the recent aforementioned advances in therapeutic avenues, it is becoming increasingly clear that one approach alone will not capture all the variance in diagnostic, prognostic, and biomarkers in DPN. A precision medicine approach, rather, will improve the development of multimodal DPN biomarkers, which can enable earlier diagnosis, before irreversible nerve damage occurs, and improve the overall sensitivity and specificity of preventive and treatment strategies (Fig. 8.6).

Precision medicine leverages an individual's variation in genes, environment, and lifestyle to define more personalized approaches of disease prevention and management. Initial insight into this strategy in diabetes derives from recent efforts in diabetic kidney disease, because kidney disease standard of care often involves collecting blood, urine, and biopsy tissue, which are amenable to pathologic, transcriptomic, proteomic, and metabolomic analyses [128–130]. As such, the Kidney Precision Initiative was launched to combine these assessments with deep clinical phenotyping over a 10-year period for individuals with kidney diseases, including diabetic nephropathy, to ultimately inform diagnosis, risk assessment, and personalized treatment opportunities [131].

Applying a similar precision medicine strategy to DPN will require developing high-throughput profiling datasets, such as the currently available genome-wide association studies (GWAS) from well-characterized clinical cohorts like DCCT/EDIC, which supported recent nephropathy risk assessments [132, 133]. DPN

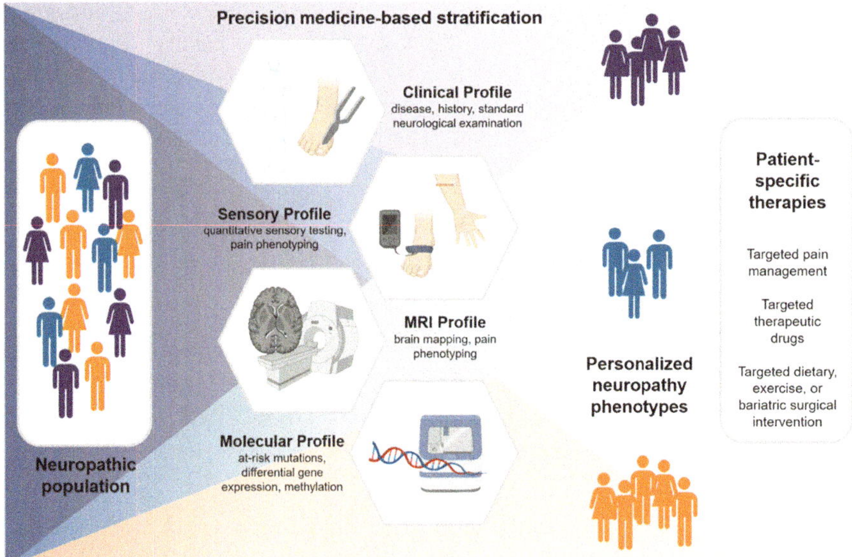

Fig. 8.6 Precision medicine-based approach to diabetic peripheral neuropathy. A precision-based medicine approach to DPN calls for the subclassification of the general DPN population into more specific subgroups, classified by clinical and pain phenotype. Such classification is guided by patient clinical presentation, QST, functional MR imaging, and genetic profile, which lead to more targeted pain management and disease-modifying interventions. (Created in part with BioRender.com)

likewise has been the focus of recent GWAS [134, 135] and epigenomic assessments [136] to establish and understand polygenic risk and mechanisms. Pairing such data with robust deep clinical phenotyping and advanced machine learning has the power to offer precision medicine-based metadata to support personalized pharmacologic therapies and improve diagnostic and prognostic strategies, risk assessment, and clinical trial designs, which account for both DPN genetics and clinical classification. Importantly, the value of subject stratification based on clinical subtypes, neuroimaging, and genetic data is beginning to be explored in painful DPN [137, 138], as discussed above. Thus, given the dichotomy of pathogenic differences in T1DPN and T2DPN, the prevalence and variability of neuropathy in obesity, prediabetes, and MetS and the occurrence of both painful and painless phenotypes, precision medicine holds great promise for more targeted, effective treatments for DPN.

Acknowledgements LD, AMS, SAS, and ELF are supported by the NeuroNetwork for Emerging Therapies at the University of Michigan

References

1. Callaghan BC, Gao L, Li Y, Zhou X, Reynolds E, Banerjee M, et al. Diabetes and obesity are the main metabolic drivers of peripheral neuropathy. Ann Clin Transl Neurol. 2018;5(4):397–405.
2. Callaghan BC, Xia R, Reynolds E, Banerjee M, Rothberg AE, Burant CF, et al. Association between metabolic syndrome components and polyneuropathy in an obese population. JAMA Neurol. 2016;73(12):1468–76.
3. Callaghan BC, Xia R, Banerjee M, de Rekeneire N, Harris TB, Newman AB, et al. Metabolic syndrome components are associated with symptomatic polyneuropathy independent of glycemic status. Diabetes Care. 2016;39(5):801–7.
4. Hanewinckel R, Drenthen J, Ligthart S, Dehghan A, Franco OH, Hofman A, et al. Metabolic syndrome is related to polyneuropathy and impaired peripheral nerve function: a prospective population-based cohort study. J Neurol Neurosurg Psychiatry. 2016;87(12):1336–42.
5. Lu B, Hu J, Wen J, Zhang Z, Zhou L, Li Y, et al. Determination of peripheral neuropathy prevalence and associated factors in Chinese subjects with diabetes and pre-diabetes - ShangHai diabetic neuRopathy epidemiology and molecular genetics study (SH-DREAMS). PLoS One. 2013;8(4):e61053.
6. Schlesinger S, Herder C, Kannenberg JM, Huth C, Carstensen-Kirberg M, Rathmann W, et al. General and abdominal obesity and incident distal sensorimotor polyneuropathy: insights into inflammatory biomarkers as potential mediators in the KORA F4/FF4 cohort. Diabetes Care. 2019;42(2):240–7.
7. Callaghan BC, Hur J, Feldman EL. Diabetic neuropathy: one disease or two? Curr Opin Neurol. 2012;25(5):536–41.
8. Eid S, Sas KM, Abcouwer SF, Feldman EL, Gardner TW, Pennathur S, et al. New insights into the mechanisms of diabetic complications: role of lipids and lipid metabolism. Diabetologia. 2019;62(9):1539–49.
9. Kazamel M, Stino AM, Smith AG. Metabolic syndrome and peripheral neuropathy. Muscle Nerve. 2021;63(3):285–93.
10. Smith AG, Rose K, Singleton JR. Idiopathic neuropathy patients are at high risk for metabolic syndrome. J Neurol Sci. 2008;273(1–2):25–8.

11. Hinder LM, O'Brien PD, Hayes JM, Backus C, Solway AP, Sims-Robinson C, et al. Dietary reversal of neuropathy in a murine model of prediabetes and metabolic syndrome. Dis Model Mech. 2017;10(6):717–25.
12. Hur J, Dauch JR, Hinder LM, Hayes JM, Backus C, Pennathur S, et al. The metabolic syndrome and microvascular complications in a murine model of type 2 diabetes. Diabetes. 2015;64(9):3294–304.
13. McGregor BA, Eid S, Rumora AE, Murdock B, Guo K, de Anda-Jáuregui G, et al. Conserved transcriptional signatures in human and murine diabetic peripheral neuropathy. Sci Rep. 2018;8(1):17678.
14. O'Brien PD, Hinder LM, Rumora AE, Hayes JM, Dauch JR, Backus C, et al. Juvenile murine models of prediabetes and type 2 diabetes develop neuropathy. Dis Model Mech. 2018;18:11(12).
15. Stino AM, Rumora AE, Kim B, Feldman EL. Evolving concepts on the role of dyslipidemia, bioenergetics, and inflammation in the pathogenesis and treatment of diabetic peripheral neuropathy. J Peripher Nerv Syst JPNS. 2020;25(2):76–84.
16. Kobayashi M, Zochodne DW. Diabetic polyneuropathy: bridging the translational gap. J Peripher Nerv Syst JPNS. 2020;25(2):66–75.
17. Malik RA, Calcutt NA. Translating diabetic peripheral neuropathy. J Peripher Nerv Syst JPNS. 2020;25(2):64–5.
18. Dyck PJ, Kratz KM, Karnes JL, Litchy WJ, Klein R, Pach JM, et al. The prevalence by staged severity of various types of diabetic neuropathy, retinopathy, and nephropathy in a population-based cohort: the Rochester diabetic neuropathy study. Neurology. 1993;43(4):817–24.
19. Franklin GM, Kahn LB, Baxter J, Marshall JA, Hamman RF. Sensory neuropathy in non-insulin-dependent diabetes mellitus. The San Luis Valley diabetes study. Am J Epidemiol. 1990;131(4):633–43.
20. Partanen J, Niskanen L, Lehtinen J, Mervaala E, Siitonen O, Uusitupa M. Natural history of peripheral neuropathy in patients with non-insulin-dependent diabetes mellitus. N Engl J Med. 1995;333(2):89–94.
21. Pop-Busui R, Boulton AJM, Feldman EL, Bril V, Freeman R, Malik RA, et al. Diabetic neuropathy: a position statement by the American Diabetes Association. Diabetes Care. 2017;40(1):136–54.
22. Ang L, Jaiswal M, Martin C, Pop-Busui R. Glucose control and diabetic neuropathy: lessons from recent large clinical trials. Curr Diab Rep. 2014;14(9):528.
23. Martin CL, Albers JW, Pop-Busui R, DCCT/EDIC Research Group. Neuropathy and related findings in the diabetes control and complications trial/epidemiology of diabetes interventions and complications study. Diabetes Care. 2014;37(1):31–8.
24. Boulton AJ, Knight G, Drury J, Ward JD. The prevalence of symptomatic, diabetic neuropathy in an insulin-treated population. Diabetes Care. 1985;8(2):125–8.
25. Control D, Complications Trial Research Group, Nathan DM, Genuth S, Lachin J, Cleary P, Crofford O, et al. The effect of intensive treatment of diabetes on the development and progression of long-term complications in insulin-dependent diabetes mellitus. N Engl J Med. 1993;329(14):977–86.
26. Albers JW, Herman WH, Pop-Busui R, Feldman EL, Martin CL, Cleary PA, et al. Effect of prior intensive insulin treatment during the diabetes Control and complications trial (DCCT) on peripheral neuropathy in type 1 diabetes during the epidemiology of diabetes interventions and complications (EDIC) study. Diabetes Care. 2010;33(5):1090–6.
27. Callaghan BC, Little AA, Feldman EL, Hughes RAC. Enhanced glucose control for preventing and treating diabetic neuropathy. Cochrane Database Syst Rev. 2012;6:CD007543.
28. Duckworth W, Abraira C, Moritz T, Reda D, Emanuele N, Reaven PD, et al. Glucose control and vascular complications in veterans with type 2 diabetes. N Engl J Med. 2009;360(2):129–39.

29. Ismail-Beigi F, Craven T, Banerji MA, Basile J, Calles J, Cohen RM, et al. Effect of intensive treatment of hyperglycaemia on microvascular outcomes in type 2 diabetes: an analysis of the ACCORD randomised trial. Lancet Lond Engl. 2010;376(9739):419–30.
30. Tesfaye S, Vileikyte L, Rayman G, Sindrup SH, Perkins BA, Baconja M, et al. Painful diabetic peripheral neuropathy: consensus recommendations on diagnosis, assessment and management. Diabetes Metab Res Rev. 2011;27(7):629–38.
31. Smith AG, Singleton JR. Obesity and hyperlipidemia are risk factors for early diabetic neuropathy. J Diabetes Complicat. 2013;27(5):436–42.
32. Andersson C, Guttorp P, Särkkä A. Discovering early diabetic neuropathy from epidermal nerve fiber patterns. Stat Med. 2016;35(24):4427–42.
33. Devigili G, Tugnoli V, Penza P, Camozzi F, Lombardi R, Melli G, et al. The diagnostic criteria for small fibre neuropathy: from symptoms to neuropathology. Brain J Neurol. 2008;131(Pt 7):1912–25.
34. Vinik AI, Erbas T. Diabetic autonomic neuropathy. Handb Clin Neurol. 2013;117:279–94.
35. Moore JX, Chaudhary N, Akinyemiju T. Metabolic syndrome prevalence by race/ethnicity and sex in the United States, National Health and nutrition examination survey, 1988-2012. Prev Chronic Dis. 2017;14:E24.
36. Christensen DH, Knudsen ST, Gylfadottir SS, Christensen LB, Nielsen JS, Beck-Nielsen H, et al. Metabolic factors, lifestyle habits, and possible polyneuropathy in early type 2 diabetes: a Nationwide study of 5,249 patients in the Danish Centre for Strategic Research in type 2 diabetes (DD2) cohort. Diabetes Care. 2020;43(6):1266–75.
37. Callaghan BC, Reynolds E, Banerjee M, Chant E, Villegas-Umana E, Feldman EL. Central obesity is associated with neuropathy in the severely obese. Mayo Clin Proc. 2020;95(7):1342–53.
38. Reynolds EL, Callaghan BC, Banerjee M, Feldman EL, Viswanathan V. The metabolic drivers of neuropathy in India. J Diabetes Complicat. 2020;34(10):107653.
39. Hughes RAC, Umapathi T, Gray IA, Gregson NA, Noori M, Pannala AS, et al. A controlled investigation of the cause of chronic idiopathic axonal polyneuropathy. Brain J Neurol. 2004;127(Pt 8):1723–30.
40. Wiggin TD, Sullivan KA, Pop-Busui R, Amato A, Sima AAF, Feldman EL. Elevated triglycerides correlate with progression of diabetic neuropathy. Diabetes. 2009;58(7):1634–40.
41. Callaghan BC, Feldman E, Liu J, Kerber K, Pop-Busui R, Moffet H, et al. Triglycerides and amputation risk in patients with diabetes: ten-year follow-up in the DISTANCE study. Diabetes Care. 2011;34(3):635–40.
42. Smith AG, Russell J, Feldman EL, Goldstein J, Peltier A, Smith S, et al. Lifestyle intervention for pre-diabetic neuropathy. Diabetes Care. 2006;29(6):1294–9.
43. Look AHEAD Research Group. Effects of a long-term lifestyle modification programme on peripheral neuropathy in overweight or obese adults with type 2 diabetes: the look AHEAD study. Diabetologia. 2017;60(6):980–8.
44. Kristensen FP, Christensen DH, Callaghan BC, Kahlert J, Knudsen ST, Sindrup SH, et al. Statin therapy and risk of polyneuropathy in type 2 diabetes: a Danish cohort study. Diabetes Care. 2020;43(12):2945–52.
45. Rajamani K, Colman PG, Li LP, Best JD, Voysey M, D'Emden MC, et al. Effect of fenofibrate on amputation events in people with type 2 diabetes mellitus (FIELD study): a prespecified analysis of a randomised controlled trial. Lancet Lond Engl. 2009;373(9677):1780–8.
46. Müller-Stich BP, Fischer L, Kenngott HG, Gondan M, Senft J, Clemens G, et al. Gastric bypass leads to improvement of diabetic neuropathy independent of glucose normalization--results of a prospective cohort study (DiaSurg 1 study). Ann Surg. 2013;258(5):760–5; discussion 765-766.
47. Davis TME, Yeap BB, Davis WA, Bruce DG. Lipid-lowering therapy and peripheral sensory neuropathy in type 2 diabetes: the Fremantle diabetes study. Diabetologia. 2008;51(4):562–6.

48. Sjöström L, Peltonen M, Jacobson P, Sjöström CD, Karason K, Wedel H, et al. Bariatric surgery and long-term cardiovascular events. JAMA. 2012;307(1):56–65.
49. Ziegler D, Rathmann W, Dickhaus T, Meisinger C, Mielck A, KORA Study Group. Neuropathic pain in diabetes, prediabetes and normal glucose tolerance: the MONICA/ KORA Augsburg surveys S2 and S3. Pain Med Malden Mass. 2009;10(2):393–400.
50. Lee CC, Perkins BA, Kayaniyil S, Harris SB, Retnakaran R, Gerstein HC, et al. Peripheral neuropathy and nerve dysfunction in individuals at high risk for type 2 diabetes: the PROMISE cohort. Diabetes Care. 2015;38(5):793–800.
51. Sumner CJ, Sheth S, Griffin JW, Cornblath DR, Polydefkis M. The spectrum of neuropathy in diabetes and impaired glucose tolerance. Neurology. 2003;60(1):108–11.
52. Pourhamidi K, Dahlin LB, Englund E, Rolandsson O. No difference in small or large nerve fiber function between individuals with normal glucose tolerance and impaired glucose tolerance. Diabetes Care. 2013;36(4):962–4.
53. Thaisetthawatkul P, Lyden E, Americo Fernandes J, Herrmann DN. Prediabetes, diabetes, metabolic syndrome, and small fiber neuropathy. Muscle Nerve. 2020;61(4):475–9.
54. Dyck PJ, Clark VM, Overland CJ, Davies JL, Pach JM, Dyck PJB, et al. Impaired glycemia and diabetic polyneuropathy: the OC IG survey. Diabetes Care. 2012;35(3):584–91.
55. Kassardjian CD, Dyck PJB, Davies JL, Carter RE, Dyck PJ. Does prediabetes cause small fiber sensory polyneuropathy? Does it matter? J Neurol Sci. 2015;355(1–2):196–8.
56. American Diabetes Association. 13. children and adolescents: standards of medical care in diabetes-2020. Diabetes Care. 2020;43(Suppl 1):S163–82.
57. Divers J, Mayer-Davis EJ, Lawrence JM, Isom S, Dabelea D, Dolan L, et al. Trends in incidence of type 1 and type 2 diabetes among youths - selected counties and Indian reservations, United States, 2002-2015. MMWR Morb Mortal Wkly Rep. 2020;69(6):161–5.
58. Pettitt DJ, Talton J, Dabelea D, Divers J, Imperatore G, Lawrence JM, et al. Prevalence of diabetes in U.S. youth in 2009: the SEARCH for diabetes in youth study. Diabetes Care. 2014;37(2):402–8.
59. Dabelea D, Mayer-Davis EJ, Saydah S, Imperatore G, Linder B, Divers J, et al. Prevalence of type 1 and type 2 diabetes among children and adolescents from 2001 to 2009. JAMA. 2014;311(17):1778–86.
60. Mayer-Davis EJ, Lawrence JM, Dabelea D, Divers J, Isom S, Dolan L, et al. Incidence trends of type 1 and type 2 diabetes among youths, 2002-2012. N Engl J Med. 2017;376(15):1419–29.
61. Patterson CC, Gyürüs E, Rosenbauer J, Cinek O, Neu A, Schober E, et al. Trends in childhood type 1 diabetes incidence in Europe during 1989-2008: evidence of non-uniformity over time in rates of increase. Diabetologia. 2012;55(8):2142–7.
62. Zeitler P. Progress in understanding youth-onset type 2 diabetes in the United States: recent lessons from clinical trials. World J Pediatr WJP. 2019;15(4):315–21.
63. Imperatore G, Boyle JP, Thompson TJ, Case D, Dabelea D, Hamman RF, et al. Projections of type 1 and type 2 diabetes burden in the U.S. population aged <20 years through 2050: dynamic modeling of incidence, mortality, and population growth. Diabetes Care. 2012;35(12):2515–20.
64. Maser RE, Steenkiste AR, Dorman JS, Nielsen VK, Bass EB, Manjoo Q, et al. Epidemiological correlates of diabetic neuropathy. Report from Pittsburgh epidemiology of diabetes complications study. Diabetes. 1989;38(11):1456–61.
65. Tesfaye S, Stevens LK, Stephenson JM, Fuller JH, Plater M, Ionescu-Tirgoviste C, et al. Prevalence of diabetic peripheral neuropathy and its relation to glycaemic control and potential risk factors: the EURODIAB IDDM complications study. Diabetologia. 1996;39(11):1377–84.
66. Olsen BS, Johannesen J, Sjølie AK, Borch-Johnsen K, Hougarrdss P, Thorsteinsson B, et al. Metabolic control and prevalence of microvascular complications in young Danish patients with type 1 diabetes mellitus. Danish study Group of Diabetes in childhood. Diabet Med J Br Diabet Assoc. 1999;16(1):79–85.

67. Nelson D, Mah JK, Adams C, Hui S, Crawford S, Darwish H, et al. Comparison of conventional and non-invasive techniques for the early identification of diabetic neuropathy in children and adolescents with type 1 diabetes. Pediatr Diabetes. 2006;7(6):305–10.
68. Eppens MC, Craig ME, Cusumano J, Hing S, Chan AKF, Howard NJ, et al. Prevalence of diabetes complications in adolescents with type 2 compared with type 1 diabetes. Diabetes Care. 2006;29(6):1300–6.
69. Jaiswal M, Divers J, Dabelea D, Isom S, Bell RA, Martin CL, et al. Prevalence of and risk factors for diabetic peripheral neuropathy in youth with type 1 and type 2 diabetes: SEARCH for diabetes in youth study. Diabetes Care. 2017;40(9):1226–32.
70. Moser J, Lipman T, Langdon DR, Bevans KB. Development of a youth-report measure of DPN symptoms: conceptualization and content validation. J Clin Transl Endocrinol. 2017;9:55–60.
71. Arslanian S, Bacha F, Grey M, Marcus MD, White NH, Zeitler P. Evaluation and Management of Youth-Onset Type 2 diabetes: a position statement by the American Diabetes Association. Diabetes Care. 2018;41(12):2648–68.
72. NCD Risk Factor Collaboration (NCD-RisC). Worldwide trends in body-mass index, underweight, overweight, and obesity from 1975 to 2016: a pooled analysis of 2416 population-based measurement studies in 128·9 million children, adolescents, and adults. Lancet Lond Engl. 2017;390(10113):2627–42.
73. Janssen I, Katzmarzyk PT, Boyce WF, Vereecken C, Mulvihill C, Roberts C, et al. Comparison of overweight and obesity prevalence in school-aged youth from 34 countries and their relationships with physical activity and dietary patterns. Obes Rev Off J Int Assoc Study Obes. 2005;6(2):123–32.
74. Akinci G, Savelieff MG, Gallagher G, Callaghan BC, Feldman EL. Diabetic neuropathy in children and youth: new and emerging risk factors. Pediatr Diabetes. 2021;22(2):132–47.
75. Thamotharampillai K, Chan AKF, Bennetts B, Craig ME, Cusumano J, Silink M, et al. Decline in neurophysiological function after 7 years in an adolescent diabetic cohort and the role of aldose reductase gene polymorphisms. Diabetes Care. 2006;29(9):2053–7.
76. Monastiriotis C, Papanas N, Trypsianis G, Karanikola K, Veletza S, Maltezos E. The ε4 allele of the APOE gene is associated with more severe peripheral neuropathy in type 2 diabetic patients. Angiology. 2013;64(6):451–5.
77. Rudofsky G, Schroedter A, Schlotterer A, Voron'ko OE, Schlimme M, Tafel J, et al. Functional polymorphisms of UCP2 and UCP3 are associated with a reduced prevalence of diabetic neuropathy in patients with type 1 diabetes. Diabetes Care. 2006;29(1):89–94.
78. Strokov IA, Bursa TR, Drepa OI, Zotova EV, Nosikov VV, Ametov AS. Predisposing genetic factors for diabetic polyneuropathy in patients with type 1 diabetes: a population-based case-control study. Acta Diabetol. 2003;40(Suppl 2):S375–9.
79. Chistiakov DA, Zotova EV, Savost'anov KV, Bursa TR, Galeev IV, Strokov IA, et al. The 262T>C promoter polymorphism of the catalase gene is associated with diabetic neuropathy in type 1 diabetic Russian patients. Diabetes Metab. 2006;32(1):63–8.
80. Guo K, Eid SA, Elzinga SE, Pacut C, Feldman EL, Hur J. Genome-wide profiling of DNA methylation and gene expression identifies candidate genes for human diabetic neuropathy. Clin Epigenetics. 2020;12(1):123.
81. Fernyhough P. Mitochondrial dysfunction in diabetic neuropathy: a series of unfortunate metabolic events. Curr Diab Rep. 2015;15(11):89.
82. Rumora AE, Lentz SI, Hinder LM, Jackson SW, Valesano A, Levinson GE, et al. Dyslipidemia impairs mitochondrial trafficking and function in sensory neurons. FASEB J Off Publ Fed Am Soc Exp Biol. 2018;32(1):195–207.
83. O'Brien PD, Guo K, Eid SA, Rumora AE, Hinder LM, Hayes JM, et al. Integrated lipidomic and transcriptomic analyses identify altered nerve triglycerides in mouse models of prediabetes and type 2 diabetes. Dis Model Mech. 2020;24:13(2).

84. Viader A, Sasaki Y, Kim S, Strickland A, Workman CS, Yang K, et al. Aberrant Schwann cell lipid metabolism linked to mitochondrial deficits leads to axon degeneration and neuropathy. Neuron. 2013;77(5):886–98.
85. Hur J, Sullivan KA, Pande M, Hong Y, Sima AAF, Jagadish HV, et al. The identification of gene expression profiles associated with progression of human diabetic neuropathy. Brain J Neurol. 2011;134(Pt 11):3222–35.
86. Vincent AM, Hayes JM, McLean LL, Vivekanandan-Giri A, Pennathur S, Feldman EL. Dyslipidemia-induced neuropathy in mice: the role of oxLDL/LOX-1. Diabetes. 2009;58(10):2376–85.
87. Nowicki M, Müller K, Serke H, Kosacka J, Vilser C, Ricken A, et al. Oxidized low-density lipoprotein (oxLDL)-induced cell death in dorsal root ganglion cell cultures depends not on the lectin-like oxLDL receptor-1 but on the toll-like receptor-4. J Neurosci Res. 2010;88(2):403–12.
88. Vincent AM, Perrone L, Sullivan KA, Backus C, Sastry AM, Lastoskie C, et al. Receptor for advanced glycation end products activation injures primary sensory neurons via oxidative stress. Endocrinology. 2007;148(2):548–58.
89. Shoelson SE, Lee J, Goldfine AB. Inflammation and insulin resistance. J Clin Invest. 2006;116(7):1793–801.
90. Elzinga S, Murdock BJ, Guo K, Hayes JM, Tabbey MA, Hur J, et al. Toll-like receptors and inflammation in metabolic neuropathy; a role in early versus late disease? Exp Neurol. 2019;320:112967.
91. Shevalye H, Yorek MS, Coppey LJ, Holmes A, Harper MM, Kardon RH, et al. Effect of enriching the diet with menhaden oil or daily treatment with resolvin D1 on neuropathy in a mouse model of type 2 diabetes. J Neurophysiol. 2015;114(1):199–208.
92. Hinder LM, Park M, Rumora AE, Hur J, Eichinger F, Pennathur S, et al. Comparative RNA-Seq transcriptome analyses reveal distinct metabolic pathways in diabetic nerve and kidney disease. J Cell Mol Med. 2017;21(9):2140–52.
93. Eid SA, O'Brien PD, Hinder LM, Hayes JM, Mendelson FE, Zhang H, et al. Differential effects of Empagliflozin on microvascular complications in murine models of type 1 and type 2 diabetes. Biology. 2020;22:9(11).
94. Kellogg AP, Wiggin TD, Larkin DD, Hayes JM, Stevens MJ, Pop-Busui R. Protective effects of cyclooxygenase-2 gene inactivation against peripheral nerve dysfunction and intraepidermal nerve fiber loss in experimental diabetes. Diabetes. 2007;56(12):2997–3005.
95. Asea A, Kraeft SK, Kurt-Jones EA, Stevenson MA, Chen LB, Finberg RW, et al. HSP70 stimulates cytokine production through a CD14-dependant pathway, demonstrating its dual role as a chaperone and cytokine. Nat Med. 2000;6(4):435–42.
96. Truini A, Spallone V, Morganti R, Tamburin S, Zanette G, Schenone A, et al. A cross-sectional study investigating frequency and features of definitely diagnosed diabetic painful polyneuropathy. Pain. 2018;159(12):2658–66.
97. Themistocleous AC, Ramirez JD, Shillo PR, Lees JG, Selvarajah D, Orengo C, et al. The pain in neuropathy study (PiNS): a cross-sectional observational study determining the somatosensory phenotype of painful and painless diabetic neuropathy. Pain. 2016;157(5):1132–45.
98. Raputova J, Srotova I, Vlckova E, Sommer C, Üçeyler N, Birklein F, et al. Sensory phenotype and risk factors for painful diabetic neuropathy: a cross-sectional observational study. Pain. 2017;158(12):2340–53.
99. Shillo P, Sloan G, Greig M, Hunt L, Selvarajah D, Elliott J, et al. Painful and painless diabetic neuropathies: what is the difference? Curr Diab Rep. 2019;19(6):32.
100. Sloan G, Selvarajah D, Tesfaye S. Pathogenesis, diagnosis and clinical management of diabetic sensorimotor peripheral neuropathy. Nat Rev End. In Press.
101. Finnerup NB, Attal N, Haroutounian S, McNicol E, Baron R, Dworkin RH, et al. Pharmacotherapy for neuropathic pain in adults: a systematic review and meta-analysis. Lancet Neurol. 2015;14(2):162–73.

102. Woolf CJ, Bennett GJ, Doherty M, Dubner R, Kidd B, Koltzenburg M, et al. Towards a mechanism-based classification of pain? Pain. 1998;77(3):227–9.
103. Edwards RR, Dworkin RH, Turk DC, Angst MS, Dionne R, Freeman R, et al. Patient phenotyping in clinical trials of chronic pain treatments: IMMPACT recommendations. Pain. 2016;157(9):1851–71.
104. Maier C, Baron R, Tölle TR, Binder A, Birbaumer N, Birklein F, et al. Quantitative sensory testing in the German research network on neuropathic pain (DFNS): somatosensory abnormalities in 1236 patients with different neuropathic pain syndromes. Pain. 2010;150(3):439–50.
105. Shy ME, Frohman EM, So YT, Arezzo JC, Cornblath DR, Giuliani MJ, et al. Quantitative sensory testing: report of the therapeutics and technology assessment Subcommittee of the American Academy of neurology. Neurology. 2003;60(6):898–904.
106. Rolke R, Magerl W, Campbell KA, Schalber C, Caspari S, Birklein F, et al. Quantitative sensory testing: a comprehensive protocol for clinical trials. Eur J Pain Lond Engl. 2006;10(1):77–88.
107. Tesfaye S, Boulton AJM, Dickenson AH. Mechanisms and management of diabetic painful distal symmetrical polyneuropathy. Diabetes Care. 2013;36(9):2456–65.
108. Birbaumer N, Lutzenberger W, Montoya P, Larbig W, Unertl K, Töpfner S, et al. Effects of regional anesthesia on phantom limb pain are mirrored in changes in cortical reorganization. J Neurosci. 1997;17(14):5503–8.
109. Flor H, Elbert T, Knecht S, Wienbruch C, Pantev C, Birbaumer N, et al. Phantom-limb pain as a perceptual correlate of cortical reorganization following arm amputation. Nature. 1995;375(6531):482–4.
110. Wrigley PJ, Press SR, Gustin SM, Macefield VG, Gandevia SC, Cousins MJ, et al. Neuropathic pain and primary somatosensory cortex reorganization following spinal cord injury. Pain. 2009;141(1–2):52–9.
111. Wilkinson ID, Teh K, Heiberg-Gibbons F, Awadh M, Kelsall A, Shillo P, et al. Determinants of treatment response in painful diabetic peripheral neuropathy: a combined deep sensory phenotyping and multimodal brain MRI study. Diabetes. 2020;69(8):1804–14.
112. Campbell CM, Kipnes MS, Stouch BC, Brady KL, Kelly M, Schmidt WK, et al. Randomized control trial of topical clonidine for treatment of painful diabetic neuropathy. Pain. 2012;153(9):1815–23.
113. Bouhassira D, Wilhelm S, Schacht A, Perrot S, Kosek E, Cruccu G, et al. Neuropathic pain phenotyping as a predictor of treatment response in painful diabetic neuropathy: data from the randomized, double-blind. COMBO-DN study Pain. 2014;155(10):2171–9.
114. Demant et al. The effect of oxcarbazepine in peripheral neuropathic pain depends on pain phenotype: a randomised, double-blind, placebo-controlled phenotype-stratified study. Pain. 2014;155(11):2263–73.
115. Yarnitsky D, Granot M, Nahman-Averbuch H, Khamaisi M, Granovsky Y. Conditioned pain modulation predicts duloxetine efficacy in painful diabetic neuropathy. Pain. 2012;153(6):1193–8.
116. Haroutounian S, Nikolajsen L, Bendtsen TF, Finnerup NB, Kristensen AD, Hasselstrøm JB, et al. Primary afferent input critical for maintaining spontaneous pain in peripheral neuropathy. Pain. 2014;155(7):1272–9.
117. Feldman et al. Diabetic neuropathy. Nature reviews disease primers. 2019;5(1):1–8.
118. Wager TD, Atlas LY, Lindquist MA, Roy M, Woo C-W, Kross E. An fMRI-based neurologic signature of physical pain. N Engl J Med. 2013;368(15):1388–97.
119. Tracey I. "Seeing" how our drugs work brings translational added value. Anesthesiology. 2013;119(6):1247–8.
120. Selvarajah D, Wilkinson ID, Emery CJ, Harris ND, Shaw PJ, Witte DR, et al. Early involvement of the spinal cord in diabetic peripheral neuropathy. Diabetes Care. 2006;29(12):2664–9.

121. Selvarajah D, Wilkinson ID, Maxwell M, Davies J, Sankar A, Boland E, et al. Magnetic resonance neuroimaging study of brain structural differences in diabetic peripheral neuropathy. Diabetes Care. 2014;37(6):1681–8.
122. Selvarajah D, Wilkinson ID, Fang F, Sankar A, Davies J, Boland E, et al. Structural and functional abnormalities of the primary somatosensory cortex in diabetic peripheral neuropathy: a multimodal MRI study. Diabetes. 2019;68(4):796–806.
123. Buxton RB. Interpreting oxygenation-based neuroimaging signals: the importance and the challenge of understanding brain oxygen metabolism. Front Neuroenerg. 2010;2:8.
124. Pereira F, Mitchell T, Botvinick M. Machine learning classifiers and fMRI: a tutorial overview. NeuroImage. 2009;45(1 Suppl):S199–209.
125. Wager TD, Lindquist MA, Nichols TE, Kober H, Van Snellenberg JX. Evaluating the consistency and specificity of neuroimaging data using meta-analysis. NeuroImage. 2009;45(1 Suppl):S210–21.
126. Alger JR, Ellingson BM, Ashe-McNalley C, Woodworth DC, Labus JS, Farmer M, et al. Multisite, multimodal neuroimaging of chronic urological pelvic pain: methodology of the MAPP research network. NeuroImage Clin. 2016;12:65–77.
127. Zunhammer M, Bingel U, Wager TD. Placebo imaging consortium. Placebo effects on the neurologic pain signature: a meta-analysis of individual participant functional magnetic resonance imaging data. JAMA Neurol. 2018;75(11):1321–30.
128. Eddy S, Mariani LH, Kretzler M. Integrated multi-omics approaches to improve classification of chronic kidney disease. Nat Rev Nephrol. 2020;16(11):657–68.
129. Heerspink HJL, de Zeeuw D. Treating diabetic complications; from large randomized clinical trials to precision medicine. Diabetes Obes Metab. 2018;20(Suppl 3):3–5.
130. Idzerda NMA, Pena MJ, Heerspink HJL. Personalized medicine in diabetic kidney disease: a novel approach to improve trial design and patient outcomes. Curr Opin Nephrol Hypertens. 2018;27(6):426–32.
131. de Boer IH, Alpers CE, Azeloglu EU, Balis UGJ, Barasch JM, Barisoni L, et al. Rationale and design of the kidney precision medicine project. Kidney Int. 2021;99(3):498–510.
132. van Zuydam NR, Ahlqvist E, Sandholm N, Deshmukh H, Rayner NW, Abdalla M, et al. A genome-wide association study of diabetic kidney disease in subjects with type 2 diabetes. Diabetes. 2018;67(7):1414–27.
133. Pezzolesi MG, Poznik GD, Mychaleckyj JC, Paterson AD, Barati MT, Klein JB, et al. Genome-wide association scan for diabetic nephropathy susceptibility genes in type 1 diabetes. Diabetes. 2009;58(6):1403–10.
134. Lan D, Jiang H-Y, Su X, Zhao Y, Du S, Li Y, et al. Transcriptome-wide association study identifies genetically dysregulated genes in diabetic neuropathy. Comb Chem High Throughput Screen. 2021;24(2):319–25.
135. Ustinova M, Peculis R, Rescenko R, Rovite V, Zaharenko L, Elbere I, et al. Novel susceptibility loci identified in a genome-wide association study of type 2 diabetes complications in population of Latvia. BMC Med Genet. 2021;14(1):18.
136. Guo K, Elzinga S, Eid S, Figueroa-Romero C, Hinder LM, Pacut C, et al. Genome-wide DNA methylation profiling of human diabetic peripheral neuropathy in subjects with type 2 diabetes mellitus. Epigenetics. 2019;14(8):766–79.
137. Yang H, Sloan G, Ye Y, Wang S, Duan B, Tesfaye S, et al. New perspective in diabetic neuropathy: from the periphery to the brain, a call for early detection, and precision medicine. Front Endocrinol. 2019;10:929.
138. Themistocleous AC, Crombez G, Baskozos G, Bennett DL. Using stratified medicine to understand, diagnose, and treat neuropathic pain. Pain. 2018;159(Suppl 1):S31–42.
139. Chen W-T, Yuan R-Y, Chiang S-C, Sheu J-J, Yu J-M, Tseng I-J, et al. OnabotulinumtoxinA improves tactile and mechanical pain perception in painful diabetic polyneuropathy. Clin J Pain. 2013;29(4):305–10.

140. Ghasemi M, Ansari M, Basiri K, Shaigannejad V. The effects of intradermal botulinum toxin type a injections on pain symptoms of patients with diabetic neuropathy. J Res Med Sci Off J Isfahan Univ Med Sci. 2014;19(2):106–11.
141. Nawfar SA, Yacob NBM. Effects of monochromatic infrared energy therapy on diabetic feet with peripheral sensory neuropathy: a randomised controlled trial. Singap Med J. 2011;52(9):669–72.
142. Jude EB, Dang C, Boulton AJM. Effect of L-arginine on the microcirculation in the neuropathic diabetic foot in type 2 diabetes mellitus: a double-blind, placebo-controlled study. Diabet Med J Br Diabet Assoc. 2010;27(1):113–6.
143. Syngle A, Verma I, Krishan P, Garg N, Syngle V. Minocycline improves peripheral and autonomic neuropathy in type 2 diabetes: MIND study. Neurol Sci Off J Ital Neurol Soc Ital Soc Clin Neurophysiol. 2014;35(7):1067–73.
144. Fraser DA, Diep LM, Hovden IA, Nilsen KB, Sveen KA, Seljeflot I, et al. The effects of long-term oral benfotiamine supplementation on peripheral nerve function and inflammatory markers in patients with type 1 diabetes: a 24-month, double-blind, randomized, placebo-controlled trial. Diabetes Care. 2012;35(5):1095–7.

Chapter 9
Inpatient Precision Medicine for Diabetes

Georgia Davis, Guillermo E. Umpierrez, and Francisco J. Pasquel

Introduction

The pursuit of precision medicine in diabetes surrounds numerous efforts to assemble and understand complex genetic, phenotypic, and environmental data and its associated impact on disease risk, progression, and therapeutic responses [1, 2]. There has been significant movement along the path from *personalized* to *precision* diabetes management, but many current diagnostic, risk stratification, and treatment strategies have yet to fully integrate genomic factors and other "-omics" data into targeted precise therapies for diabetes management, including in the hospital setting [3]. However, continued advancement of precision diagnostics, monitoring, and pharmacologic therapy for diabetes applicable to the outpatient setting can inform individualized management for hospitalized patients. Additionally, the inpatient setting may confer unique insight into other dimensions of precision diabetes care, including (1) patient stratification by metabolic phenotype and severity of illness on admission, (2) optimal inpatient glucose monitoring strategies, and (3) individualized glycemic targets and pharmacologic therapy. The next evolution in inpatient precision diabetes care surrounds the ability to leverage the diverse networks of patient-specific phenotypic background data, dynamic inpatient clinical data, and large-scale public data to guide hospital diabetes management.

Extraordinary advances in diabetes pharmacotherapeutics and technology have emerged over the past two decades, allowing for more personalized care particularly in the outpatient setting. These more individualized management strategies have moved into the inpatient setting and include the use of non-insulin antihyperglycemic agents, as well as the implementation of diabetes technology for inpatient

G. Davis · G. E. Umpierrez · F. J. Pasquel (✉)
Division of Endocrinology, Department of Medicine, Emory University School of Medicine, Atlanta, GA, USA
e-mail: fpasque@emory.edu; geumpie@emory.edu

R. Basu (ed.), *Precision Medicine in Diabetes*,
https://doi.org/10.1007/978-3-030-98927-9_9

glucose monitoring. Existing background phenotypic data in combination with data obtained during treatment of acute illness (i.e., biomarker changes, glycemic control trends) may provide a deeper understanding of the dynamic clinical and metabolic conditions underlying an individual's disease process and response to diabetes therapy. Expansion of the inpatient knowledge base moving forward will allow for the generation of more comprehensive data sets applicable to inpatient diabetes management. To date, true *precision* medicine has not been realized for inpatient diabetes care, but with continued data acquisition, we are moving toward this goal.

Patient Heterogeneity and Complexity in Factors Affecting Metabolism

Glucose metabolism is influenced by multiple factors in the hospital, including intrinsic patient factors, severity of illness, and hospital treatment. Intrinsic patient characteristics such as background metabolic status (obesity, prediabetes, type 1 or type 2 diabetes) significantly influence insulin-dependent glucose disposal. In patients with diabetes, the complexity of the home management regimen and the duration of diabetes, as well as relevant comorbidities (e.g., chronic kidney disease), can also significantly influence inpatient glycemic control. Furthermore, glucose metabolism is influenced by the severity of illness, which is associated with hormonal activation (cortisol, catecholamines) and an immunometabolic response mediated by cytokines and other tissue injury-related factors associated with changes in insulin sensitivity [4–6].

Even though hyperglycemia and diabetes are primarily considered disorders of glucose metabolism, analyses of large cohorts using high-resolution metabolomics (HRM) techniques have reported positive associations of branched-chain amino acids (BCAAs) and products of fatty acid metabolism (i.e., acylcarnitines) with insulin resistance, insulin secretion defects, and incident diabetes [7–12]. These relationships suggest that circulating and increased release of amino acids and acylcarnitines during hormone-mediated catabolism during stress could mediate insulin resistance and beta-cell dysfunction.

Furthermore, common hospital factors including the type of nutrition (oral, enteral, parenteral) or medications (e.g., steroids, vasopressors) can significantly influence glucose metabolism. Figure 9.1 shows the complexity of glucose metabolism in the hospital related to intrinsic patient factors, severity of illness, and hospital factors (nutrition, medications).

Automated evaluation of clinical data through deep learning with medical applications is becoming a recent reality [13] and is laying the groundwork for the integration of clinical data, computation, and likely systems biology data in the near future. Integrating underlying metabolic phenotypic information, severity of illness biomarkers, glucose metabolism biomarkers (glucose, A1c, CGM-derived metrics), hospital factors (nutrition, medications), individual- and population-derived data,

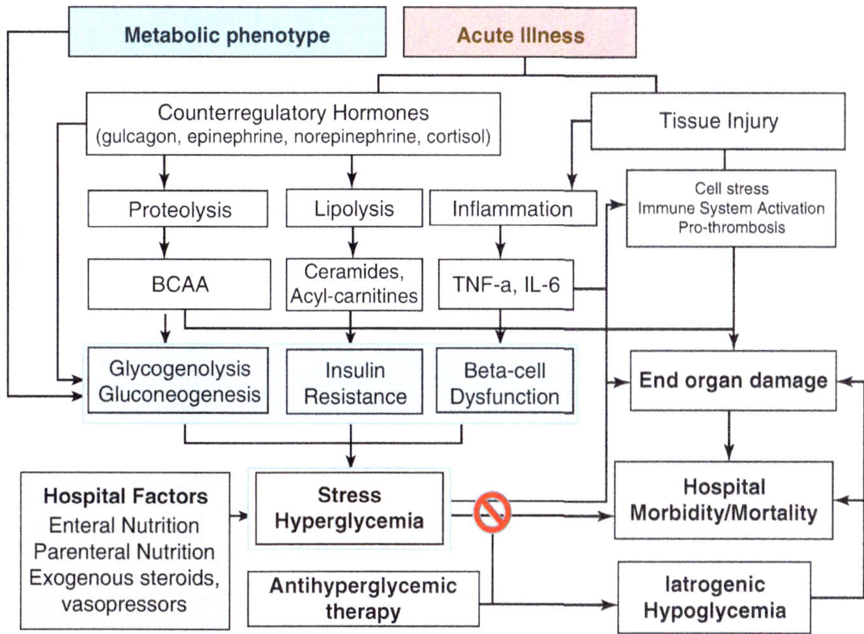

Fig. 9.1 Multiple factors influence glucose metabolism in acutely ill patients. Patient-specific factors including the metabolic phenotype (normoglycemia, obesity, prediabetes, type 1 or type 2 diabetes), the severity of disease (counterregulatory response and the severity of disease), as well as hospital factors (medical nutrition therapy, steroids, vasopressors). Potential mediators of dysglycemia include metabolites originating from catabolism and inflammation during the acute illness that have been associated with increase hepatic glucose output, insulin resistance, and beta-cell dysfunction including BCAA (branched-chain amino acids), ceramides, and acylcarnitines

social factors, and patient preferences may further facilitate the generation of precise recommendations to improve care at the individual and population level (Fig. 9.2). Furthermore, the integration of systems biology and the digital revolution are transforming healthcare toward a P7 medicine concept [14, 15] where care is more *personalized, predictive, precise, preventive, pervasive, participatory, and protective* (Table 9.1).

Hospital Glucose Monitoring and Data Acquisition

Optimizing glycemic control in the inpatient setting has been limited by infrequent glucose testing, most often relying on point-of-care finger-stick blood samples. In utilizing this method of glucose monitoring, a desire for increased frequency of glucose testing increases the work burden of staff responsible for the POC glucose testing. Even with an increased number of POC glucose values, the glycemic

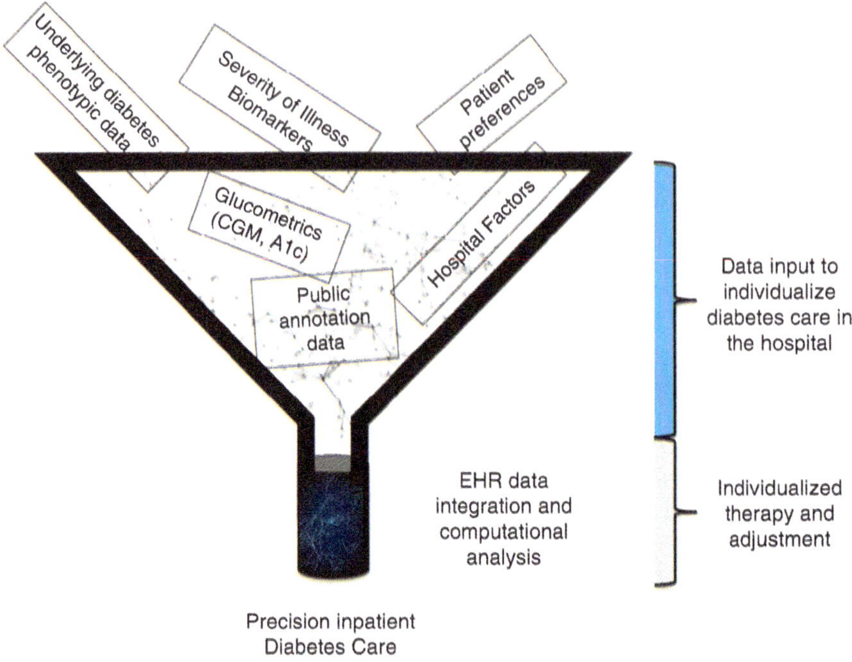

Fig. 9.2 Integrating multidimensional data for precision medicine in the hospital. Advances in bioinformatics that integrate multidimensional data and the use of artificial intelligence with deep learning techniques may facilitate personalized and adaptive diabetes management

Table 9.1 Adapting the elements of the P7 concept to the future of inpatient diabetes care [14, 15]

Personalized medicine	Individualized inpatient therapy strategies that work should be standardized
Predictive	Development of risk prediction tools using EHR data and -omics data may help determine susceptibility to additional diseases and hospital complications in patients with diabetes
Precise	The information obtained from multidimensional data may be used to precisely determine inpatient regimens and appropriate transitions of care
Preventive	Personalized approaches using machine learning and decision analytical tools can be used to develop strategies to prevent severe glycemic excursions and medication interactions and reduce the risk of readmissions
Pervasive	The information for inpatient care utilizing dynamic metrics should be available at any time and at any location
Participatory	Patient preferences should be included in the decision-making for inpatient care and at time of discharge
Protective	Cybersecurity measures should be implemented to ensure confidentiality of all patient data

control data generated still provides only a limited snapshot of glucose trends and fluctuations. Accordingly, there has been much interest in moving continuous glucose monitoring (CGM) into the hospital setting. During the coronavirus 2019 (COVID-19) pandemic, efforts to implement real-time CGM (rt-CGM) for inpatient use were rapidly put in place to minimize viral exposures while maintaining adequate monitoring of glycemic control. While these devices were able to be used in the hospital without objection from the Food and Drug Administration during a public health crisis [4, 16], there are limited studies and data on the use of CGM in the inpatient setting, with ongoing studies continuing to investigate reliability and functionality of CGM in hospitalized patients. However, the rapid and widespread implementation of hospital CGM use during COVID-19 has provided a snapshot of the potential benefits of CGM for hospital monitoring of glucose values and trends [16–18]. The most frequently used CGM systems employ subcutaneous monitoring of interstitial glucose values every few minutes with a corresponding glucose trend arrow, as well as alerts that can be set to detect hypoglycemia, hyperglycemia, and rapid changes in glucose trend. Real-time CGM generates exponentially more glycemic control data than that from POC glucose testing alone and addresses prior limitations in hospital glucose monitoring through closer observation of glucose values and the use of glucose trends and alerts to prevent severe glycemic excursions and hypoglycemic events [4, 19].

Though inpatient rt-CGM implementation is a crucial step forward in guiding personalized diabetes management in the hospital, further consideration on how CGM data can be accurately and meaningfully recorded for incorporation into larger diverse data sets will be required to move toward precision diabetes care. As CGM data from hospitalized patients becomes available, infrequent discrete glucose measurements are being replaced by glucose values every few minutes during hospitalization. This wealth of glucose data affords the opportunity to aggregate data on hospital glucose measurements and glycemic control metrics (time in glucose ranges, glycemic variability) for the creation of comprehensive databases with information on individual-level inpatient glycemic control [20]. Previous studies have proposed that more comprehensive subtyping of diabetes classification is needed to inform precision diabetes care [21], with one study suggesting the use of individual-level CGM data related to other glucose control and clinical characteristics to classify patterns and underlying mechanisms of glucose dysregulation ("glucotypes") potentially associated with early type 2 diabetes or cardiovascular risk [22]. However, this glucose excursion-based classification from CGM data combined with other risk stratification phenotypes, inpatient clinical metrics and pharmacotherapeutic data, could be a powerful technique to help predict treatment responses and individualize glucose monitoring. Current efforts to translate CGM to the hospital setting are allowing an opportunity to define patterns of glycemia in heterogeneous populations with acute illnesses. A detailed assessment of glucose patterns with CGM integrated with other clinical parameters, such as ECG, may in the near future continue to facilitate optimal individualized glucose monitoring and prevention of hypoglycemia [23].

Individualized Management Strategies: Glycemic Targets and Pharmacotherapy

Current recommended glycemic targets for both noncritical and critical care settings have been derived from clinical trials and observational studies with the goal of limiting hyperglycemic and hypoglycemic excursions known to be associated with poor hospital outcomes [24]. Some of the largest studies from which the recommendations are derived included heterogeneous populations that did not account for individual-level patient characteristics, including a diagnosis of diabetes, which could impact determination of clinically appropriate target glucose ranges [25, 26]. Still, it is not well-known (a) who are the most vulnerable patients to extreme glucose fluctuations, (b) how diabetes phenotypes and severity of illness impact glycemic control patterns, (c) the actual biological impact and reversibility of both hyperglycemia- and hypoglycemia-associated complications, and (d) the most optimal diabetes treatment strategies during acute illness for diverse populations.

Recent clinical trials have shown that even in controlled hospital settings not all patients are able to reach recommended glucose targets [27, 28] and worse control is expected in real-world inpatient scenarios. The landscape of available therapies for the management of diabetes has significantly expanded in the last decade, and new agents have emerged as potential alternatives to insulin, considered for many years the ideal treatment strategy in the hospital. Recent data documented with CGM has shown that even with subcutaneous insulin therapy, the proportion of time spent in target glucose range (defined as 70–180 mg/dL) is often suboptimal [18, 27–30]. Additionally, data from inpatient hospitalizations, nursing homes, and rehabilitation facilities have consistently shown increased hypoglycemia risk with insulin therapy [25, 31–33]. Recent studies including vulnerable patients with diabetes (such as those with older age and/or renal failure) have shown, as expected, that less insulin is associated with a lower risk of hypoglycemia and that the use of non-insulin agents may be appropriate in certain circumstances to achieve glycemic control in the inpatient setting [4].

The individualization of inpatient diabetes management strategies is evolving to include new pharmacotherapeutic agents, insulin delivery systems, and glucose monitoring strategies. In choosing patient-specific therapy, glycemic targets will also be personalized based on patient factors as well as risks associated with these individualized therapeutic strategies. Recent clinical trials have started to delineate the characteristics of patients more likely to benefit from insulin and non-insulin therapy regimens. Figure 9.3 shows a framework utilizing clinical patient data, admission biometrics, and severity of disease to individualized therapy with insulin and non-insulin agents.

Even though insulin therapy with fixed insulin dosing regimens has been considered standard of care for patients with type 2 diabetes in the hospital, recent observational studies have shown that oral agents (i.e., metformin or sulfonylureas) are commonly used in the hospital. A basal-bolus insulin regimen [with a total daily dose usually delivered as basal insulin (50%) along with scheduled prandial insulin

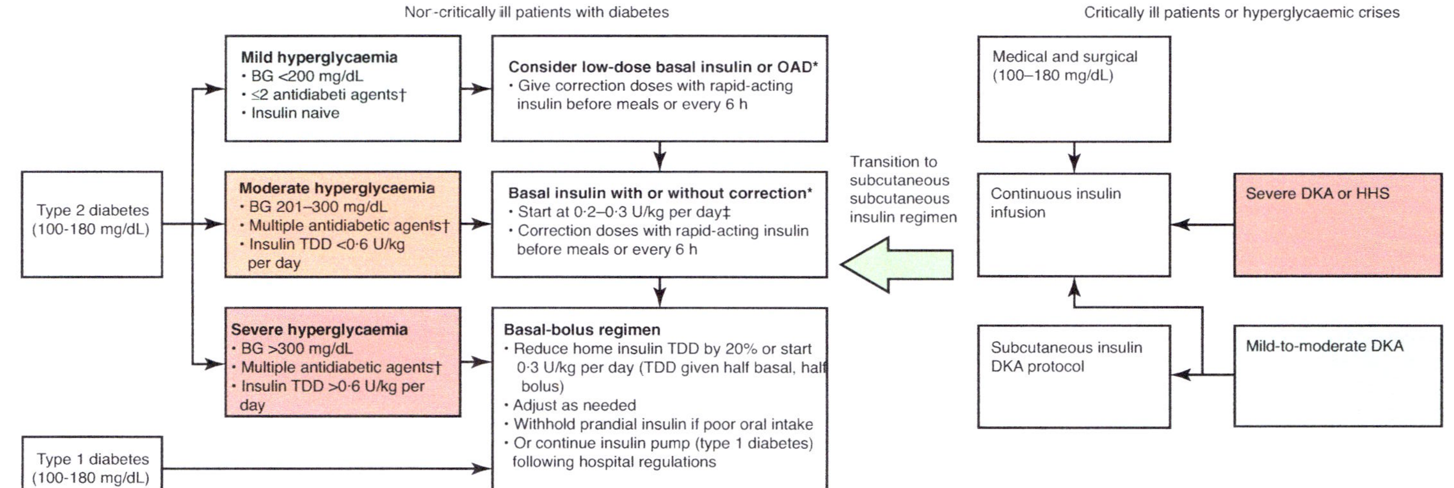

Fig. 9.3 Individualized antihyperglycemic therapy in hospitalized patients with diabetes. In critically ill patients, continuous insulin infusion is recommended followed by transition to subcutaneous insulin regimens once patients are stable and close to discharge from the intensive care unit. Subcutaneous insulin DKA protocols might be considered in patients with mild-to-moderate DKA (subcutaneous insulin protocol examples adapted for COVID-19 are available online). We discourage the widespread use of premixed insulin regimens in the hospital setting. (BG, blood glucose. DKA, diabetic ketoacidosis. HHS, hyperosmolar hyperglycemic state. OAD, oral antidiabetic drug. TDD, total daily dose. U, units. *Consider OAD if no contraindications (only DPP-4 inhibitors have been studied in randomized controlled trials); metformin is commonly used in the hospital setting but might be associated with lactic acidosis in high-risk patients (e.g., sepsis, shock, renal or liver failure). †Antidiabetic agents include OADs and GLP-1 receptor agonists. ‡In patients with hypoglycemia risk (frail, elderly, acute kidney injury), reduce starting dose to 0·15 U/kg per day (basal alone) or TDD 0·3 U/kg per day (basal-bolus). From Pasquel FJ et al. with permission [4])

before meals (50% divided in three doses)] can lead to lower average BG levels compared to sliding-scale insulin (SSI). This approach, however, is labor-intensive, requiring multiple injections per day, and is associated with increased risk of iatrogenic hypoglycemia [34]. More recently, RCTs have consistently shown that DPP-4 inhibitors with SSI are safe in hospitalized patients with mild hyperglycemia (<200 mg/dl) [35]. For patients with BG 140–400 mg/dL treated at home with oral agents or insulin at a dose <0.6 units/kg/day, a DPP-4 inhibitor and basal insulin combination is as effective as a basal-bolus regimen [35]. Currently, individualization of care approaches unfortunately demand clinical experience of inpatient providers familiar with the field. Data integration using technology for systematic decision-making with precise regimens may alleviate the burden for providers taking care of patients with diabetes in the hospital.

Diabetes technology may become an integral part of diabetes care in the future. In addition to rt-CGM, other technologies are emerging in the inpatient setting. These technologies include various computerized decision support systems and EHR enhancements for glucose management implemented to systematically initiate therapy in patients with diabetes or hyperglycemia [36]. In addition, current technology allows for individualized care (CGM-based insulin delivery) along with population health management (cloud-based platforms). We recently showed feasibility of integrating remote rt-CGM technology with a protocol incorporating EHR validation of glucose values (confirmation of sensor accuracy compared to POC) with a computerized algorithm for continuous insulin infusion to care for critically ill patients with COVID-19 [17].

Furthermore, the use of automated insulin delivery (AID) systems, or artificial pancreas technology, has been rapidly expanding in the outpatient setting and is becoming more common in the hospital; however, the infrastructure is not readily available for the inpatient use of AID. Initial studies with AID have shown improvement in glycemic control in diverse populations of noncritically ill patients [29, 30]. A recent retrospective analyses of inpatient studies with closed-loop showed a high variability of exogenous insulin requirements in hospitalized patients, particularly overnight, confirming the need for personalized glucose-responsive approaches to achieve glucose targets while minimizing hypoglycemia risk [37]. Further development of this technology for inpatient therapy will likely integrate more individualized algorithms through the use of artificial intelligence to adapt care during acute illness.

Conclusions

As precision medicine continues to advance through ongoing initiatives for those living with diabetes, it must also include the expansion of inpatient knowledge bases and data analytics to inform more comprehensive, patient-specific hospital diabetes management. Although there have been significant advances made in understanding individual-level genetic, metabolic, environmental, and lifestyle factors pertaining to diabetes risk, glycemic control, and responses to pharmacologic therapy, there are opportunities to develop more complete inpatient-specific data to guide care during acute illness. It is important to understand not only how baseline patient phenotypes can be employed to guide inpatient diabetes therapy but also how the interplay of other clinical parameters, such as illness severity, can modify metabolism and therapeutic response. Future efforts need to ensure this extensive knowledge can be translated into meaningful treatment strategies associated with improved clinical outcomes in the hospital setting.

Developing inpatient precision diabetes medicine includes aspects of *precision diagnostics* (characterization of unique individual-level genetic, metabolic, and clinical phenotypes for more accurate disease-state classification and inpatient risk stratification), *precision monitoring* (real-time continuous glucose data with remote monitoring capabilities and patient-specific glycemic control targets), and *precision therapeutics* (addition of non-insulin agents with associated benefits beyond glycemic control, computer-based decision algorithms, and automated insulin delivery). To date, there is advancing but limited application of these concepts of precision medicine in the hospital setting, but also a clear need to combine acute and chronic disease-state data to better comprehend individual-level responses to diabetes treatment and help guide care during acute illness.

References

1. Fradkin JE, Hanlon MC, Rodgers GP. NIH precision medicine initiative: implications for diabetes research: table 1. Diabetes Care. 2016;39(7):1080–4.
2. Meyer RJ. Precision medicine, diabetes, and the U.S. Food and Drug Administration. Diabetes Care. 2016;39(11):1874–8.
3. Klonoff DC. Precision medicine for managing diabetes. J Diabetes Sci Technol. 2015;9(1):3–7.
4. Pasquel FJ, Lansang MC, Dhatariya K, Umpierrez GE. Management of diabetes and hyperglycaemia in the hospital. Lancet Diabetes Endocrinol. 2021;9(3):174–88.
5. Reyes-Umpierrez D, Davis G, Cardona S, et al. Inflammation and oxidative stress in cardiac surgery patients treated to intensive vs. conservative glucose targets. J Clin Endocrinol Metabol. 2016:jc.2016–3197.
6. Hotamisligil G. Molecular mechanisms of insulin resistance and the role of the adipocyte. Int J Obes. 2000;24(S4):S23–7.
7. Guasch-Ferre M, Hruby A, Toledo E, et al. Metabolomics in prediabetes and diabetes: a systematic review and meta-analysis. Diabetes Care. 2016;39(5):833–46.
8. Menni C, Fauman E, Erte I, et al. Biomarkers for type 2 diabetes and impaired fasting glucose using a nontargeted metabolomics approach. Diabetes. 2013;62(12):4270–6.
9. Wang TJ, Larson MG, Vasan RS, et al. Metabolite profiles and the risk of developing diabetes. Nat Med. 2011;17(4):448–53.
10. Batchuluun B, Al Rijjal D, Prentice KJ, et al. Elevated medium chain-Acylcarnitines are associated with gestational diabetes, and early progression to Type-2 diabetes, and induce pancreatic beta-cell dysfunction. Diabetes. 2018.
11. Sun L, Liang L, Gao X, et al. Early prediction of developing type 2 diabetes by plasma Acylcarnitines: a population-based study. Diabetes Care. 2016;39(9):1563–70.
12. Ruiz-Canela M, Toledo E, Clish CB, et al. Plasma branched-chain amino acids and incident cardiovascular disease in the PREDIMED trial. Clin Chem. 2016;62(4):582–92.

13. Ardila D, Kiraly AP, Bharadwaj S, et al. End-to-end lung cancer screening with three-dimensional deep learning on low-dose chest computed tomography. Nat Med. 2019;25(6):954–61.
14. Hood L, Flores M. A personal view on systems medicine and the emergence of proactive P4 medicine: predictive, preventive, personalized and participatory. New Biotechnol. 2012;29(6):613–24.
15. Sriram RD, Reddy SSK. Artificial intelligence and digital tools. Clin Geriatr Med. 2020;36(3):513–25.
16. Galindo RJ, Aleppo G, Klonoff DC, et al. Implementation of continuous glucose monitoring in the hospital: emergent considerations for remote glucose monitoring during the COVID-19 pandemic. J Diabetes Sci Technol. 2020;14(4):822–32.
17. Davis GM, Faulds E, Walker T, et al. Remote continuous glucose monitoring with a computerized insulin infusion protocol for critically ill patients in a COVID-19 medical ICU: proof of concept. Diabetes Care. 2021;44(4):1055–8.
18. Agarwal S, Mathew J, Davis GM, et al. Continuous glucose monitoring in the intensive care unit during the COVID-19 pandemic. Diabetes Care. 2021;44(3):847–9.
19. Singh LG, Satyarengga M, Marcano I, et al. Reducing inpatient hypoglycemia in the general wards using real-time continuous glucose monitoring: the glucose telemetry system, a randomized clinical trial. Diabetes Care. 2020;43(11):2736–43.
20. Vettoretti M, Cappon G, Acciaroli G, Facchinetti A, Sparacino G. Continuous glucose monitoring: current use in diabetes management and possible future applications. J Diabetes Sci Technol. 2018;12(5):1064–71.
21. Ahlqvist E, Storm P, Käräjämäki A, et al. Novel subgroups of adult-onset diabetes and their association with outcomes: a data-driven cluster analysis of six variables. Lancet Diabetes Endocrinol. 2018;6(5):361–9.
22. Hall H, Perelman D, Breschi A, et al. Glucotypes reveal new patterns of glucose dysregulation. PLoS Biol. 2018;16(7):e2005143.
23. Porumb M, Stranges S, Pescapè A, Pecchia L. Precision medicine and artificial intelligence: a pilot study on deep learning for hypoglycemic events detection based on ECG. Sci Rep. 2020;10(1):170.
24. 15. Diabetes care in the hospital: standards of medical care in diabetes—2021. Diabetes Care. 2021;44(Supplement 1):S211–20.
25. Intensive versus conventional glucose control in critically ill patients. New England J Med. 2009;360(13):1283–97.
26. Moghissi ES, Korytkowski MT, Dinardo M, et al. American Association of Clinical Endocrinologists and American Diabetes Association Consensus Statement on inpatient glycemic control. Diabetes Care. 2009;32(6):1119–31.
27. Fortmann AL, Spierling Bagsic SR, Talavera L, et al. Glucose as the fifth vital sign: a randomized controlled trial of continuous glucose monitoring in a non-ICU hospital setting. Diabetes Care. 2020;43(11):2873–7.
28. Pasquel FJ, Lansang MC, Khowaja A, et al. A randomized controlled trial comparing glargine U300 and glargine U100 for the inpatient Management of Medicine and Surgery Patients with Type 2 diabetes: glargine U300 hospital trial. Diabetes Care. 2020;43(6):1242–8.
29. Bally L, Thabit H, Hartnell S, et al. Closed-loop insulin delivery for glycemic control in noncritical care. N Engl J Med. 2018;379(6):547–56.
30. Boughton CK, Bally L, Martignoni F, et al. Fully closed-loop insulin delivery in inpatients receiving nutritional support: a two-Centre, open-label, randomised controlled trial. Lancet Diabetes Endocrinol. 2019;7(5):368–77.
31. Pasquel FJ, Powell W, Peng L, et al. A randomized controlled trial comparing treatment with oral agents and basal insulin in elderly patients with type 2 diabetes in long-term care facilities. BMJ Open Diabetes Res Care. 2015;3(1):e000104.
32. Umpierrez GE, Cardona S, Chachkhiani D, et al. A randomized controlled study comparing a DPP4 inhibitor (Linagliptin) and basal insulin (Glargine) in Patients with type 2 diabetes

in long-term care and skilled nursing facilities: linagliptin-LTC trial. J Am Med Directors Associat. 2018;19(5):399–404.e393.
33. Umpierrez GE, Hor T, Smiley D, et al. Comparison of inpatient insulin regimens with Detemir plus Aspart versus neutral protamine Hagedorn plus regular in medical patients with type 2 diabetes. J Clin Endocrinol Metabol. 2009;94(2):564–9.
34. Umpierrez GE, Hellman R, Korytkowski MT, et al. Management of hyperglycemia in hospitalized patients in non-critical care setting: an endocrine society clinical practice guideline. J Clin Endocrinol Metab. 2012;97(1):16–38.
35. Pasquel FJ, Gianchandani R, Rubin DJ, et al. Efficacy of sitagliptin for the hospital management of general medicine and surgery patients with type 2 diabetes (Sita-Hospital): a multicentre, prospective, open-label, non-inferiority randomised trial. Lancet Diabetes Endocrinol. 2017;5(2):125–33.
36. Davis GM, Galindo RJ, Migdal AL, Umpierrez GE. Diabetes Technology in the Inpatient Setting for Management of Hyperglycemia. Endocrinol Metab Clin N Am. 2020;49(1):79–93.
37. Boughton CK, Daly A, Thabit H, et al. Day-to-day variability of insulin requirements in the inpatient setting: observations during fully closed-loop insulin delivery. Diabetes Obesity Metabol. 2021.

Chapter 10
Precision Medical Management Strategies for Diabetes Remission

Sangeetha R. Kashyap and Saif M. Borgan

Definition of Remission in Type 2 DM

Remission of type 2 diabetes mellitus refers to normalization of blood glucose levels to levels below the threshold at which diabetes is diagnosed, in the absence of active pharmacological agents, for a period of at least 6–12 months [1]. The duration of normalization has been an area of controversy, which has caused some degree of heterogeneity across studies [2]. The term remission is usually adopted, rather than cure, as the genetic and environmental factors that led to the development of this chronic disease still exist in many patients who achieve remission. Thus, the risk of redeveloping diabetes is still considered greater than in the general population [1]. Partial remission refers to patients whose hyperglycemia improves to the prediabetic but does not reach normal glucose threshold, while those who achieve normal glucose parameters have complete remission [1].

Twin Cycle Hypothesis and Remission Window: Clinical Inertia

Grasping the pathophysiology and timeline underlining the development of type 2 DM is crucial to understanding proposed mechanisms for its reversal [3]. According to the "twin cycle hypothesis," in the right environment, usually a prolonged positive energy balance with genetic predisposition, the developing insulin resistance at

S. R. Kashyap (✉)
Cleveland Clinic Lerner College of Medicine, Cleveland, OH, USA
e-mail: kashyas@ccf.org

S. M. Borgan
Endocrinology and Metabolism Institute, Cleveland Clinic Foundation, Cleveland, OH, USA

R. Basu (ed.), *Precision Medicine in Diabetes*,
https://doi.org/10.1007/978-3-030-98927-9_10

the level of muscles and hepatic fat deposition cause reduced uptake of glucose from the blood, as well as abnormally increased hepatic glucose production [4]. In response to hyperglycemia, pancreatic B cells produce excess amounts of insulin which further lead to the favored processing of triacylglycerol in the liver into either storage (leading to worsened fatty liver, hepatic insulin resistance, and increased hepatic glucose production) or transportation in blood (which contributes to fatty acid deposition in the pancrease, eventually contributing to permanent reduced B-cell function and reduced sensitivity in response to hyperglycemia) [3].

Peripheral insulin resistance and hepatic glucose production occur early in the pathophysiological state, usually spanning years before clinical diabetes becomes evident [5]. In the years of hyperinsulinemia, elevated plasma triacylglycerol leads to progressive decompensation of beta cells. In fact, there is evidence that this B-cell dysfunction begins before the development of diabetes, as defined by our thresholds [5]. It is not thought to become irreversible until at least 2–3 years from the initial diagnosis [3]. While the exact duration is unclear, based on clinical data from prospective studies, 50% of patients with type 2 diabetes will require insulin at 10 years, likely reflecting irreversible B-cell loss [6].

Inducing remission early is important for a number of reasons. Firstly, the duration of hyperglycemia has a linear relationship with the development of microvascular and macrovascular complications of diabetes [6]. Additionally, as described earlier, the likelihood of remission success relies on the reversibility of B-cell dysfunction, which is time-dependent. Recognizing this narrow time window is important for successful attempts to induce remission. Unfortunately, clinical inertia is widely prevalent among physicians treating type 2 diabetes, especially early in diabetes [7]. This may stem from physicians' historic perspective that type 2 diabetes is a chronic lifelong disorder, in which Hba1c control is achieved by addition of anti-hyperglycemic agents in a stepwise reactive fashion.

Negative Energy Balance, How It Can Induce Remission, and Clinical Trials Showing Practicality

A negative energy balance either through medically supervised hypocaloric diet or facilitated through bariatric surgery has been the most successful intervention in inducing remission from type 2 diabetes mellitus. During a hypocaloric diet, the mobilization of liver fat occurs at a disproportionately greater rate than subcutaneous and visceral fat [8]. Thus, the reduction in liver overall size and fat content is expected to begin within days of negative energy balance diet [9, 10]. The change in hepatic fat corresponds to normalization of hyperglycemia. As demonstrated in a trial of hypocaloric diet (330 calorie/day) in 30 subjects with type 2 diabetes mellitus, 87% of the plasma glucose reduction happened in the first 10 days of the trial, compared with 13% additional decline in hyperglycemia across the remaining 30 days [11]. Interestingly, the degree of plasma glucose reduction was not associated with the rate or extent of the weight loss, but rather associated with a reduction in hepatic glucose output. While this study did not evaluate diabetes remission per se, it does provide important insight into the effect of low-calorie diet on hepatic glucose output and the speed of improvement of plasma glucose. A more recent study using a less restrictive diet (600 calorie/day diet) has subsequently confirmed these findings, including normalization of fasting plasma levels within 1 week of diet initiation, reduction of hepatic glucose output, reduced hepatic triacylglycerol content, and improved first-phase insulin response at week 8 [12]. While these studies show short-term changes in glycemic indices with very low-calorie diets, they do not confirm longitudinal remission of type 2 diabetes, especially after return to long-term isocaloric feeding.

To address this, a prospective study measured the maintenance of remission of type 2 diabetes 6 months after resumption of isocaloric feeding. Thirty patients with type 2 diabetes (duration 0.5–23 years) underwent an 8-week course of very low caloric diet (624–700 calorie per day through liquid meal replacement with 240 g of non-starchy vegetables) followed by 2-week gradual reintroduction of solid food and then a 6-month weight loss management program. At 6 months' follow-up visit, 13 out of 30 patients (40%) had achieved remission (partial or complete). Duration of diabetes was significantly shorter in responders compared to nonresponders (M3.8 (±1) vs M9.8 (±1.6)), while weight loss was similar between both groups [13]. Another study randomized 83 patients with recently diagnosed type 2 diabetes (<3 year duration) into 8- and 16-week "intensive metabolic intervention" (negative 500–750 calories from daily requirement and exercise) or standard care and established a 21.4% and 40.7% remission rates at the 3-month follow-up visit in the two intervention groups [14].

A less restrictive diet may be unhelpful in terms of remission especially in those with more prolonged diabetes duration, as shown in a parallel arm study of 215 patients with type 2 diabetes (mean duration 5.1 years) randomized either to low-carb Mediterranean diet (1500 cal/day for females, 1800 cal/day for males) or to low-fat diet. Remission rates were 4.6% and 0.9% at 1 year, respectively [15]. In a retrospective analysis of 88 obese patients with type 2 diabetes who underwent a 12-week multidisciplinary weight loss program ("Why WAIT"; 1200–1800 calories per day, along with exercise and other interventions), many had improved glycemic control, but only four were able to meet criteria for partial or complete remission at 1-year follow-up visit [16]. The "Look AHEAD study" randomized 5145 patients with type 2 diabetes (median duration 5 years) into either "intensive lifestyle intervention" (target calorie consumption 1200–1800 per day, exercise, counseling, and twice monthly contact) or diabetes support and education, with complete remission prevalence being 1.3% at 1 year in the intensive lifestyle intervention group (any remission prevalence 11.5%) [17].

Considering the need for very low-calorie diet, the real-world applicability of inducing remission in type 2 diabetics in the ambulatory setting, aside from bariatric surgery or intensive clinical trials, has come into question. The latest of the remission trials was meant to address this. The "DiRECT" study randomized 306 participants with type 2 diabetes across 49 primary centers to either "weight loss management program" or best practice (control). The intervention group received meal replacement through formula (825–853 calorie/day for 3–5 months), followed by a gradual reintroduction of food spanning 2–8 weeks and monthly visits to maintain weight loss, with a total of 8 hours of structured counseling by dieticians/nurses trained in "Counterweight-Plus" weight management program. Remission of diabetes at 12 months was achieved in 46% ($n = 68$) of patients in the intervention group (mean duration of diabetes 3.0 years, SD 1.7), with mean weight loss of 10.0 kg (SD = 8) [18]. In a subsequent durability measure of that study, patients were followed for an additional of 12 months, and while the intervention group continued to receive 30-minute monthly counseling sessions, they were offered a "rescue" partial meal replacement course for 2–4 weeks if they had gained more than 2 kg and full meal replacement course for 4 weeks if they gained more than 4 kg. At 24 months, remission rates dropped to 36% ($n = 53$) in the intervention group, with remission being directly linked to the extent of sustained weight loss among participants [19]. A subset of patients who achieved remission underwent functional B-cell capacity testing and were shown to have normalization of indices, confirming remission at the physiological as well as the clinical levels [20].

Pharmacotherapy with Oral Hypoglycemics, Insulin, and Appetite Suppressants

The use of pharmacotherapy and insulin to induce remission from type 2 diabetes has been investigated, with mixed but perhaps promising results. Theoretically, eliminating glucotoxicity early through intensive control of plasma glucose is expected to reduce B-cell decompensation. Pharmacological interventions in these settings were performed alongside weight loss management. A multicenter study in China investigated the utility of intensive glucose management in early diabetes on long-term remission rates. Patients (n = 382) with newly diagnosed type 2 diabetes were randomized to intensive insulin therapy through continuous subcutaneous infusion (CSI), multiple daily insulin (MDI) injections, or oral hypoglycemics (either metformin, gliclazide, or a combination of both upon escalation) with a goal of reducing fasting glucose to <6.1 mmol/L (<110 mg/dL) dubbed "euglycemia." Two weeks after attainment of euglycemia, treatments were discontinued, and patients were asked to continue diet and exercise. Mean duration to euglycemia was less than 10 days in all groups but significantly shorter in the insulin groups. Remission rates at 12 months were 51.1% in the CSI group, 44.9% in the MDI group, and 26.7% in the oral hypoglycemic group [21]. While the glycemic goals reached in the insulin and oral hypoglycemic groups were similar, the reason for improved remission rates in the insulin groups was postulated to be secondary to insulin-induced "B-cell rest," among other insulin-induced effects [21]. In another intensive therapy study, the REMIT-DAPA study from Canada, 154 patients with established type 2 diabetes, most of whom were already on oral hypoglycemics with a mean diabetes duration of 3 years, were randomized into "intensive intervention" or standard care. The intensive intervention group stopped their home oral hypoglycemic and received a 12-week course of "induction" treatment with basal insulin (titration for morning glucose of 70–95), maximal doses of metformin and dapagliflozin, as well as weight reduction and exercise counseling. Intervention continued until attainment of Hba1c of <7.3%, at which point all their hypoglycemic agents and insulin were stopped and they were asked to continue diet and exercise and were followed for 64 weeks. By 12 weeks, 49% of the intensive group reached morning glucose of <95, and all of them had Hba1c of <7.3% and stopped therapy, compared to 5.2% and 68.8% in the standard care group, respectively. Remission rates at 24 weeks not significantly different between the two groups [22]. While more research is needed to confirm the utility of intensive glucose management on type 2 diabetes remission, previous studies challenge the dogma of the stepwise approach that is usually used to manage uncontrolled diabetes [2].

There is a paucity of studies evaluating the utility of using pharmacological weight loss agents to induce remission from type 2 diabetes. In one study evaluating glycemic indices with orlistat treatment, 39 patients with type 2 diabetes were randomized to nutritional counseling (500 calorie negative balance) with orlistat or with placebo. At 6 months' follow-up, both groups have similar rates of weight loss and Hba1c reduction, but the orlistat group had statistically significant improvement in free fatty acids and insulin sensitivity. The combination of weight loss medications phentermine and topiramate has been investigated in the "OB202" and "DM-230"studies, each 28-week studies evaluating the safety and efficiency of once-daily phentermine/topiramate in weight loss and glycemic control of patients with type 2 diabetes. At the end of the 56-week intervention, patients on phentermine/topiramate had lower weight (−9.6% vs −2.6%) and lower Hba1c compared to placebo (−1.6% vs −1.2%) with 32% reaching target Hba1c <6.5% compared to 16% in the placebo group. However, the study was not meant to address remission, and antidiabetic agents were not discontinued prior to study initiation.

In summary, remission of type 2 diabetes requires reversal of the conditions that led to its development. Namely, a large negative energy balance early in the diagnosis is the most effective way to induce medical remission. The ability of pharmacotherapy to induce remission is an area of active research.

References

1. Buse JB, Caprio S, Cefalu WT, et al. How do we define cure of diabetes? Diabetes Care. 2009;32:2133–5.
2. Rasouli N. An escape from diabetes. J Clin Endocrinol Metab. 2020;105:3460–1.
3. Taylor R. Pathogenesis of type 2 diabetes: tracing the reverse route from cure to cause. Diabetologia. 2008;51:1781–9.
4. Cersosimo E, Triplitt C, Mandarino LJ, DeFronzo RA. Pathogenesis of type 2 diabetes mellitus – endotext – NCBI Bookshelf. Endotext, Compr. Free online Endocrinol B. 2015.

5. Ferrannini E, Gastaldelli A, Miyazaki Y, Matsuda M, Mari A, DeFronzo RA. β-Cell function in subjects spanning the range from normal glucose tolerance to overt diabetes: a new analysis. J Clin Endocrinol Metab. 2005;90:493–500.
6. U.K. prospective diabetes study 16: overview of 6 years' therapy of Type II diabetes: a progressive disease. Diabetes. 1995;44:1249–58.
7. Pantalone KM, Wells BJ, Chagin KM, Ejzykowicz F, Yu C, Milinovich A, Bauman JM, Kattan MW, Rajpathak S, Zimmerman RS. Intensification of diabetes therapy and time until A1C goal attainment among patients with newly diagnosed type 2 diabetes who fail metformin monotherapy within a large integrated health system. Diabetes Care. 2016;39:1527–34.
8. Petersen KF, Dufour S, Befroy D, Lehrke M, Hendler RE, Shulman GI. Reversal of nonalcoholic hepatic steatosis, hepatic insulin resistance, and hyperglycemia by moderate weight reduction in patients with type 2 diabetes. Diabetes. 2005;54:603–8.
9. Dixon JB, Bhathal PS, O'Brien PE. Nonalcoholic fatty liver disease: predictors of nonalcoholic steatohepatitis and liver fibrosis in the severely obese. Gastroenterology. 2001;121:91–100.
10. Hollingsworth KG, Abubacker MZ, Joubert I, Allison MED, Lomas DJ. Low-carbohydrate diet induced reduction of hepatic lipid content observed with a rapid non-invasive MRI technique. Br J Radiol. 2006;79:712–5.
11. Henry RR, Scheaffer L, Olefsky JM. Glycemic effects of intensive caloric restriction and isocaloric refeeding in noninsulin-dependent diabetes mellitus*. J Clin Endocrinol Metab. 1985;61:917–25.
12. Lim EL, Hollingsworth KG, Aribisala BS, Chen MJ, Mathers JC, Taylor R. Reversal of type 2 diabetes: normalisation of beta cell function in association with decreased pancreas and liver triacylglycerol. Diabetologia. 2011;54:2506–14.
13. Steven S, Hollingsworth KG, Al-Mrabeh A, Avery L, Aribisala B, Caslake M, Taylor R. Very low-calorie diet and 6 months of weight stability in type 2 diabetes: pathophysiological changes in responders and nonresponders. Diabetes Care. 2016;39:808–15.
14. McInnes N, Smith A, Otto R, Vandermey J, Punthakee Z, Sherifali D, Balasubramanian K, Hall S, Gerstein HC. Piloting a remission strategy in type 2 diabetes: results of a randomized controlled trial. J Clin Endocrinol Metab. 2017;102:1596–605.
15. Esposito K, Maiorino MI, Petrizzo M, Bellastella G, Giugliano D. The effects of a Mediterranean diet on the need for diabetes drugs and remission of newly diagnosed type 2 diabetes: follow-up of a randomized trial. Diabetes Care. 2014;37:1824–30.
16. Mottalib A, Sakr M, Shehabeldin M, Hamdy O. Diabetes remission after nonsurgical intensive lifestyle intervention in obese patients with type 2 diabetes. J Diabetes Res. 2015;2015:10–3.
17. Gregg EW, Chen H, Wagenknecht LE, et al. Association of an intensive lifestyle intervention with remission of type 2 diabetes. JAMA. 2012;308(23):2489–96. https://doi.org/10.1001/jama.2012.67929.
18. Lean ME, Leslie WS, Barnes AC, et al. Primary care-led weight management for remission of type 2 diabetes (DiRECT): an open-label, cluster-randomised trial. Lancet. 2018;391:541–51.
19. Lean MEJ, Leslie WS, Barnes AC, et al. Durability of a primary care-led weight-management intervention for remission of type 2 diabetes: 2-year results of the DiRECT open-label, cluster-randomised trial. Lancet Diabetes Endocrinol. 2019;7:344–55.
20. Zhyzhneuskaya SV, Al-Mrabeh A, Peters C, Barnes A, Aribisala B, Hollingsworth KG, McConnachie A, Sattar N, Lean MEJ, Taylor R. Time course of normalization of functional β-cell capacity in the diabetes remission clinical trial after weight loss in type 2 diabetes. Diabetes Care. 2020;43:813–20.
21. Weng J, Li Y, Xu W, et al. Effect of intensive insulin therapy on β-cell function and glycaemic control in patients with newly diagnosed type 2 diabetes: a multicentre randomised parallel-group trial. Lancet. 2008;371:1753–60.
22. McInnes N, Hall S, Sultan F, Aronson R, Hramiak I, Harris S, Sigal RJ, Woo V, Liu YY, Gerstein HC. Remission of type 2 diabetes following a short-term intervention with insulin glargine, metformin, and dapagliflozin. J Clin Endocrinol Metab. 2020;105:2532–40.

Chapter 11
Surgical Management for Diabetes Remission

A. Maria Daniela Hurtado and Maria Collazo-Clavell

Introduction

Diabetes mellitus type 2 (DM2) is a multifactorial, complex, and progressive disease. In 2017, the worldwide prevalence of DM2 was 6.3%, which was equivalent to a staggering 462 million people [1]. A significant proportion of patients with DM2 has disease-related comorbidities and overall decreased lifespan. The underlying chronic hyperglycemia characteristic of this disease leads to macrovascular and microvascular complications. As a matter of fact, diabetes is the leading cause of amputations of the lower extremities, kidney failure, and blindness. As such, DM2 is the ninth leading cause of death globally [2, 3]. DM2 also poses an economic burden: in the United States alone, the estimated cost of DM2 in 2017 was $327 billion [4]. Consequently, DM2 is recognized as a global public health problem.

Excess weight is one of the most important risk factors for DM2. The prevalence of overweight and obesity among patients with DM2 is almost double compared to the overall prevalence of these conditions in the general population (90% vs 50%, respectively) [2]. This health crisis is known as the "twin pandemic." Lifestyle interventions with the goal of weight reduction are the cornerstone of DM2 management. Weight loss of 5–10% of the total body weight with intensive lifestyle modification has been associated with improved glycemic control and even DM2

A. Maria Daniela Hurtado
Division of Endocrinology, Diabetes, Metabolism, and Nutrition, Department of Medicine, Mayo Clinic Health System, La Crosse, WI, USA

Division of Endocrinology, Diabetes, Metabolism, and Nutrition, Department of Medicine, Mayo Clinic, Rochester, MN, USA

M. Collazo-Clavell (✉)
Division of Endocrinology, Diabetes, Metabolism, and Nutrition, Department of Medicine, Mayo Clinic, Rochester, MN, USA
e-mail: collazoclavell.maria@mayo.edu

R. Basu (ed.), *Precision Medicine in Diabetes*,
https://doi.org/10.1007/978-3-030-98927-9_11

remission in patients with obesity [5]. However, sustained weight loss with conservative measures such as lifestyle interventions and medications is challenging to achieve. Thus, bariatric surgeries, the gold standard treatment for achieving sustained weight loss, have become accepted therapeutic options to treat DM2, especially when DM2 is refractory to lifestyle and pharmacologic interventions. Furthermore, because of the progressive nature of DM2 resulting in multiple complications and the overall improvement of the cardiovascular risk after bariatric surgery, modeling analyses suggest that bariatric surgery may be a cost-saving and practical therapeutic option for patients with DM2 [6, 7].

The beneficial effects of bariatric surgery on glycemic control have been known for the past three decades [8]. Given the strong evidence surrounding the role of bariatric surgery on DM2 remission, the American Diabetes Association in conjunction with many other international organizations has consistently recommended bariatric surgery consideration for the treatment of DM2 in patients with a body mass index (BMI) as low as 30 kg/m^2 (27.5 kg/m^2 for Asians), particularly when DM2 control is not achieved with lifestyle or pharmacologic interventions [9–12].

In this chapter, first, we will define DM2 remission; second, we will briefly describe the bariatric surgeries that have been associated with DM2 remission; third, we will summarize the supporting evidence of the role of bariatric surgery on DM2 remission; finally, we will discuss the mechanisms involved in DM2 remission.

DM2 Cure Versus Remission

Medical dictionaries define cure as the restoration of health. Remission, on the other hand, is defined as a state or period during which the symptoms of a disease subside but may recur [13]. With respect to DM2, the definitions of cure and remission have not been consistently delineated over the years. Although therapies with curative intent have been developed, evidence suggests that given the complex pathophysiology of DM2, there is always a chance of relapse. Consequently, a consensus group in 2009 concluded that for DM2, it would be more accurate to use the term remission than cure [14].

The consensus group defined DM2 remission based on:

1. Glucose levels below the diabetes range.
2. The absence of glucose-lowering medications and/or ongoing procedures to maintain glucose homeostasis.
3. Sustainability over time (for at least 1 year).

Conventionally, complete remission is defined as an HbA1c below 6% or <42 mmol/mol, and partial remission is defined by an HbA1c below 6.5% or <48 mmol/mol. Prolonged remission is defined as complete remission for at least 5 years [14].

Although complete remission is the most coveted outcome, partial remission has clinical significance. Partial remission has also been associated with a reduced risk of developing microvascular and macrovascular complications, and an overall decreased mortality, protection that is carried over even if patients experience relapse of their DM2 [15, 16].

Bariatric Surgeries Associated with DM2 Remission

Figure 11.1 shows a schematic representation of the types of bariatric surgeries that have been associated with DM2 remission which include laparoscopic adjustable gastric banding (LAGB), vertical sleeve gastrectomy (VSG), Roux-en-Y gastric bypass (RYGB), and biliopancreatic diversion (BPD) with or without duodenal switch (BPD-DS).

The first two procedures, the LAGB and the VSG, are purely restrictive procedures, i.e., they do not encompass rerouting of the food through the gastrointestinal tract. The LAGB consists of a band like tube that encircles the upper part of the stomach, immediately after the gastroesophageal junction. When the tube is filled with saline solution, it creates a small gastric pouch that results in restriction of the stomach volume. The VSG is characterized by the removal of the greater curvature and fundus of the stomach that results in a significantly decreased gastric capacity.

The RYGB, the BPD, and BPD-DS are all surgeries characterized by bypasses, i.e., they encompass rerouting of the food through the gastrointestinal tract in addition to their restrictive component. The RYGB involves a partial horizontal gastrectomy resulting in a small functional gastric pouch that is then connected to the jejunum; consequently, food bypasses 95% of the stomach, the entire duodenum, and a small portion of the jejunum. The BPD is similar to the RYGB as it involves a partial horizontal gastrectomy leaving a variable sized functional gastric pouch that is anastomosed to the ileum; thus, this procedure bypasses a significant part of the stomach, the duodenum, and the jejunum and a portion of the ileum. The BPD-DS is characterized by a vertical sleeve gastrectomy and preservation of the

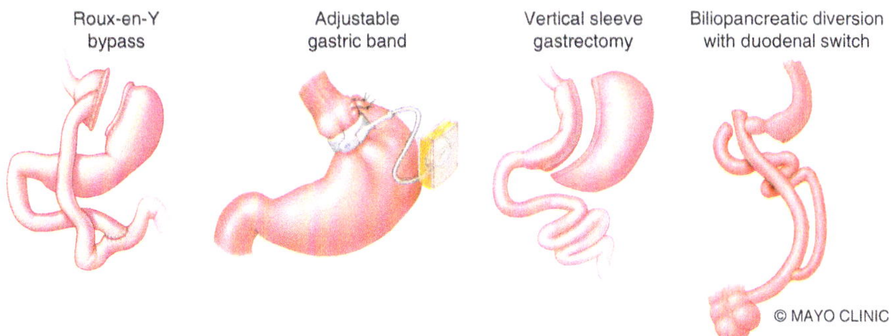

Fig. 11.1 Bariatric surgeries associated with DM2 remission

proximal duodenum that is then anastomosed to the ileum resulting in a bypass of most of the duodenum, the jejunum, and a portion of the ileum.

At present, the most commonly utilized bariatric surgeries are the VSG and the RYGB [17].

DM2 Remission After Bariatric Surgery

The beneficial effects of bariatric surgery on glucose control were first anecdotally described in the 1970s. It was not until the mid-1990s that a seminal paper by Pories et al. reported impressive DM2 remission rates after RYGB: at the end of the 14-year follow-up (mean 7.6 years), 83% of patients with DM2 who had undergone RYGB were in remission [8]. Since then, strong evidence has continued to emerge about the role of bariatric surgery on DM2 remission and the underlying mechanisms that are involved.

Among the different bariatric procedures, the BPD-DS results in a higher degree and length of DM2 remission, followed by the RYGB, the VSG, and finally the LAGB [18–20]. Multiple randomized controlled trials and observational studies have consistently demonstrated remission rates of 30–95% between 1 and 5 years postoperatively [21–39]. Table 11.1 summarizes the evidence to date on DM2

Table 11.1 Studies supporting the role of bariatric surgery on DM2 remission

Study	Type of surgery	Definition of DM2 remission	Mean or median time of follow-up time (years)	Rate of DM2 remission
Pories et al. (1995) [8]	RYGB	"Normal" FPG and HbA1c	7.6	82.9%
Schauer et al. (2003) [19]	RYGB	FPG ≤110 mg/dL, a normal HbA1c on no medications	5	82%
Dixon et al. (2008) [24]	LAGB	FPG <126 mg/dL, HbA1c <6.2% on no medications	2	76%
Iaconelli et al. (2011) [36]	BPD	ADA criteria for complete remission[a]	10	100%
Schauer et al. (2012) [34]	RYGB and VSG	ADA criteria for complete remission[a]	1	42% for RYGB 37% for VSG
Adams et al. (2012) [37]	RYGB	"Normal" FPG and HbA1c on no medications	2 and 6	75% at 2 years 62% at 6 years
Mingrone et al. (2012) [33]	RYGB and BPD	ADA criteria for partial remission[a]	2	75% for RYGB 95% for BPD
Liang et al. (2013) [35]	RYGB	"Normal" FPG and HbA1c on no medications	1	90%
Arterburn et al. (2013) [45]	RYGB	ADA criteria for complete remission[a]	1, 3, and 5	37% at 1 year 63% at 3 years 68% at 5 years

Table 11.1 (continued)

Study	Type of surgery	Definition of DM2 remission	Mean or median time of follow-up time (years)	Rate of DM2 remission
Wentworth et al. (2014) [27]	LAGB	FPG <16 mg/dL and less than <200 mg/dL 2 h after oral glucose	2	52%
Courcoulas et al. (2014) [25]	RYGB and LAGB	ADA criteria for complete remission[a]	1	17% for RYGB 23% for LAGB
Halperin et al. (2014) [26]	RYGB	FPG <126 mg/dL and HbA1c <6.5% ± medications	1	58%
Courcoulas et al. (2015) [30]	RYGB and LAGB	ADA criteria for complete remission[a]	3	15% for RYGB 5% for LAGB
Ding et al. (2015) [28]	LAGB	HbA1c <6.5% and FPG <126 mg/dl ± medications	1	33%
Mingrone et al. (2015) [21]	RYGB and BPD	ADA criteria for partial remission[a]	5	37% for RYGB 63% for BPD
Yska et al. (2015) [18]	RYGB, VSG, and LAGB	ADA criteria for complete remission[a]	2.4	94.5/1000 person-years
Cummings et al. (2016) [29]	RYGB	ADA criteria for complete remission[a]	1	60%
Purnell et al. (2016)	RYGB and LAGB	ADA criteria for partial remission[a]	3	69% for RYGB 30% for LAGB
Ikramuddin et al. (2016) [23]	RYGB	ADA criteria for complete remission[a]	3	17%
Gulliford et al. (2016) [44]	RYGB, VSG, and LAGB	ADA criteria for partial remission[a]	2	34% for RYGB 38% for VSG 20% for LAGB
Schauer et al. (2017) [22]	RYGB and VSG	ADA criteria for complete remission[a]	5	22% for RYGB 15% for VSG
Madsen et al. (2019) [39]	RYGB	HbA1c <6.5% on no medications or <6% on metformin only	1	74%
Jans et al. (2019) [32]	RYGB and VSG	ADA criteria for complete remission[a]	2 and 5	58% at 2 years 47% at 5 years

Abbreviations used: *ADA* American Diabetes Association, *BPD* biliopancreatic diversion, *DM2* type 2 diabetes mellitus, *FPG* fasting plasma glucose, *HbA1c* hemoglobin A1c, *LAGB* laparoscopic adjustable gastric banding, *RYGB* Roux-en-Y gastric bypass, *VSG* vertical sleeve gastrectomy

[a]ADA criteria: Complete remission is defined as an HbA1c below 6% or <42 mmol/mol on no medications and maintained for at least 1 year; Partial remission is defined by an HbA1c below 6.5% or <48 mmol/mol on no medications and maintained for at least 1 year

remission rates after bariatric surgery. Overall, the rate of partial remission is, on average, 10% higher compared to the rate of complete remission in studies that have reported both [40]. Several meta-analyses have echoed these findings [41, 42]. The largest meta-analysis included 621 studies with a total of 135,246 patients, with more than 3000 patients with DM2. This study showed that the overall DM2 remission rate after bariatric procedures was 78.1%, 95.1% after BPD-DS, 80.3% after RYGB, and 56.7% after LAGB, with consistent rates among studies up to approximately 2 years after surgery [20].

In spite of the increasing evidence of the effect of bariatric surgery in patients with DM2, there are data showing that postoperative DM2 remission is not always durable. Studies have shown that the maximum cumulative incidence of DM2 remission occurs 3 years after bariatric surgery. After 3 years, relapses begin to accumulate [21, 23, 30, 37, 39, 43, 44]. Studies estimate that at 5 years after RYGB, 35–50% of patients in remission experience a relapse [21, 45–47]. The rate of relapse is higher after VSG and reported at 80% at 5 years [48].

Several preoperative and postoperative factors play a role in the probability of postoperative DM2 remission. A Swedish nationwide register-based cohort study including more than 8000 patients demonstrated that preoperative factors strongly associated with a higher rate of DM2 remission after bariatric surgery included shorter duration of DM2 and no insulin treatment [32]. Other preoperative factors that have been shown to influence DM2 remission include younger age, male sex, higher BMI, glycemic control, and higher education [22, 32, 43, 45, 49–55]. Among Asians, visceral fat has also been found to be an important predictor [56]. Postoperative factors include higher amount of weight loss after surgery and the type of procedure, with RYGB associated with a higher rate of remission [32].

Because bariatric surgery is not a treatment without risk, the rates of DM2 after bariatric surgery are widely variable, and the risk of DM2 recurrence over time is not irrelevant, researchers have developed scoring systems to help identify the most suitable candidates for bariatric surgery aimed at DM2 remission. The most commonly used score systems are the ABCD and the DiaRem (Table 11.2). The former takes into consideration age, BMI, C-peptide, and duration of DM2. The latter takes into consideration age, HbA1c, and the use of antidiabetic medications [57, 58]. Both scoring systems have their own limitations, but validation studies suggest that the ABCD scoring system may be better predictive tool for DM2 remission after bariatric surgery [59].

Mechanisms Driving DM2 Remission

The effects of bariatric surgery on glucose homeostasis are intricate, and not all the mechanisms involved are completely understood. Bariatric surgery overall results in enhanced β-cell function, decreased hepatic glucose production, increased insulin sensitivity, and improved peripheral glucose uptake. The significant weight loss achieved after bariatric surgery is undoubtedly an important factor for DM2

Table 11.2 Scoring systems to predict the remission of DM2 after bariatric surgery

DiaRem score		
Factor		Points
Age		
	<40	0
	40–49	1
	50–59	2
	≥60	3
HbA1c		
	<6.5%	0
	6.5–6.9%	2
	7.0–8.9%	4
	≥9.0%	6
Diabetes drugs		
	No medication or metformin only	0
	Sulfonylureas and insulin-sensitizing agents other than metformin	3
Treatment with insulin		
	No	0
	Yes	10
Total score calculated by adding each of the four variables		0–22
Lower DiaRem scores predict a higher probability of DM2 remission after RYGB		
ABCD score		
Factor		Points
Age (years)		
	<40	1
	≥40	0
BMI (kg/m^2)		
	<27	0
	27–34.9	1
	35–41.9	2
	≥42	3
C-peptide (ng/mL)		
	<2	0
	2–2.9	1
	3–3.9	2
	≥5	3
Duration of DM2 (years)		
	>8	0
	4–8	1
	1–3.9	2
	<1	3
Total score calculated by adding each of the four variables		0–10

Higher ABCD scores predict a higher probability of DM2 remission after RYGB
Abbreviations used: *BMI* body mass index, *DM2*, type 2 diabetes mellitus, *HbA1c* hemoglobin A1c, *RYGB* Roux-en-Y gastric bypass

remission. However, a strong body of evidence suggests that there are weight loss-independent mechanisms that play a crucial role in DM2 remission as well.

The massive weight loss associated with bariatric procedures promotes glucose transport into the muscle and overall whole-body glucose disposal [60]. The mechanisms behind this phenomenon include increased levels of adiponectin which is an insulin-sensitizing hormone, increased insulin receptor concentration at the level of the muscle, and decreased concentrations of intramuscular lipids and fatty acyl-CoA molecules [61–63].

The following facts support the role of weight loss-independent mechanisms of DM2 remission:

1. The remission of DM2 occurs before significant and sustained weight loss occurs, generally within days to weeks after RYGB or BPD-DS, phenomenon not seen after LAGB or SVG [8, 19, 64, 65].
2. DM2 remission rate is higher in patients after RYGB compared to other interventions that result in similar weight loss such as lifestyle interventions, VSG, and LAGB [66–68].
3. Certain GI bypass procedures, such as the duodenal-jejunal bypass and the endoluminal duodenal bypass, improve glucose control disproportionately to weight loss [69–72].
4. The existence of the rare hyperinsulinemic hypoglycemia, which is a late complication of the RYGB [73].

Mechanistically, these factors are thought to play a major role in weight loss-independent DM2:

1. Significant and rapid reduction in hepatic and pancreatic fat content precipitated by caloric restriction and resulting in a rapid improvement of insulin secretion [74, 75].
2. Increased secretion of gastrointestinal peptides, mainly GLP-1 and PYY, resulting from the anatomical rearrangement and the consequent nutrient and bile acid-mediated stimulation of the distal intestinal tract (also known as hindgut hypothesis) [76, 77].
3. Intestinal adaptation characterized by mucosal hypertrophy and hyperplasia (particularly of GLP-1 and GIP producing L-enteroendocrine cells), enhanced expression of glucose transporters, and increased glucose uptake in the intestinal epithelium [78].
4. Decreased secretion of the orexigenic and prodiabetic hormone ghrelin.
5. Increase in circulating bile acids that induce GLP-1, GIP, and PYY secretion [79].
6. Alterations in the gut microbiome [80, 81].
7. Reduction of yet to be defined anti-incretins, substances secreted by the duodenum and possibly jejunum, whose role would be to counteract the effect of incretins (GLP-1 and GIP) to prevent postprandial hypoglycemia (foregut hypothesis).

Important Considerations of Bariatric Surgery in DM2 Remission and Future Directions

Although bariatric surgery is a safe surgical intervention with a low mortality rate, it is an invasive and costly procedure with potential complications. Over the last several years, less invasive endoscopic procedures have been developed and are considered cost-effective alternatives to bariatric surgery. These include the intragastric balloon, the endoscopic sleeve gastroplasty, the duodenal-jejunal bypass liner, and the gastro-duodeno-jejunal bypass sleeve. The intragastric balloon is a mechanical device that is inflated in the stomach, thereby decreasing gastric capacity. The endoscopic sleeve gastroplasty mimics the anatomic changes of the VSG by stapling the anterior and posterior walls of the stomach to decrease its size. The duodenal-jejunal bypass liner consists of an impermeable liner anchored to the duodenal bulb that extends through the proximal part of the small intestine covering the intestinal mucosa. This procedure mimics the intestinal bypass portion of the RYGB by excluding the proximal small intestine from the alimentary flow. The gastro-duodeno-jejunal bypass sleeve is a flexible plastic device anchored to the gastroesophageal junction that extends into the proximal intestine. This procedure excludes the stomach and proximal small intestine from the alimentary flow. Although these procedures and devices have demonstrated encouraging weight loss results, there is a paucity of data on safety and long-term efficacy, particularly in relation to DM2 outcomes [82–85].

Although not aimed at weight loss, the duodenal mucosal resurfacing is a novel endoscopic procedure involving the thermal ablation, and subsequent regeneration, of the duodenal mucosa with the goal of improving glucose metabolism. The duodenal mucosa has been implicated as an important regulator of glucose homeostasis, and data so far suggest a promising potential therapeutic target in DM2 control [86].

Conclusions

For a long time, DM2 had been seen as a chronic, progressive, and incurable disease. With the advent of bariatric surgery, DM2 remission has become a reality. Extensive evidence has demonstrated that bariatric surgery is the most efficient and effective therapeutic modality to achieve DM2 remission compared with any other nonsurgical modality. The rate of complete DM2 remission after bariatric surgery varies but has been overall consistently robust among studies. The BPD-DS and the RYGB have been associated with the highest DM2 remission rates (70–90%), whereas the LAGB is associated with the lowest rates of remission. There are preoperative and postoperative predictors of DM2 remission after bariatric surgery that must be taken into consideration when discussing this possible outcome with patients. It is also important to disclose that DM2 recidivism has been described after all procedures over time.

There is a substantial body of evidence demonstrating that in addition to caloric restriction and massive weight loss, other important mechanisms are involved in DM2 remission, some of which remain to be fully characterized. Some of these mechanisms include increased levels of GLP-1, PYY, and GIP, impaired ghrelin secretion, improved bile acid metabolism, and changes in the microbiome.

The utilization of bariatric surgery is hindered by the small, albeit existent, risk of complications and its cost. With the mounting evidence showing that gastrointestinal modifications from bariatric surgery influence glucose metabolism through multiple mechanisms, research has focused on developing less invasive gastrointestinal procedures. Likewise, bariatric surgery and these experimental gastrointestinal procedures have helped gained insight into the physiologic role of the different parts of the gastrointestinal system on glucose homeostasis. Eventually, this knowledge could lead to the development of pharmacologic therapies and metabolic procedures aimed at DM2 treatment and not necessarily focused on weight loss.

References

1. The International Diabetes Federation 2020 [Available from: https://www.idf.org/.
2. Prevention CfDCa. National Diabetes Statistics Repor. tAtlanta, GA: Centers for Disease Control and Prevention, U.S. Dept of Health and Human Services; 2020. 2020.
3. Khan MAB, Hashim MJ, King JK, Govender RD, Mustafa H, Al KJ. Epidemiology of type 2 diabetes - global burden of disease and forecasted trends. J Epidemiol Glob Health. 2020;10(1):107–11.
4. Association AD. Economic Costs of Diabetes in the U.S. in 2017. Diabetes Care; 2018.
5. Gregg EW, Zhuo X, Cheng YJ, Albright AL, Narayan KMV, Thompson TJ. Trends in lifetime risk and years of life lost due to diabetes in the USA, 1985–2011: a modelling study. Lancet Diabetes Endocrinol. 2014;2(11):867–74.
6. The clinical effectiveness and cost-effectiveness of bariatric (weight loss) surgery for obesity: a systematic review and economic evaluation. Clin Governance Inter J. 2010;15(1).
7. Keating C, Neovius M, Sjöholm K, Peltonen M, Narbro K, Eriksson JK, et al. Health-care costs over 15 years after bariatric surgery for patients with different baseline glucose status: results from the Swedish obese subjects study. Lancet Diabetes Endocrinol. 2015;3(11):855–65.
8. Pories WJ, Swanson MS, MacDonald KG, Long SB, Morris PG, Brown BM, et al. Who would have thought it? An operation proves to be the most effective therapy for adult-onset diabetes mellitus. Ann Surg. 1995;222(3):339–52.
9. 8. Obesity management for the treatment of type 2 diabetes: standards of medical care in diabetes—2021. Diabetes Care. 2021;44(Supplement 1):S100–10.
10. Rubino F, Kaplan LM, Schauer PR, Cummings DE. The diabetes surgery summit consensus conference: recommendations for the evaluation and use of gastrointestinal surgery to treat type 2 diabetes mellitus. Ann Surg. 2010;251(3):399–405.
11. Zimmet P, Alberti KG, Rubino F, Dixon JB. IDF's view of bariatric surgery in type 2 diabetes. Lancet. 2011;378(9786):108–10.
12. Kasama K, Mui W, Lee WJ, Lakdawala M, Naitoh T, Seki Y, et al. IFSO-APC consensus statements 2011. Obes Surg. 2012;22(5):677–84.
13. Medical Terminology. Available from: https://www.merriam-webster.com/dictionary/medicalDictionary.

14. Buse JB, Caprio S, Cefalu WT, Ceriello A, Del Prato S, Inzucchi SE, et al. How do we define cure of diabetes? Diabetes Care. 2009;32(11):2133–5.
15. Coleman KJ, Haneuse S, Johnson E, Bogart A, Fisher D, O'Connor PJ, et al. Long-term microvascular disease outcomes in patients with type 2 diabetes after bariatric surgery: evidence for the legacy effect of surgery. Diabetes Care. 2016;39(8):1400–7.
16. Sheng B, Truong K, Spitler H, Zhang L, Tong X, Chen L. The Long-term effects of bariatric surgery on type 2 diabetes remission, microvascular and macrovascular complications, and mortality: a systematic review and meta-analysis. Obes Surg. 2017;27(10):2724–32.
17. Ponce J, DeMaria EJ, Nguyen NT, Hutter M, Sudan R, Morton JM. American Society for Metabolic and Bariatric Surgery estimation of bariatric surgery procedures in 2015 and surgeon workforce in the United States. Surgery for Obesity and Related Diseases : Official Journal of the American Society for Bariatric Surgery. 2016;12(9):1637–9.
18. Yska JP, van Roon EN, de Boer A, Leufkens HG, Wilffert B, de Heide LJ, et al. Remission of type 2 diabetes mellitus in patients after different types of bariatric surgery: a population-based cohort study in the United Kingdom. JAMA Surg. 2015;150(12):1126–33.
19. Schauer PR, Burguera B, Ikramuddin S, Cottam D, Gourash W, Hamad G, et al. Effect of laparoscopic roux-en Y gastric bypass on type 2 diabetes mellitus. Ann Surg. 2003;238(4):467–85.
20. Buchwald H, Estok R, Fahrbach K, Banel D, Jensen MD, Pories WJ, et al. Weight and type 2 diabetes after bariatric surgery: systematic review and meta-analysis. Am J Med. 2009;122(3):248–56.e5.
21. Mingrone G, Panunzi S, De Gaetano A, Guidone C, Iaconelli A, Nanni G, et al. Bariatric-metabolic surgery versus conventional medical treatment in obese patients with type 2 diabetes: 5 year follow-up of an open-label, single-Centre, randomised controlled trial. Lancet. 2015;386(9997):964–73.
22. Schauer PR, Bhatt DL, Kirwan JP, Wolski K, Aminian A, Brethauer SA, et al. Bariatric surgery versus intensive medical therapy for diabetes - 5-year outcomes. N Engl J Med. 2017;376(7):641–51.
23. Ikramuddin S, Korner J, Lee W-J, Bantle JP, Thomas AJ, Connett JE, et al. Durability of addition of roux-en-Y gastric bypass to lifestyle intervention and medical management in achieving primary treatment goals for uncontrolled type 2 diabetes in mild to moderate obesity: a randomized control trial. Diabetes Care. 2016;39(9):1510–8.
24. Dixon JB, O'Brien PE, Playfair J, Chapman L, Schachter LM, Skinner S, et al. Adjustable gastric banding and conventional therapy for type 2 diabetesA randomized controlled trial. JAMA. 2008;299(3):316–23.
25. Courcoulas AP, Goodpaster BH, Eagleton JK, Belle SH, Kalarchian MA, Lang W, et al. Surgical vs medical treatments for type 2 diabetes mellitus: a randomized clinical trial. JAMA Surg. 2014;149(7):707–15.
26. Halperin F, Ding S-A, Simonson DC, Panosian J, Goebel-Fabbri A, Wewalka M, et al. Roux-en-Y gastric bypass surgery or lifestyle with intensive medical Management in Patients with Type 2 diabetes: feasibility and 1-year results of a randomized clinical trial. JAMA Surg. 2014;149(7):716–26.
27. Wentworth JM, Playfair J, Laurie C, Ritchie ME, Brown WA, Burton P, et al. Multidisciplinary diabetes care with and without bariatric surgery in overweight people: a randomised controlled trial. Lancet Diabetes Endocrinol. 2014;2(7):545–52.
28. Ding S-A, Simonson DC, Wewalka M, Halperin F, Foster K, Goebel-Fabbri A, et al. Adjustable gastric band surgery or medical management in patients with Type 2 diabetes: a randomized clinical trial. J Clin Endocrinol Metabol. 2015;100(7):2546–56.
29. Cummings DE, Arterburn DE, Westbrook EO, Kuzma JN, Stewart SD, Chan CP, et al. Gastric bypass surgery vs intensive lifestyle and medical intervention for type 2 diabetes: the CROSSROADS randomised controlled trial. Diabetologia. 2016;59(5):945–53.
30. Courcoulas AP, Belle SH, Neiberg RH, Pierson SK, Eagleton JK, Kalarchian MA, et al. Three-year outcomes of bariatric surgery vs lifestyle intervention for type 2 diabetes mellitus treatment: a randomized clinical trial. JAMA Surg. 2015;150(10):931–40.

31. Gloy VL, Briel M, Bhatt DL, Kashyap SR, Schauer PR, Mingrone G, et al. Bariatric surgery versus non-surgical treatment for obesity: a systematic review and meta-analysis of randomised controlled trials. BMJ: Br Med J. 2013;347:f5934.
32. Jans A, Näslund I, Ottosson J, Szabo E, Näslund E, Stenberg E. Duration of type 2 diabetes and remission rates after bariatric surgery in Sweden 2007–2015: a registry-based cohort study. PLoS Med. 2019;16(11):e1002985.
33. Mingrone G, Panunzi S, De Gaetano A, Guidone C, Iaconelli A, Leccesi L, et al. Bariatric surgery versus conventional medical therapy for type 2 diabetes. N Engl J Med. 2012;366(17):1577–85.
34. Schauer PR, Kashyap SR, Wolski K, Brethauer SA, Kirwan JP, Pothier CE, et al. Bariatric surgery versus intensive medical therapy in obese patients with diabetes. N Engl J Med. 2012;366(17):1567–76.
35. Liang Z, Wu Q, Chen B, Yu P, Zhao H, Ouyang X. Effect of laparoscopic roux-en-Y gastric bypass surgery on type 2 diabetes mellitus with hypertension: a randomized controlled trial. Diabetes Res Clin Pract. 2013;101(1):50–6.
36. Iaconelli A, Panunzi S, De Gaetano A, Manco M, Guidone C, Leccesi L, et al. Effects of bilio-pancreatic diversion on diabetic complications: a 10-year follow-up. Diabetes Care. 2011;34(3):561–7.
37. Adams TD, Davidson LE, Litwin SE, Kolotkin RL, LaMonte MJ, Pendleton RC, et al. Health benefits of gastric bypass surgery after 6 years. JAMA. 2012;308(11):1122–31.
38. Purnell JQ, Selzer F, Wahed AS, Pender J, Pories W, Pomp A, et al. Type 2 diabetes remission rates after laparoscopic gastric bypass and gastric banding: results of the longitudinal assessment of bariatric surgery study. Diabetes Care. 2016;39(7):1101–7.
39. Madsen LR, Baggesen LM, Richelsen B, Thomsen RW. Effect of roux-en-Y gastric bypass surgery on diabetes remission and complications in individuals with type 2 diabetes: a Danish population-based matched cohort study. Diabetologia. 2019;62(4):611–20.
40. Isaman DJM, Rothberg AE, Herman WH. Reconciliation of type 2 diabetes remission rates in studies of roux-en-Y gastric bypass. Diabetes Care. 2016;39(12):2247–53.
41. Tice JA, Karliner L, Walsh J, Petersen AJ, Feldman MD. Gastric banding or bypass? A systematic review comparing the two most popular bariatric procedures. Am J Med. 2008;121(10):885–93.
42. Chang SH, Stoll CR, Song J, Varela JE, Eagon CJ, Colditz GA. The effectiveness and risks of bariatric surgery: an updated systematic review and meta-analysis, 2003-2012. JAMA Surg. 2014;149(3):275–87.
43. Brethauer SA, Aminian A, Romero-Talamás H, Batayyah E, Mackey J, Kennedy L, et al. Can diabetes be surgically cured? Long-term metabolic effects of bariatric surgery in obese patients with type 2 diabetes mellitus. Ann Surg. 2013;258(4):628–36; discussion 36-7.
44. Gulliford MC, Booth HP, Reddy M, Charlton J, Fildes A, Prevost AT, et al. Effect of contemporary bariatric surgical procedures on type 2 diabetes remission. A population-based matched cohort study. Obes Surg. 2016;26(10):2308–15.
45. Arterburn DE, Bogart A, Sherwood NE, Sidney S, Coleman KJ, Haneuse S, et al. A multisite study of long-term remission and relapse of type 2 diabetes mellitus following gastric bypass. Obes Surg. 2013;23(1):93–102.
46. Chikunguwo SM, Wolfe LG, Dodson P, Meador JG, Baugh N, Clore JN, et al. Analysis of factors associated with durable remission of diabetes after roux-en-Y gastric bypass. Surgery for Obesity and Related Diseases: Official Journal of the American Society for Bariatric Surgery. 2010;6(3):254–9.
47. DiGiorgi M, Rosen DJ, Choi JJ, Milone L, Schrope B, Olivero-Rivera L, et al. Re-emergence of diabetes after gastric bypass in patients with mid- to long-term follow-up. Surgery for Obesity and Related Diseases : Official Journal of the American Society for Bariatric Surgery. 2010;6(3):249–53.
48. Golomb I, Ben David M, Glass A, Kolitz T, Keidar A. Long-term metabolic effects of laparoscopic sleeve gastrectomy. JAMA Surg. 2015;150(11):1051–7.

49. Panunzi S, Carlsson L, De Gaetano A, Peltonen M, Rice T, Sjöström L, et al. Determinants of diabetes remission and glycemic control after bariatric surgery. Diabetes Care. 2016;39(1):166–74.
50. Aung L, Lee WJ, Chen SC, Ser KH, Wu CC, Chong K, et al. Bariatric surgery for patients with early-onset vs late-onset type 2 diabetes. JAMA Surg. 2016;151(9):798–805.
51. Blackstone R, Bunt JC, Cortés MC, Sugerman HJ. Type 2 diabetes after gastric bypass: remission in five models using HbA1c, fasting blood glucose, and medication status. Surgery for Obesity and Related Diseases : Official Journal of the American Society for Bariatric Surgery. 2012;8(5):548–55.
52. Backman O, Bruze G, Näslund I, Ottosson J, Marsk R, Neovius M, et al. Gastric bypass surgery reduces De novo cases of type 2 diabetes to population levels: a Nationwide cohort study from Sweden. Ann Surg. 2019;269(5):895–902.
53. Sjöström L, Peltonen M, Jacobson P, Ahlin S, Andersson-Assarsson J, Anveden Å, et al. Association of bariatric surgery with long-term remission of type 2 diabetes and with microvascular and macrovascular complications. JAMA. 2014;311(22):2297–304.
54. Hariri K, Guevara D, Jayaram A, Kini SU, Herron DM, Fernandez-Ranvier G. Preoperative insulin therapy as a marker for type 2 diabetes remission in obese patients after bariatric surgery. Surg Obes Relat Dis. 2018;14(3):332–7.
55. Hall TC, Pellen MG, Sedman PC, Jain PK. Preoperative factors predicting remission of type 2 diabetes mellitus after roux-en-Y gastric bypass surgery for obesity. Obes Surg. 2010;20(9):1245–50.
56. Yu H, Di J, Bao Y, Zhang P, Zhang L, Tu Y, et al. Visceral fat area as a new predictor of short-term diabetes remission after roux-en-Y gastric bypass surgery in Chinese patients with a body mass index less than 35 kg/m2. Surgery for Obesity and Related Diseases : Official Journal of the American Society for Bariatric Surgery. 2015;11(1):6–11.
57. Lee WJ, Hur KY, Lakadawala M, Kasama K, Wong SK, Chen SC, et al. Predicting success of metabolic surgery: age, body mass index, C-peptide, and duration score. Surgery for Obesity and Related Diseases : Official Journal of the American Society for Bariatric Surgery. 2013;9(3):379–84.
58. Still CD, Wood GC, Benotti P, Petrick AT, Gabrielsen J, Strodel WE, et al. Preoperative prediction of type 2 diabetes remission after roux-en-Y gastric bypass surgery: a retrospective cohort study. Lancet Diabetes Endocrinol. 2014;2(1):38–45.
59. Lee W-J, Chong K, Chen S-C, Zachariah J, Ser K-H, Lee Y-C, et al. Preoperative prediction of type 2 diabetes remission after gastric bypass surgery: a comparison of DiaRem scores and ABCD scores. Obes Surg. 2016;26(10):2418–24.
60. Friedman JE, Dohm GL, Leggett-Frazier N, Elton CW, Tapscott EB, Pories WP, et al. Restoration of insulin responsiveness in skeletal muscle of morbidly obese patients after weight loss. Effect on muscle glucose transport and glucose transporter GLUT4. J Clin Invest. 1992;89(2):701–5.
61. Houmard JA, Tanner CJ, Yu C, Cunningham PG, Pories WJ, MacDonald KG, et al. Effect of weight loss on insulin sensitivity and intramuscular Long-chain fatty acyl-CoAs in morbidly obese subjects. Diabetes. 2002;51(10):2959–63.
62. Gray RE, Tanner CJ, Pories WJ, MacDonald KG, Houmard JA. Effect of weight loss on muscle lipid content in morbidly obese subjects. Am J Physiol Endocrinol Metabol. 2003;284(4):E726–E32.
63. Pender C, Goldfine ID, Tanner CJ, Pories WJ, MacDonald KG, Havel PJ, et al. Muscle insulin receptor concentrations in obese patients post bariatric surgery: relationship to hyperinsulinemia. Int J Obes. 2004;28(3):363–9.
64. Wickremesekera K, Miller G, Naotunne TD, Knowles G, Stubbs RS. Loss of insulin resistance after roux-en-Y gastric bypass surgery: a time course study. Obes Surg. 2005;15(4):474–81.
65. Martinussen C, Bojsen-Møller KN, Dirksen C, Jacobsen SH, Jørgensen NB, Kristiansen VB, et al. Immediate enhancement of first-phase insulin secretion and unchanged glucose

effectiveness in patients with type 2 diabetes after roux-en-Y gastric bypass. Am J Physiol Endocrinol Metabol. 2015;308(6):E535–E44.
66. Laferrère B, Teixeira J, McGinty J, Tran H, Egger JR, Colarusso A, et al. Effect of weight loss by gastric bypass surgery versus hypocaloric diet on glucose and incretin levels in patients with type 2 diabetes. J Clin Endocrinol Metabol. 2008;93(7):2479–85.
67. Lee W-J, Wang W, Lee Y-C, Huang M-T, Ser K-H, Chen J-C. Effect of laparoscopic mini-gastric bypass for type 2 diabetes mellitus: comparison of BMI >35 and <35 kg/m2. J Gastrointest Surg. 2008;12(5):945–52.
68. Pattou F, Beraud G, Arnalsteen L, Seguy D, Pigny P, Fermont C, et al. O47 La restauration de l'insulinosécrétion après Gastric bypass chez le diabétique de type 2 est indépendante de la perte de poids et corrélée à l'augmentation du GLP1. Diabetes Metab. 2008;34:H24.
69. Ramos AC, Galvão Neto MP, de Souza YM, Galvão M, Murakami AH, Silva AC, et al. Laparoscopic duodenal–Jejunal exclusion in the treatment of type 2 diabetes mellitus in patients with BMI <30 kg/m2 (LBMI). Obes Surg. 2009;19(3):307–12.
70. Cohen RV, Schiavon CA, Pinheiro JS, Correa JL, Rubino F. Duodenal-jejunal bypass for the treatment of type 2 diabetes in patients with body mass index of 22–34 kg/m2: a report of 2 cases. Surg Obes Relat Dis. 2007;3(2):195–7.
71. Tarnoff M, Rodriguez L, Escalona A, Ramos A, Neto M, Alamo M, et al. Open label, prospective, randomized controlled trial of an endoscopic duodenal-jejunal bypass sleeve versus low calorie diet for pre-operative weight loss in bariatric surgery. Surg Endosc. 2009;23(3):650–6.
72. Rodriguez L, Reyes E, Fagalde P, Oltra MS, Saba J, Aylwin CG, et al. Pilot clinical study of an endoscopic, removable duodenal-Jejunal bypass liner for the treatment of type 2 diabetes. Diabetes Technol Ther. 2009;11(11):725–32.
73. Service FJ. Hypoglycemic disorders. N Engl J Med. 1995;332(17):1144–52.
74. Lim EL, Hollingsworth KG, Aribisala BS, Chen MJ, Mathers JC, Taylor R. Reversal of type 2 diabetes: normalisation of beta cell function in association with decreased pancreas and liver triacylglycerol. Diabetologia. 2011;54(10):2506–14.
75. Steven S, Hollingsworth KG, Small PK, Woodcock SA, Pucci A, Aribisala B, et al. Weight loss decreases excess pancreatic triacylglycerol specifically in type 2 diabetes. Diabetes Care. 2016;39(1):158–65.
76. Purnell JQ, Johnson GS, Wahed AS, Dalla Man C, Piccinini F, Cobelli C, et al. Prospective evaluation of insulin and incretin dynamics in obese adults with and without diabetes for 2 years after roux-en-Y gastric bypass. Diabetologia. 2018;61(5):1142–54.
77. Yousseif A, Emmanuel J, Karra E, Millet Q, Elkalaawy M, Jenkinson AD, et al. Differential effects of laparoscopic sleeve gastrectomy and laparoscopic gastric bypass on appetite, circulating acyl-ghrelin, peptide YY3-36 and active GLP-1 levels in non-diabetic humans. Obes Surg. 2014;24(2):241–52.
78. Cavin JB, Couvelard A, Lebtahi R, Ducroc R, Arapis K, Voitellier E, et al. Differences in alimentary glucose absorption and intestinal disposal of blood glucose after roux-En-Y gastric bypass vs sleeve gastrectomy. Gastroenterology. 2016;150(2):454–64.e9.
79. Penney NC, Kinross J, Newton RC, Purkayastha S. The role of bile acids in reducing the metabolic complications of obesity after bariatric surgery: a systematic review. Int J Obes. 2015;39(11):1565–74.
80. Tremaroli V, Karlsson F, Werling M, Ståhlman M, Kovatcheva-Datchary P, Olbers T, et al. Roux-en-Y gastric bypass and vertical banded gastroplasty induce Long-term changes on the human gut microbiome contributing to fat mass regulation. Cell Metab. 2015;22(2):228–38.
81. Liou AP, Paziuk M, Luevano J-M, Machineni S, Turnbaugh PJ, Kaplan LM. Conserved shifts in the gut microbiota due to gastric bypass reduce host weight and adiposity. Sci Translat Med. 2013;5(178):178ra41.
82. Sharaiha RZ, Kumta NA, Saumoy M, Desai AP, Sarkisian AM, Benevenuto A, et al. Endoscopic sleeve Gastroplasty significantly reduces body mass index and metabolic complications in obese patients. Clin Gastroenterol Hepatol. 2017;15(4):504–10.

83. Hadefi A, Arvanitakis M, Huberty V, Devière J. Metabolic endoscopy: Today's science-tomorrow's treatment. United European Gastroenterol J. 2020;8(6):685–94.
84. Jirapinyo P, Haas AV, Thompson CC. Effect of the duodenal-Jejunal bypass liner on glycemic control in patients with type 2 diabetes with obesity: a meta-analysis with secondary analysis on weight loss and hormonal changes. Diabetes Care. 2018;41(5):1106–15.
85. Petry TZ, Fabbrini E, Otoch JP, Carmona MA, Caravatto PP, Salles JE, et al. Effect of duodenal-jejunal bypass surgery on glycemic control in type 2 diabetes: a randomized controlled trial. Obesity (Silver Spring, Md). 2015;23(10):1973–9.
86. van Baar ACG, Holleman F, Crenier L, Haidry R, Magee C, Hopkins D, et al. Endoscopic duodenal mucosal resurfacing for the treatment of type 2 diabetes mellitus: one year results from the first international, open-label, prospective, multicentre study. Gut. 2020;69(2):295–303.

Chapter 12
Precision Nutrition for Type 2 Diabetes

Orly Ben-Yacov and Michal Rein

Introduction

The prevalence of diabetes is increasing worldwide, affecting more than 10% of the global population, with the vast majority of cases classified as type 2 diabetes mellitus (T2DM) [1]. Substantial evidence indicates that T2DM can be largely prevented by adherence to healthy lifestyles, which include high-quality healthy diets, habitual exercise, and healthy body weight maintenance [2]. Once fully bloomed, T2DM is clinically managed by healthy diets and lifestyles combined with glucose-lowering pharmacological agents that aim to prevent or delay both acute symptoms of hyperglycemia and long-term complications of the disease [3]. As recommended by the Dietary Guidelines for Americans [4] and the American Diabetes Association [5], a healthy dietary pattern that protects against T2DM is rich in fruits, vegetables (except potatoes), whole grains, nuts, and legumes and low in refined grains, red or processed meats, and sugar-sweetened beverages. However, these current dietary recommendations are based on population averages and often do not take into account interpersonal variability in response to specific foods and dietary components. Although successful in reducing the population-level chronic disease burden to some extent [6], dietary guidelines based on population averages may not be best suited for a given individual, and personalization of interventions may be more effective in changing behavior that will affect health outcomes [7, 8]. In addition,

O. Ben-Yacov (✉)
Department of Computer Science and Applied Mathematics and Department of Molecular Cell Biology, Weizmann Institute of Science, Rehovot, Israel
e-mail: orlyby@weizmann.ac.il

M. Rein
Department of Computer Science and Applied Mathematics and Department of Molecular Cell Biology, Weizmann Institute of Science, Rehovot, Israel

School of Public Health, Faculty of Social Welfare and Health Sciences, University of Haifa, Haifa, Israel

R. Basu (ed.), *Precision Medicine in Diabetes*,
https://doi.org/10.1007/978-3-030-98927-9_12

T2DM is a heterogeneous disease from a genetic, pathophysiological, and clinical point of view [9]. Current understanding of the pathophysiological mechanisms of T2DM remains insufficient to explain the large variability between individuals in both the development and the clinical manifestations of the disease [10, 11]. Moreover, individual responses to dietary, lifestyle, and pharmaceutical interventions vary considerably [12–16].

Recently, the concept of precision nutrition (also known as personalized nutrition) has gained a great deal of interest in the scientific community and the general public [17–20]. Similar to precision medicine, the key mission of precision nutrition is to tailor dietary recommendations to individuals or population subgroups based on their unique characteristics, including genome sequence, microbiome composition, medical history, lifestyle, diet, and other personal factors, to prevent and manage chronic diseases. Recent advances in omics technologies [21–24], wearable devices [25, 26], and mobile technologies [27, 28] have broaden the possibilities of applying precision nutrition for prevention and management of T2DM. Integrated data from these emerging technologies along with traditional nutritional assessment allow deep phenotyping of individuals and monitoring of their metabolic state, thus promoting the development of innovative approaches in precision nutrition (Fig. 12.1). This comprehensive profiling of individuals will ultimately promote the achievement of several goals: (a) better understanding of the mechanisms underlying the variability between individuals in response to dietary exposures or interventions, (b) better assessment of dietary intakes and nutritional status in free-living populations, (c) identification of novel biomarkers that are more effective than traditional biomarkers at predicting risk of disease and its health complications, (d) identification of new targets for lifestyle and pharmacological interventions, and

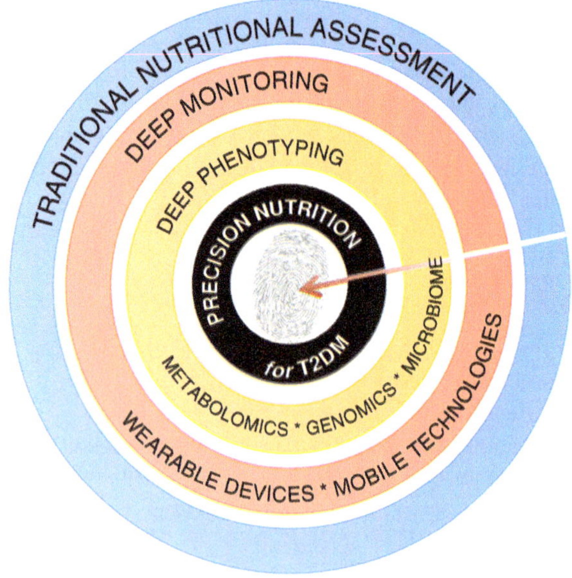

Fig. 12.1 The core components for comprehensive nutritional assessments of individuals and design of precision nutrition approaches for prevention and management of T2DM

(e) an ability to provide personalized dietary and lifestyle guidance for more effective prevention and management per person [29].

This chapter is seeking to review the current evidence from population-based studies on precision nutrition in T2DM using different technology axes and discuss promises and challenges of applying such approaches for prevention and management of T2DM in clinical practice.

Determinants of Precision Nutrition in T2DM

Deep Phenotyping (Omics Technologies)

Nutrigenetics and Nutrigenomics

The major increase in genome-wide association studies (GWAS) in the past decade has contributed extensively to the knowledge about the genetic architecture of T2DM [30]. GWAS, and more recently exome sequencing studies have identified more than 100 loci reproducibly associated with risk of T2DM and glycemic traits [31]. While most identified loci have a small effect size (risk of T2DM increased by 5–40%) and are common across populations, some causal variants have been identified for few loci [32, 33]. The GWAS loci collectively explain ~10% of the heritability of the disease [34]. Gene-environment and gene-gene interactions along with epigenetics are likely to contribute to the missing heritability of the disease. Epigenetic factors, such as DNA methylations and histone modifications, are especially important because they might mediate the effects of environmental exposures, including diet, on the risk of T2DM. Genome-wide DNA methylation studies comparing patients who have T2DM with healthy controls found varying levels of DNA methylation in pancreatic islets for thousands of CpG sites, corresponding to a large number of genes, including many known T2DM loci such as *TCF7L2*, *FTO*, and *PPARG* [35–37]. Other gene-environment studies explored the distinctive effect of dietary patterns on metabolic health depending on genetic makeup using a genetic risk score (GRS). For example, in a recent case-control study with more than 7000 participants, with or without T2DM, issued from the PREDIMED study [38], a significant interaction was observed between the adherence score to the MEDAS (Mediterranean Diet Adherence Screener) 14-item questionnaire and a GRS formed by two SNPs at the *FTO* and *MC4R* loci in determining T2DM risk ($P_{interaction} = 0.006$). Specifically, carriers of the rare alleles of these two loci had higher T2DM risk when adherence to the Mediterranean diet was low, but this association disappeared as adherence increased.

Overall, GWAS have not yet led to meaningful clinical advances in prevention or management of T2DM, and findings in this field are still relatively far from giving their fully expected potential in terms of translation and application of the genetic knowledge to precision nutrition. Nevertheless, discoveries of specific genetic variants directly related to dietary intake and nutrient metabolism may partially help to formulate effective dietary recommendations to improve nutritional status of individuals, including those with T2DM or at risk to develop the disease. This is the case for hypolactasia [39], celiac disease [40], and phenylketonuria [41] diagnoses, for example, which allowed the implementation of tailored dietary advices based on genetic makeup for years. Other, more recent, discoveries include genetic variants related to caffeine metabolism [42–44], predisposition to weight gain by saturated fat intake [45, 46], increased risk of developing hypertension by high salt intake [47, 48], zinc transport [49], alcohol metabolism [50], macronutrient intake [51], and predisposition to obesity by macronutrient intake [52], among others. On the private sector, many companies are already offering genetic tests to customize dietary recommendations based on individual response to specific nutrients, such as those mentioned above. However, the scientific community generally agrees that the future of precision nutrition cannot rely solely on nutrigenetics/nutrigenomics [53] and other factors beyond genetics must be considered in order to establish comprehensive and dynamic nutritional recommendations based on shifting, interacting parameters in a person's internal and external environment throughout life. In this regard, two large randomized controlled trials initiated about a decade ago, PREDIMED [54] and Food4Me [55], were among the most stimulating wide-scale approaches which aimed to broaden the knowledge about factors involved in the different response to a given nutritional intervention, utilizing a constellation of omics technologies (transcriptomics, genomics, epigenomics, and metabolomics), deep phenotyping and genotyping, and robust dietary adherence assessment.

Taken together, it seems that precision nutrition approaches must include, in addition to genetics, other deep phenotyping factors such as omics technologies (e.g., microbiome, metabolomics) and comprehensive assessment of dietary habits, food behavior, and physical activity to establish a comprehensive framework for prevention and management of T2DM [56–58].

Microbiome

The gut microbiota, which consists of trillions of bacterial microorganisms, has a central role in human health and disease. Emerging evidence suggests that the gut microbiome profile, which is unique to each individual, should be included as a key feature of precision nutrition [59, 60]. Specifically, the role of microbiome in the interpersonal variability of host metabolism and glycemic status is being under intense research in the last decade [12, 13]. In that sense, it was shown that part of the variability between people in postprandial glucose responses (PPGR) to foods can be explained by microbiome features in both healthy individuals and subjects with an elevated glycemic status [13, 61].

Gut bacterial abundances are influenced by dietary intakes and are representative of the habitual diet and metabolic state of individuals. A recent study by Asnicar et al. suggested that many significant associations between gut microbes and specific dietary components are driven by the presence and diversity of healthy and plant-based foods. The authors further demonstrated that a panel of intestinal species found to be associated with healthy dietary habits also overlapped with those associated with favorable cardio-metabolic and postprandial markers, suggesting potential stratification of the gut microbiome into generalizable health levels even in individuals without clinically manifest disease [62]. With respect to diabetes, alterations in gut microbiome composition and function, including changes in microbial richness, diversity, and specific bacterial taxa, have been repeatedly linked to glycemic status and T2DM [63–70]. Importantly, a recent study by Wu et al. indicated that overall gut microbiota shifts in parallel with glycemic status in humans, independent of diabetes medications. In addition, microbial functional changes of the gut microbiota, such as biotin biosynthesis and butyrate production, within heterogeneous populations of glycemic status, also suggest potential interactions between the gut microbiota and the diet that could be important for the onset of T2DM [71]. As such, the gut microbiota represents an important modifiable factor to consider when developing precision nutrition approaches for prevention of T2DM.

Several recent studies incorporated multiple data sources, including microbiome data, and applied big data analytics to inform personalized nutrition interventions [12, 13, 72]. In a pioneering work by Zeevi et al., the researchers devised a machine learning algorithm that integrates blood parameters, dietary habits, anthropometrics, physical activity, and gut microbiota, measured in an 800-person cohort, to predict personalized postprandial glycemic response (PPGR) to real-life meals. Short-term personalized dietary interventions based on this algorithm successfully lowered PPGRs in healthy individuals and individuals with prediabetes [13]. Following that study, a recently completed randomized clinical trial (RCT) for further evaluating the long-term clinical efficacy of the algorithm-based diet in adults with prediabetes showed that the personalized algorithm-based diet, aimed at lowering PPGR, improved glycemic control more than a standard Mediterranean-style diet, as measured by blood HbA1c levels and average daily time of glucose levels above 140 mg/dl in a 6-month dietary intervention and additional follow-up at 12 months [73]. Additionally, in a small-scale dietary intervention in individuals with newly diagnosed T2DM and naïve to diabetes medications, the personalized algorithm-based diet improved multiple metabolic parameters, including glycemic control, blood lipid profile, and body composition measurements, and resulted in diabetes remission in 61% of the participants, as measured by HbA1c [74]. The PREDICT 1 study, another large-scale and high-resolution study, also suggested that part of the interindividual variability in postprandial responses is explained by person-specific factors, including gut microbiome. Using gut microbiome data as well as other informative personal and meal features, the researchers further developed machine learning models that were able to predict triglycerides and glycemic responses to meals [12]. Lastly, a recent large-scale study (n = 4132) by Reitmeier et al. demonstrated that specific microbiota members show 24-hour oscillations in their relative abundance and identified 13 taxa with disrupted rhythmicity in T2DM patients. The researchers applied cross-validation prediction models based on this signature which enabled risk classification and prediction of T2DM, suggesting a functional link between circadian rhythms and the microbiome in T2DM [75].

Several other nutritional studies identified some metabolic phenotypes related to glycemic control and diabetes, typically in response to a dietary intervention, which were associated with some aspects of the gut microbiome. For example, in an RCT of a dietary intervention in subjects with T2DM, Zhao et al. found that adopting a high-fiber diet promoted the growth of a select group of 15 bacterial strains that produce short-chain fatty acids (SCFA), while other potential SCFA producers were either diminished or unchanged. The high-fiber diet induced changes to the entire gut microbiome that correlated with elevated levels of glucagon-like peptide-1 (GLP-1), a reduction in HbA1c and improved blood-glucose regulation [69]. Importantly, the production of SCFA through bacterial fermentation of dietary carbohydrates is considered beneficial to the host since it provides an energy substrate to colonocytes, mitigates inflammation, and regulates satiety [76, 77]. Deficiency in SCFA production has been repeatedly associated with various metabolic conditions, including T2DM [65–67, 78]. Notably, in the context of a fiber-type intervention, various studies have highlighted several associations of microbiome features with response to dietary fiber, including the ratio of *Prevotella* to *Bacteroides* (P/B ratio) or enterotype, diversity and richness, functional gene content within groups of taxa, abundance and diversity of SCFA-producing bacteria, and abundance of certain groups of taxa such as *Bifidobacteria*, *Bacteroides*, *Ruminococcus*, *Dialister* and *Coriobacteriaceae*, *Eubacterium*, *Clostridium*, and *Coprobacter fastidiosus* and *Lachnospiraceae* [79].

Another pioneering work, which indicates causality of the microbiome in determining host metabolic phenotype, is the work by Kootte et al. which showed that fecal microbiota transplantation (FMT) from lean donors to obese patients with metabolic syndrome improved insulin sensitivity, a transient effect associated with changes in microbiota composition and fasting plasma metabolites. Furthermore, the researchers demonstrated that baseline fecal microbiota composition in recipients was able to predict the response to lean donor FMT [80]. This important result suggests that individual microbiome-targeting dietary interventions prior to FMT may potentially improve treatment success.

Taken together, there is considerably increasing evidence that gut microbiome represents an important factor in precision nutrition and that targeted promotion of certain microbiome features via precision nutrition may present a novel ecological approach for manipulating the gut microbiota to prevent or manage T2DM and its metabolic manifestations.

Metabolomics

Metabolomics, defined as the comprehensive assessment of small molecules in biological specimens (usually blood or urine), is based on high-throughput metabolite profiling technologies such as mass spectrometry (MS) and nuclear magnetic resonance (NMR) for individual assessment of dietary intake and metabolic state [81,

82]. Recently, metabolomics has emerged as a potential valuable tool for diabetes prevention [83–85] and treatment [84, 86, 87]. The individual metabolomics fingerprint consists of some endogenously produced metabolites and some that have been taken up from the environment [88, 89]. Specifically, it is affected by diet, suggesting that metabolite profiles can be used to accurately and objectively characterize short-term [90, 91] or long-term dietary patterns [85, 92–94], evaluate adherence to dietary interventions [95], and unveil dietary biomarkers related to metabolic health and diabetes progression. Therefore, metabolomics research has become an important component in the field of precision nutrition [29, 96].

Some studies indicated that the metabolome responds to diet before other deep phenotyping strategies, such as transcriptome and proteome [87], which suggests a role for metabolomics in early diagnosis and enable targeted interventions for diabetes prevention, with dietary modifications and increased physical activity [81, 97]. For example, levels of 2-aminoadipic acid (2-AAA), an intermediate metabolite of lysine metabolism associated with insulin resistance, were enriched up to 12 years before the onset of overt diabetes, in two long-term follow-up cohorts [98]. Furthermore, branched-chain amino acids, aromatic amino acids (BCAA/As), and lipids (phospholipids and triglycerides) were suggested as promising biomarkers for diagnosis of T2DM, as their serum concentrations have been found to be higher in individuals with prediabetes and T2DM as compared to healthy individuals in several studies [83, 84, 99, 100]. Notably, the positive associations of BCAA/As levels with the risk of diabetes were attenuated after adjusting for clinical measures, such as baseline body mass index (BMI) and fasting plasma glucose (FPG), in obese subjects with increased risk for developing T2DM as reported in the Diabetes Prevention Program (DPP) trial [100].

Interventional studies in mice or humans that investigated the metabolomics fingerprint associated with a single metabolite supplementation or a full dietary plan are particularly important as they improve our understanding of the molecular factors that mediate metabolic outcomes [69, 97, 101–103]. For example, in a study originated from the DPP trial, it was suggested that serum levels of betaine, a metabolite of choline that can also be obtained directly from the diet, were independently associated with reduced incidence of T2DM and were able to predict a successful response to prevention strategies [100]. Interestingly, 16 weeks of betaine supplementation to mice improved metabolic status including glucose homeostasis and hepatic lipid accumulation [101]. On a dietary intervention aimed for weight loss in obese subjects, average protein diets (15% of total daily energy) lowered BCAA/As concentration, more than high-protein diets (25% of total daily energy). Importantly, the improved amino acid profiles, especially reductions in alanine and the tyrosine levels, were related to reduced insulin resistance independent of weight loss [103]. Another work by Thaiss et al. [102] investigated microbiome dynamics in mice in response to post-dieting weight regain cycles, also known as the "yoyo effect." The authors suggested that the microbiome contributes to diminished post-dieting levels of a flavonoid metabolite and reduced energy expenditure and further demonstrate that flavonoid-based "post-biotic" intervention ameliorates excessive secondary weight gain in susceptible mice [102].

Overall, metabolomics platform may serve as a complementary tool, in parallel to other traditional tools, for more accurate and objective assessment of disease progression and patient response to a nutritional treatment. As such, metabolomics may help to attain the goal of precision nutrition to usefully tailor dietary advice based on anticipated individual responses to a nutritional intake.

Deep Monitoring

In addition to deep phenotyping by different types of omics data, precision nutrition should integrate patients' information from both traditional sources (validated questionnaires, standard clinical tests, etc.) and modern sources (electronic health records and deep monitoring from mobile applications and wearable devices). This integration of data from multiple disparate sources requires the use of bioinformatics tools, such as big data analytics, to be able to analyze and interpret the high volume and complexity of available data. However, the field is still in its infancy, and researchers using these methods face different challenges, such as incomplete and unreliable input data as well as misleading interpretations of findings owing to a lack of expert knowledge.

Mobile Technologies for Nutritional Assessment and Diabetes Management

Mobile applications have the potential to improve real-time assessment of dietary intake and provide feedback, thus encouraging individuals to actively participate in their own behavior change and disease management. Therefore, it may provide a useful tool for monitoring and implementing precision nutrition for improving glycemic control among individuals with prediabetes or T2DM. Diabetes mobile phone applications (hereafter referred to as diabetes apps) are defined as mobile phone software that accept data (transmitted or manual entry) and provide feedback to patients on improved management (automated or by a healthcare professional [HCP]). In a systematic review and meta-analysis, which included ten studies that examined diabetes app use in individuals with T2DM ($n = 586$), a significant mean reduction of 0.49% in HbA1c was reported among participants using diabetes apps as compared with controls (95% CI 0.30, 0.68; $I^2 = 10\%$). Subgroup analyses indicated that younger patients were more likely to benefit from the use of diabetes apps, and the effect size was enhanced with HCP feedback [27]. Indeed, recent healthcare concerns are rapidly expanding the use of technology-based services, including mobile applications, to advance traditional approaches of diabetes self-management education and support (DSMES) [104]. This issue also deserved a specific highlight in a recent expert consensus report [105] and in the 2021 ADA's Standards of Medical Care in Diabetes [106].

The use of mobile apps for food logging and real-time assessment of dietary intake has been utilized in several research settings. Large-scale population-based studies, such as the studies by Zeevi et al. and Berry et al., previously described in this chapter, utilized real-time self-recorded dietary intake using designated mobile applications to accurately assess metabolic responses to food intakes, evaluate eating behaviors, and further use these data to predict personalized metabolic responses to standardized and real-world meals [12, 13]. In other studies, such as several dietary interventions, self-recording of dietary intake by study participants allowed to both accurately characterize dietary habits prior to the intervention and during the intervention and monitor participants' compliance to dietary regimes and distinguish de facto between different dietary treatments. As such, it allowed to draw more precise conclusions about health outcomes of different dietary changes for different people [73, 107]. Notably, in the recently completed dietary interventions for personalized nutrition by prediction of glycemic responses in subjects with prediabetes and T2DM (previously described in this chapter), the utilization of a designated mobile application for delivering personalized dietary recommendations and real-time feedback on predicted PPGRs to real-life meals was a unique feature in study design that may have contributed to participants' engagement with the dietary treatment and high satisfaction [74].

Taken together, the utilization of mobile technologies to effectively collect personal data and provide feedback to individuals is emerging as a potential important tool for implementation of precision nutrition in T2DM.

Wearable Devices for Metabolic Assessment

Wearable devices for real-time assessment of physiological variables are emerging as potential valuable tools for discovering authentic physiological and behavioral patterns that are relevant for accurate tailoring of personalized diets. In particular, physiological variables such as blood-glucose levels, heart rate, physical activity, and sleep quality, traditionally tested in clinical settings only, are now available for use in free-living populations. The integration of deep and continuous data collected by wearable devices with comprehensive nutritional assessments can be used to discover metabolic and behavioral patterns [108, 109], estimate predicted physiological responses to specific lifestyle interventions [12, 13, 110], and potentially help individuals in adopting better lifestyle habits and dietary choices [111–113]. Together with recent advances in technologies and the fact that wearable devices are relatively inexpensive, it is not surprising that the use of wearable devices has become more prevalent in research and clinical settings as well as personal use in the private sector.

Wearable devices for tracking physical activity are commonly used for continuous measurement of activity levels and intensity, which provide the ability to calculate energy expenditure and improve lifestyle habits [114]. Other widely used wearable devices are continuous glucose monitoring (CGM) sensors, which estimate blood-glucose levels with high accuracy through measurement of interstitial glucose concentrations in several minute intervals [115]. The data extracted from CGMs provide the ability to identify undetected glucose dysregulations, like hypoglycemia and hyperglycemia, and unveil individual responses to a variety of foods or meals [13, 68]. For example, by grouping nondiabetic individuals into subgroups of glucose fluctuation patterns, based on CGM data, Hall and colleagues could define "glucotypes" (low, moderate, and severe) which were correlated with other metabolic parameters such as fasting plasma glucose, HbA1c, and BMI [109]. Likewise, by using 7-day-long CGM data from 1000 individuals, Zeevi and colleagues were able to predict with high accuracy personalized PPGRs of individuals to any meal [13]. In the PREDICT 1 study, participants were connected to several wearable devices, including physical activity sensors, CGM, and sleep monitors, as part of the study design. Interestingly, dietary and lifestyle features extracted from these wearables and from food recordings in a mobile logging application, such as meal composition and timing, physical activity, and sleep were reported as core determinants in prediction of glucose responses to meals [12]. Another unique wearable device is seeking to track eating patterns such as nocturnal eating, overeating, and snacking habits, which may also help to assess energy intake and add a different point of view on lifestyle behaviors. The device is a wrist motion sensor coupled with a micro-electro-mechanical gyroscope that estimates caloric intake by monitoring food bites and provides information about individuals' eating habits or adherence to a given dietary intervention [20, 25]. Despite its potential to provide accurate assessments of energy intake, further studies are needed to validate its accuracy and overcome different confounders in measurement such as eating speed of different food types.

Taken together, wearable devices measure physiological parameters in a real-time and continuous manner, thus providing complementary information about individuals' lifestyle habits and physiological responses. Integrating data from wearable devices with other deep phenotyping methods allows in-depth exploration of human physiological responses in research settings and may facilitate decision-making by HCPs in clinical care settings, both highly valuable for promoting precision nutrition solutions in T2DM.

From Science to Practice: Clinical Translation

As described thoroughly in the previous sections of this chapter, the cutting-edge omics technologies and ever developing mobile applications and wearable devices are emerging as promising tools for advancing the field of precision nutrition toward the design of personalized and unbiased nutritional solutions for prevention and management of T2DM. The translation of the growing evidence emerging from basic nutritional science into meaningful and clinically relevant dietary advices represents nowadays one of the main challenges of clinical nutrition.

While mobile apps and wearable devices are already implemented to some extent in clinical care and facilitate decision-making by HCPs for T2DM management, the use of omics technologies in clinical practice is still scarce, due to cost-effectiveness considerations and lack of sufficient clinical evidence base. In particular, the omics technologies have not yet provided clinically scalable biomarkers for predicting both disease outcomes and interpersonal variability to specific dietary exposures. For example, when biomarkers recently identified by GWAS and metabolomics studies were added to a risk prediction model of traditional risk factors, the model showed only a modest improvement in predicting risk of T2DM [116]. Likewise, metabolomics and microbiome technologies are not yet incorporated into comprehensive frameworks for broad use in clinical and public health settings, although they are rapidly evolving and might be incorporated in the future into personalized nutrition in clinical care, as demonstrated by several proof-of-concept studies [12, 13, 74].

In the private sector, there are some direct-to-consumer nutrigenomics companies that advocate customized dietary recommendations, but scientific evidence suggests that these approaches are not comprehensive enough and it is unlikely that prediction algorithms using DNA variant data alone would be sufficiently effective in improving metabolic outcomes. Broader approaches that integrate personal data from other omics axes, such as microbiome and metabolomics, for tailoring dietary recommendations, are still rare in the private sector, and the evidence regarding the clinical efficacy of such commercial products for improving metabolic outcomes among customers is limited. In that sense, one company that uses microbiome and other personal data to guide personalized meal planning recommendations for controlling postprandial glycemic responses [110] recently reported a mean reduction of 0.97% in HbA1c among subjects with T2DM following a 3-month pilot intervention conducted in real-world settings with five different employer groups ($n = 125$). Another commercial company is offering personalized nutrition plans as well as personal recommendations for probiotic and prebiotic supplementation based on comprehensive gut microbiome activity profiling, using meta-transcriptomic methods [117]. According to the company website, there is an ongoing research conducted to study the adherence of customers to their recommended personalized nutrition programs and determine impacts on metabolic health and wellness.

Another resource for potential developments of precision nutrition solutions for prevention and management of T2DM may rise from governments and/or industry-backed biobank initiatives that contain in-depth genetic and other health information in large population-based cohorts. The large-scale biological and physiological datasets generated by these initiatives may be harnessed for precision nutritional diagnostics and therapeutics. Pragmatic studies of decision support systems utilizing rich information in healthcare systems, particularly those with biobank-linked electronic healthcare records, will be needed to guide implementation of precision nutrition in diabetes into clinical practice and to generate the much needed cost-efficacy data for broader adoption [118].

Taken together, the field of precision nutrition has rapidly evolved in recent years, thanks to major advances in omics, mobile, and wearable technologies that allow in-depth phenotyping and monitoring of individuals. Despite these advances, major challenges exist in applying precision nutrition approaches for broad use in clinical and public health settings for the prevention and management of T2DM. One major challenge is the integration of high-dimensional data from multiple disparate sources and application of big data analytics, to provide valuable and clinically scalable biomarkers, along with expert knowledge for accurate interpretation and assimilation of findings into clinical practice. This field is in its infancy and still awaits clinically robust and reproducible results. Other important challenges that need to be overcome in order to successfully translate basic nutritional science into an effective precision nutrition care in T2DM include the high costs of omics technologies as well as feasibility and accessibility of technology-based services to wide-range populations. Lastly, as demonstrated in the latest consensus report from the American Diabetes Association (ADA) and the European Association for the Study of Diabetes (EASD) about precision medicine in diabetes [118], there is a need to establish partnerships between the scientific community, patients, healthcare systems, providers, payors, and industry and regulatory bodies involved in the development, evaluation, approval, adoption, and implementation of precision nutritional diagnostics, monitoring, and therapeutics that are deemed acceptable for safe, efficacious, and cost-effective use in precision diabetes care.

Bibliography

1. Ogurtsova K, da Rocha Fernandes JD, Huang Y, Linnenkamp U, Guariguata L, Cho NH, Cavan D, Shaw JE, Makaroff LE. IDF diabetes atlas: global estimates for the prevalence of diabetes for 2015 and 2040. Diabetes Res ClinPract. 2017;128:40–50.
2. Hu FB, Manson JE, Stampfer MJ, Colditz G, Liu S, Solomon CG, Willett WC. Diet, lifestyle, and the risk of type 2 diabetes mellitus in women. N Engl J Med. 2001;345:790–7.
3. Inzucchi SE, Bergenstal RM, Buse JB, et al. Management of hyperglycemia in type 2 diabetes: a patient-centered approach: position statement of the American Diabetes Association (ADA) and the European Association for the Study of diabetes (EASD). Diabetes Care. 2012;35:1364–79.
4. McGuire S. Dietary guidelines for Americans. 2010.
5. Evert AB, Boucher JL, Cypress M, et al. Nutrition therapy recommendations for the management of adults with diabetes. Diabetes Care. 2013;36:3821–42.
6. Wang DD, Li Y, Afshin A, Springmann M, Mozaffarian D, Stampfer MJ, Hu FB, Murray CJL, Willett WC. Global improvement in dietary quality could lead to substantial reduction in premature death. J Nutr. 2019;149:1065–74.
7. Celis-Morales C, Lara J, Mathers JC. Personalising nutritional guidance for more effective behaviour change. ProcNutrSoc. 2015;74:130–8.
8. Woolf SH, Purnell JQ. The good life: working together to promote opportunity and improve population health and well-being. JAMA. 2016;315:1706–8.
9. Scheen AJ. Precision medicine: the future in diabetes care? Diabetes Res Clin Pract. 2016;117:12–21.
10. Reddy SSK. Evolving to personalized medicine for type 2 diabetes. Endocrinol Metab Clin North Am. 2016;45:1011–20.
11. Florez JC. Precision medicine in diabetes: is it time? Diabetes Care. 2016;39:1085–8.
12. Berry SE, Valdes AM, Drew DA, et al. Human postprandial responses to food and potential for precision nutrition. Nat Med. 2020;26:964–73.
13. Zeevi D, Korem T, Zmora N, et al. Personalized nutrition by prediction of glycemic responses. Cell. 2015;163:1079–94.
14. DeFronzo RA, Goodman AM. Efficacy of metformin in patients with non-insulin-dependent diabetes mellitus. N Engl J Med. 1995;333(9):541–9.

15. Effect of intensive blood-glucose control with metformin on complications in overweight patients with type 2 diabetes (UKPDS 34). Lancet. 1998;352:854–65.
16. Zhou K, Donnelly L, Yang J, et al. Heritability of variation in glycaemic response to metformin: a genome-wide complex trait analysis. Lancet Diabetes Endocrinol. 2014;2:481–7.
17. Mills S, Stanton C, Lane JA, Smith GJ, Ross RP. Precision nutrition and the microbiome, part I: current state of the science. Nutrients. 2019; https://doi.org/10.3390/nu11040923.
18. Ramos-Lopez O, Milagro FI, Allayee H. Guide for current nutrigenetic, nutrigenomic, and nutriepigenetic approaches for precision nutrition involving the prevention and management of chronic diseases associated with obesity. J Nutrigenet Nutrigenomics. 2017;10(1-2):43–62.
19. Ordovas JM, Ferguson LR, Tai ES, Mathers JC. Personalised nutrition and health. BMJ. 2018;361:bmj.k2173.
20. de Toro-Martín J, Arsenault BJ, Després J-P, Vohl M-C. Precision nutrition: a review of personalized nutritional approaches for the prevention and management of metabolic syndrome. Nutrients. 2017; https://doi.org/10.3390/nu9080913.
21. Franks PW, Poveda A. Lifestyle and precision diabetes medicine: will genomics help optimise the prediction, prevention and treatment of type 2 diabetes through lifestyle therapy? Diabetologia. 2017;60:784–92.
22. Zhernakova A, Kurilshikov A, Bonder MJ, et al. Population-based metagenomics analysis reveals markers for gut microbiome composition and diversity. Science. 2016;352:565–9.
23. Wu GD, Compher C, Chen EZ, et al. Comparative metabolomics in vegans and omnivores reveal constraints on diet-dependent gut microbiota metabolite production. Gut. 2016;65:63–72.
24. Den Ouden H, Pellis L, Rutten GEHM, Geerars-van Vonderen IK, Rubingh CM, van Ommen B, van Erk MJ, Beulens JWJ. Metabolomic biomarkers for personalised glucose lowering drugs treatment in type 2 diabetes. Metabolomics. 2016;12:27.
25. Dong Y, Hoover A, Scisco J, Muth E. A new method for measuring meal intake in humans via automated wrist motion tracking. Appl Psychophysiol Biofeedback. 2012;37(3):205–15.
26. Fontana JM, Farooq M, Sazonov E. Automatic ingestion monitor: a novel wearable device for monitoring of ingestive behavior. IEEE Trans Biomed Eng. 2014;61:1772–9.
27. Hou C, Carter B, Hewitt J, Francisa T, Mayor S. Do Mobile phone applications improve Glycemic control (HbA1c) in the self-management of diabetes? A systematic review, meta-analysis, and GRADE of 14 randomized trials. Diabetes Care. 2016;39:2089–95.
28. McGloin AF, Eslami S. Digital and social media opportunities for dietary behaviour change. Proc Nutr Soc. 2015;74:139–48.
29. Wang DD, Hu FB. Precision nutrition for prevention and management of type 2 diabetes. Lancet Diabetes Endocrinol. 2018;6:416–26.
30. Fuchsberger C, Flannick J, Teslovich TM, Mahajan A, et al. The genetic architecture of type 2 diabetes. Nature. 2017;536(7614):41–7.
31. Stančáková A, Laakso M. Genetics of type 2 diabetes. Novelties in Diabetes. Endocr Dev. 2016;31:203–20.
32. Steinthorsdottir V, Thorleifsson G, Sulem P, et al. Identification of low-frequency and rare sequence variants associated with elevated or reduced risk of type 2 diabetes. Nat Genet. 2014;46:294–8.
33. SIGMA Type 2 Diabetes Consortium, Estrada K, Aukrust I, et al. Association of a low-frequency variant in HNF1A with type 2 diabetes in a Latino population. JAMA. 2014;311:2305–14.
34. Manolio TA, Collins FS, Cox NJ, et al. Finding the missing heritability of complex diseases. Nature. 2009;461:747–53.
35. Volkov P, Bacos K, Ofori JK, Esguerra JLS, Eliasson L, Rönn T, Ling C. Whole-genome Bisulfite sequencing of human pancreatic islets reveals novel differentially methylated regions in type 2 diabetes pathogenesis. Diabetes. 2017;66:1074–85.
36. Dayeh T, Volkov P, Salö S, et al. Genome-wide DNA methylation analysis of human pancreatic islets from type 2 diabetic and non-diabetic donors identifies candidate genes that influence insulin secretion. PLoS Genet. 2014;10:e1004160.

37. Volkmar M, Dedeurwaerder S, Cunha DA, et al. DNA methylation profiling identifies epigenetic dysregulation in pancreatic islets from type 2 diabetic patients. EMBO J. 2012;31:1405–26.
38. Ortega-Azorín C, Sorlí JV, Asensio EM, et al. Associations of the FTO rs9939609 and the MC4R rs17782313 polymorphisms with type 2 diabetes are modulated by diet, being higher when adherence to the Mediterranean diet pattern is low. Cardiovasc Diabetol. 2012;11:137.
39. Rasinperä H, Savilahti E, Enattah NS, Kuokkanen M, Tötterman N, Lindahl H, Järvelä I, Kolho KL. A genetic test which can be used to diagnose adult-type hypolactasia in children. Gut. 2004;53:1571–6.
40. Ludvigsson JF, Bai JC, Biagi F, et al. Diagnosis and management of adult coeliac disease: guidelines from the British Society of Gastroenterology. Gut. 2014;63:1210–28.
41. DiLella AG, Huang WM, Woo SL. Screening for phenylketonuria mutations by DNA amplification with the polymerase chain reaction. Lancet. 1988;1:497–9.
42. Cornelis MC, El-Sohemy A, Campos H. Genetic polymorphism of the adenosine A2A receptor is associated with habitual caffeine consumption. Am J Clin Nutr. 2007;86:240–4.
43. Cornelis MC, El-Sohemy A, Kabagambe EK, Campos H. Coffee, CYP1A2 genotype, and risk of myocardial infarction. JAMA. 2006;295:1135–41.
44. Cornelis MC, Kacprowski T, Menni C, et al. Genome-wide association study of caffeine metabolites provides new insights to caffeine metabolism and dietary caffeine-consumption behavior. Hum Mol Genet. 2016;25:5472–82.
45. Corella D, Peloso G, Arnett DK, et al. APOA2, dietary fat, and body mass index: replication of a gene-diet interaction in 3 independent populations. Arch Intern Med. 2009;169:1897–906.
46. Corella D, Tai ES, Sorlí JV, Chew SK, Coltell O, Sotos-Prieto M, García-Rios A, Estruch R, Ordovas JM. Association between the APOA2 promoter polymorphism and body weight in Mediterranean and Asian populations: replication of a gene-saturated fat interaction. Int J Obes. 2011;35:666–75.
47. Giner V, Poch E, Bragulat E, Oriola J, González D, Coca A, De La Sierra A. Renin-angiotensin system genetic polymorphisms and salt sensitivity in essential hypertension. Hypertension. 2000;35:512–7.
48. Poch E, González D, Giner V, Bragulat E, Coca A, de La Sierra A. Molecular basis of salt sensitivity in human hypertension. Evaluation of renin-angiotensin-aldosterone system gene polymorphisms. Hypertension. 2001;38:1204–9.
49. Cauchi S, Del Guerra S, Choquet H, D'Aleo V, Groves CJ, Lupi R, McCarthy MI, Froguel P, Marchetti P. Meta-analysis and functional effects of the SLC30A8 rs13266634 polymorphism on isolated human pancreatic islets. Mol Genet Metab. 2010;100:77–82.
50. Schumann G, Liu C, O'Reilly P, et al. KLB is associated with alcohol drinking, and its gene product β-klotho is necessary for FGF21 regulation of alcohol preference. Proc Natl Acad Sci USA. 2016;113:14372–7.
51. Tanaka T, Ngwa JS, van Rooij FJA, et al. Genome-wide meta-analysis of observational studies shows common genetic variants associated with macronutrient intake. Am J Clin Nutr. 2013;97:1395–402.
52. Goni L, Cuervo M, Milagro FI, Martínez JA. A genetic risk tool for obesity predisposition assessment and personalized nutrition implementation based on macronutrient intake. Genes Nutr. 2015;10:445.
53. Ferguson LR, De Caterina R, Görman U, Allayee H. Guide and position of the international society of nutrigenetics/nutrigenomics on personalised nutrition: part 1-fields of precision nutrition. J Nutrigenet Nutrigenomics. 2016;9(1):*12*–27.
54. Estruch R, Ros E, Salas-Salvadó J, et al. Primary prevention of cardiovascular disease with a Mediterranean diet. N Engl J Med. 2013;368:1279–90.
55. Ryan NM, O'Donovan CB, Forster H. New tools for personalised nutrition: the Food4Me project. Nutr Bull. 2015;40:134–9.
56. Allison DB, Bassaganya-Riera J, Burlingame B, et al. Goals in nutrition science 2015-2020. Front Nutr. 2015;2:26.

57. Corella D, Coltell O, Mattingley G, Sorlí JV, Ordovas JM. Utilizing nutritional genomics to tailor diets for the prevention of cardiovascular disease: a guide for upcoming studies and implementations. Expert Rev Mol Diagn. 2017;17:1–19.
58. Srinivasan B, Lee S, Erickson D, Mehta S. Precision nutrition - review of methods for point-of-care assessment of nutritional status. Curr Opin Biotechnol. 2017;44:103–8.
59. Kang JX. Gut microbiota and personalized nutrition. J Nutrigenet Nutrigenomics. 2013;6:I-II.
60. Hughes RL, Kable ME, Marco M, Keim NL. The role of the gut microbiome in predicting response to diet and the development of precision nutrition models. Part II: results. Adv Nutr. 2019;10:979–98.
61. Mendes-Soares H, Raveh-Sadka T, Azulay S, et al. Assessment of a personalized approach to predicting postprandial glycemic responses to food among individuals without diabetes. JAMA Netw Open. 2019;2:e188102.
62. Asnicar F, Berry SE, Valdes AM, et al. Microbiome connections with host metabolism and habitual diet from 1,098 deeply phenotyped individuals. Nat Med. 2021; https://doi.org/10.1038/s41591-020-01183-8.
63. Janssen AWF, Kersten S. The role of the gut microbiota in metabolic health. FASEB J. 2015;29:3111–23.
64. Allin KH, Tremaroli V, Caesar R, et al. Aberrant intestinal microbiota in individuals with prediabetes. Diabetologia. 2018;61:810–20.
65. Karlsson FH, Tremaroli V, Nookaew I, Bergström G, Behre CJ, Fagerberg B, Nielsen J, Bäckhed F. Gut metagenome in European women with normal, impaired and diabetic glucose control. Nature. 2013;498:99–103.
66. Larsen N, Vogensen FK, van den Berg FWJ, Nielsen DS, Andreasen AS, Pedersen BK, Al-Soud WA, Sørensen SJ, Hansen LH, Jakobsen M. Gut microbiota in human adults with type 2 diabetes differs from non-diabetic adults. PLoS One. 2010;5:e9085.
67. Qin J, Li Y, Cai Z, et al. A metagenome-wide association study of gut microbiota in type 2 diabetes. Nature. 2012;490:55–60.
68. Schüssler-Fiorenza Rose SM, Contrepois K, Moneghetti KJ, et al. A longitudinal big data approach for precision health. Nat Med. 2019;25:792–804.
69. Zhao L, Zhang F, Ding X, et al. Gut bacteria selectively promoted by dietary fibers alleviate type 2 diabetes. Science. 2018;359:1151–6.
70. Pallister T, Spector TD. Food: a new form of personalised (gut microbiome) medicine for chronic diseases? J R Soc Med. 2016;109:331–6.
71. Wu H, Tremaroli V, Schmidt C, Lundqvist A, Olsson LM, Krämer M, Gummesson A, Perkins R, Bergström G, Bäckhed F. The gut microbiota in prediabetes and diabetes: a population-based cross-sectional study. Cell Metab. 2020;32:379–390.e3.
72. Price ND, Magis AT, Earls JC, et al. A wellness study of 108 individuals using personal, dense, dynamic data clouds. Nat Biotechnol. 2017;35:747–56.
73. Ben-Yacov O, Godneva A, Rein M, et al. Personalized postprandial glucose response-targeting diet versus Mediterranean diet for glycemic control in prediabetes. Diabetes Care. 2021;44(9):1980–91.
74. Rein M, Ben-Yacov O, Godneva A, et al. Effects of personalized diets by prediction of glycemic responses on glycemic control and metabolic health in newly diagnosed T2DM: a randomized dietary intervention pilot trial. BMC Med. 2022;20:56.
75. Reitmeier S, Kiessling S, Clavel T, et al. Arrhythmic gut microbiome signatures predict risk of type 2 diabetes. Cell Host Microbe. 2020;28:258–272.e6.
76. Koh A, De Vadder F, Kovatcheva-Datchary P, Bäckhed F. From dietary Fiber to host physiology: short-chain fatty acids as key bacterial metabolites. Cell. 2016;165:1332–45.
77. Sawicki CM, Livingston KA, Obin M, Roberts SB, Chung M, McKeown NM. Dietary fiber and the human gut microbiota: application of evidence mapping methodology. Nutrients. 2017; https://doi.org/10.3390/nu9020125.
78. Forslund K, Hildebrand F, Nielsen T, et al. Disentangling type 2 diabetes and metformin treatment signatures in the human gut microbiota. Nature. 2015;528:262–6.

79. Hughes RL, Marco ML, Hughes JP, Keim NL, Kable ME. The role of the gut microbiome in predicting response to diet and the development of precision nutrition models-part I: overview of current methods. Adv Nutr. 2019;10:953–78.
80. Kootte RS, Levin E, Salojärvi J, et al. Improvement of insulin sensitivity after lean donor Feces in metabolic syndrome is driven by baseline intestinal microbiota composition. Cell Metab. 2017;26:611–619.e6.
81. Roberts LD, Koulman A, Griffin JL. Towards metabolic biomarkers of insulin resistance and type 2 diabetes: progress from the metabolome. Lancet Diabetes Endocrinol. 2014;2:65–75.
82. Menni C, Zhai G, Macgregor A, et al. Targeted metabolomics profiles are strongly correlated with nutritional patterns in women. Metabolomics. 2013;9:506–14.
83. Long J, Yang Z, Wang L, Han Y, Peng C, Yan C, Yan D. Metabolite biomarkers of type 2 diabetes mellitus and pre-diabetes: a systematic review and meta-analysis. BMC Endocr Disord. 2020;20:174.
84. Guasch-Ferré M, Hruby A, Toledo E, Clish CB, Martínez-González MA, Salas-Salvadó J, Hu FB. Metabolomics in prediabetes and diabetes: a systematic review and meta-analysis. Diabetes Care. 2016;39:833–46.
85. Eriksen R, Perez IG, Posma JM, et al. Dietary metabolite profiling brings new insight into the relationship between nutrition and metabolic risk: an IMI DIRECT study. EBioMedicine. 2020;58:102932.
86. Gonzalez-Franquesa A, Burkart AM, Isganaitis E, Patti M-E. What have metabolomics approaches taught us about type 2 diabetes? Curr Diab Rep. 2016;16:74.
87. O'Gorman A, Brennan L. The role of metabolomics in determination of new dietary biomarkers. Proc Nutr Soc. 2017;76:295–302.
88. Bar N, Korem T, Weissbrod O, et al. A reference map of potential determinants for the human serum metabolome. Nature. 2020; https://doi.org/10.1038/s41586-020-2896-2.
89. Tebani A, Bekri S. Paving the way to precision nutrition through metabolomics. Front Nutr. 2019;6:41.
90. Llorach R, Urpi-Sarda M, Tulipani S, Garcia-Aloy M, Monagas M, Andres-Lacueva C. Metabolomic fingerprint in patients at high risk of cardiovascular disease by cocoa intervention. Mol Nutr Food Res. 2013;57:962–73.
91. Garcia-Perez I, Posma JM, Gibson R, et al. Objective assessment of dietary patterns by use of metabolic phenotyping: a randomised, controlled, crossover trial. Lancet Diabetes Endocrinol. 2017;5:184–95.
92. Floegel A, von Ruesten A, Drogan D, Schulze MB, Prehn C, Adamski J, Pischon T, Boeing H. Variation of serum metabolites related to habitual diet: a targeted metabolomic approach in EPIC-Potsdam. Eur J Clin Nutr. 2013;67:1100–8.
93. O'Sullivan A, Gibney MJ, Brennan L. Dietary intake patterns are reflected in metabolomic profiles: potential role in dietary assessment studies. Am J Clin Nutr. 2011;93:314–21.
94. Hernández-Alonso P, Papandreou C, Bulló M, et al. Plasma metabolites associated with frequent red wine consumption: a metabolomics approach within the PREDIMED study. Mol Nutr Food Res. 2019;63:e1900140.
95. Andersen M-BS, Rinnan Å, Manach C, Poulsen SK, Pujos-Guillot E, Larsen TM, Astrup A, Dragsted LO. Untargeted metabolomics as a screening tool for estimating compliance to a dietary pattern. J Proteome Res. 2014;13:1405–18.
96. Clish CB. Metabolomics: an emerging but powerful tool for precision medicine. Cold Spring Harb Mol Case Stud. 2015;1:a000588.
97. Lee HJ, Jang HB, Kim W-H, Park KJ, Kim KY, Park SI, Lee H-J. 2-Aminoadipic acid (2-AAA) as a potential biomarker for insulin resistance in childhood obesity. Sci Rep. 2019;9:13610.
98. Wang TJ, Ngo D, Psychogios N, et al. 2-Aminoadipic acid is a biomarker for diabetes risk. J Clin Invest. 2013;123(10):4309–17.
99. Drogan D, Dunn WB, Lin W, et al. Untargeted metabolic profiling identifies altered serum metabolites of type 2 diabetes mellitus in a prospective, nested case control study. Clin Chem. 2015;61:487–97.

100. Walford GA, Ma Y, Clish C, Florez JC, Wang TJ, Gerszten RE, Diabetes Prevention Program Research Group. Metabolite profiles of diabetes incidence and intervention response in the diabetes prevention program. Diabetes. 2016;65:1424–33.
101. Ejaz A, Martinez-Guino L, Goldfine AB, et al. Dietary betaine supplementation increases fgf21 levels to improve glucose homeostasis and reduce hepatic lipid accumulation in mice. Diabetes. 2016;65:902–12.
102. Thaiss CA, Itav S, Rothschild D, et al. Persistent microbiome alterations modulate the rate of post-dieting weight regain. Nature. 2016;540:544–51.
103. Zheng Y, Ceglarek U, Huang T, et al. Weight-loss diets and 2-y changes in circulating amino acids in 2 randomized intervention trials. Am J Clin Nutr. 2016;103:505–11.
104. Greenwood DA, Gee PM, Fatkin KJ, Peeples M. A systematic review of reviews evaluating technology-enabled diabetes self-management education and support. J Diabetes Sci Technol. 2017;11:1015–27.
105. Powers MA, Bardsley JK, Cypress M, et al. Diabetes Self-management Education and Support in Adults with Type 2 Diabetes: a consensus report of the American Diabetes Association, the Association of Diabetes Care & Education Specialists, the Academy of Nutrition and Dietetics, the American Academy of Family Physicians, the American Academy of PAs, the American Association of Nurse Practitioners, and the American Pharmacists Association. Diabetes Care. 2020;43:1636–49.
106. American Diabetes Association. 5. Facilitating behavior change and well-being to improve health outcomes: standards of medical care in diabetes-2021. Diabetes Care. 2021;44:S53–72.
107. Korem T, Zeevi D, Zmora N, et al. Bread affects clinical parameters and induces gut microbiome-associated personal Glycemic responses. Cell Metab. 2017;25:1243–1253.e5.
108. Cassidy S, Chau JY, Catt M, Bauman A, Trenell MI. Cross-sectional study of diet, physical activity, television viewing and sleep duration in 233,110 adults from the UK biobank; the behavioural phenotype of cardiovascular disease and type 2 diabetes. BMJ Open. 2016;6:e010038.
109. Hall H, Perelman D, Breschi A, Limcaoco P, Kellogg R, McLaughlin T, Snyder M. Glucotypes reveal new patterns of glucose dysregulation. PLoS Biol. 2018;16:e2005143.
110. Mendes-Soares H, Raveh-Sadka T, Azulay S, et al. Model of personalized postprandial glycemic response to food developed for an Israeli cohort predicts responses in Midwestern American individuals. Am J Clin Nutr. 2019;110:63–75.
111. Yoo HJ, An HG, Park SY, et al. Use of a real time continuous glucose monitoring system as a motivational device for poorly controlled type 2 diabetes. Diabetes Res Clin Pract. 2008;82:73–9.
112. Ehrhardt N, Al Zaghal E. Behavior modification in prediabetes and diabetes: potential use of real-time continuous glucose monitoring. J Diabetes Sci Technol. 2019;13:271–5.
113. Vigersky RA, Fonda SJ, Chellappa M, Walker MS, Ehrhardt NM. Short- and long-term effects of real-time continuous glucose monitoring in patients with type 2 diabetes. Diabetes Care. 2012;35:32–8.
114. Kooiman TJM, de Groot M, Hoogenberg K, Krijnen WP, van der Schans CP, Kooy A. Self-tracking of physical activity in people with type 2 diabetes: a randomized controlled trial. Comput Inform Nurs. 2018;36:340–9.
115. Bailey TS, Ahmann A, Brazg R, Christiansen M, Garg S, Watkins E, Welsh JB, Lee SW. Accuracy and acceptability of the 6-day Enlite continuous subcutaneous glucose sensor. Diabetes Technol Ther. 2014;16:277–83.
116. Walford GA, Porneala BC, Dauriz M, Vassy JL, Cheng S, Rhee EP, Wang TJ, Meigs JB, Gerszten RE, Florez JC. Metabolite traits and genetic risk provide complementary information for the prediction of future type 2 diabetes. Diabetes Care. 2014;37:2508–14.
117. Tily H, Perlina A, Patridge E, et al. Gut microbiome activity contributes to individual variation in glycemic response in adults. BioRxiv. 2019; https://doi.org/10.1101/641019.
118. Chung WK, Erion K, Florez JC, et al. Precision medicine in diabetes: a consensus report from the American Diabetes Association (ADA) and the European Association for the Study of diabetes (EASD). Diabetologia. 2020;63:1671–93.

Chapter 13
Precision Exercise and Physical Activity for Diabetes

Normand G. Boulé and Jane E. Yardley

Definitions and Considerations

Physical Activity Definitions

Movement comes in a variety of forms. The most basic of these is referred to as physical activity, which essentially includes all movement that increases energy use above that of a resting body. The subcategory of "activities of daily living" encompasses all of the movements required to care for oneself independently and includes such things as eating, dressing, and bathing (basic activities of daily living) [1]. It can also include such things as cleaning, laundry, shopping, meal preparation, and other household tasks. Physical activity can also include any type of active transportation (walking, cycling, etc.). Finally, the term "exercise" is used to describe physical activities that are planned and structured.

Aerobic exercise includes activities such as walking, swimming, cycling, and jogging where large muscle groups are involved in repeated and continuous movement [2]. Regular moderate aerobic exercise enhances insulin sensitivity, increases the muscles' ability to burn fuels in the presence of oxygen (due to a greater availability of enzymes and mitochondria), improves several aspects of lung function, and boosts the immune system (provided that exercise duration is not extensive). In

N. G. Boulé
Faculty of Kinesiology, Sport, and Recreation, University of Alberta, Edmonton, AB, Canada

Alberta Diabetes Institute, Edmonton, AB, Canada

J. E. Yardley (✉)
Faculty of Kinesiology, Sport, and Recreation, University of Alberta, Edmonton, AB, Canada

Alberta Diabetes Institute, Edmonton, AB, Canada

Augustana Faculty, University of Alberta, Edmonton, AB, Canada

Women's and Children's Health Research Institute, Edmonton, AB, Canada
e-mail: jeyardle@ualberta.ca

R. Basu (ed.), *Precision Medicine in Diabetes*,
https://doi.org/10.1007/978-3-030-98927-9_13

addition, it increases cardiovascular health, by augmenting cardiac output, while also improving the reactivity and compliance of blood vessels. Further benefits can include improved nerve conduction, muscle mass, and bone mineral density, depending on the type of activity selected [3]. This type of activity is generally considered "aerobic," where much of the fuel provided to the working muscles is produced through oxidation of glucose and fatty acids.

Resistance exercise, also referred to as strength training, can include any type of exercise that involves the contraction of muscles against a moveable or immovable force. This type of exercise can include lifting, pushing, or pulling of weights (free weights, body weight, or machines) or working against an elastic resistance band [4]. Regular resistance exercise improves body composition by increasing muscle mass and decreasing fat mass, enhances strength, promotes mental health, increases bone mineral density, improves blood pressure, ameliorates lipid profiles, and generally benefits cardiovascular health [3]. This type of activity is usually considered "anaerobic" or high intensity, where much of the fuel provided to the working muscles is produced through glycolysis.

During *high-intensity interval exercise (HIIE)*, the participant will alternate short bursts of high to maximal intensity activity with periods of recovery. The recovery intervals can consist of rest or a certain amount of time spent performing low- to moderate-intensity aerobic exercise. The duration and intensity of the work and recovery periods vary greatly depending on the desired training response. These types of programs tend to enhance cardiovascular health, insulin sensitivity, and muscle oxidative aerobic capacity to a greater extent than aerobic exercise if an equal amount of work is performed [5].

Precision Medicine

The concept of "precision medicine" generally involves an understanding that the *right therapy* should be provided for the *right patient*, at the *right time* [6], and that a one-size-fits-all solution does not exist. The same can be said with exercise/physical activity as an essential part of management for individuals with diabetes. A great deal more success will result if the right treatment, in this case exercise and/or physical activity, is provided to individual patients with recommendations for appropriate type, timing, duration, and intensity based on their goals, preferences, and physiology. In order to be as precise as possible in these prescriptions, it will be essential to understand the acute and training effects associated with different types of exercise for both type 1 and type 2 diabetes, along with the individual patient characteristics that might mediate some of these short- and long-term outcomes.

Type 1 Diabetes

Type 1 diabetes is an autoimmune condition in which the immune system attacks the insulin-producing beta cells of the pancreas. The destruction of these cells leads to a need for insulin replacement, either via multiple daily injections or subcutaneous infusion (insulin pump) of synthetic insulin. It has recently been recognized that what has generally been classified as "type 1" diabetes actually encompasses a spectrum, where some individuals continue to produce a certain amount of insulin (usually measured by residual c-peptide), while others become completely insulin-deficient [7, 8]. Latent autoimmune diabetes in adults (LADA) is another insulin-requiring form of diabetes where patients tend to present at a slightly older age, develop insulin deficiency at a much slower rate, and also tend to possess varying degrees of insulin resistance [9]. In addition, the term "double diabetes" [10] has been used to describe a growing subpopulation of individuals with type 1 diabetes having clinical features of insulin resistance, often related to obesity, older age, and longer diabetes duration [11]. As a result, each patient requires an individualized insulin regimen in order to maintain blood glucose levels in as close to a euglycemic range as possible, and, consequently, there is a great deal of variability in individual responses to exercise [12].

The Right Treatment: Adaptations to Exercise Training and Habitual Physical Activity in People with Type 1 Diabetes

In general, being physically active is associated with increased longevity [13, 14] and a decreased risk of microvascular and macrovascular complications [13, 15–17] in individuals with type 1 diabetes. In large longitudinal studies of individuals with type 1 diabetes, performing physical activity with greater frequency and/or intensity is associated with a lower risk and/or slower progression of complications such as neuropathy [15], nephropathy [15, 18], and retinopathy [16, 19]. Training intervention studies involving individuals with type 1 diabetes are few and have generally failed to show any improvement in mean blood glucose levels (as measured by hemoglobin A1c) although this could be due to overcompensation (in terms of insulin adjustments and carbohydrate intake [20]) on the part of the participants or due to inadequate exercise "dose" (frequency, intensity, duration) in many studies [21].

The vast majority of training studies involving participants with type 1 diabetes have involved aerobic exercise with variable dosage timing, frequency, intensity, and duration. Many of these studies have shown that aerobic training leads to an increase in aerobic fitness in individuals with type 1 diabetes [22–27], along with increases in capillary density [28] and improvements in endothelial function [25, 28, 29]. While not universal, some studies of aerobic training have resulted in a decrease in insulin dosage [24, 25, 30] and/or insulin resistance [24, 26, 31] among the participants. Similar to aerobic training in adults without diabetes, several studies involving participants with type 1 diabetes show an improvement in blood lipid levels as a result of performing regular aerobic exercise [22, 24, 25, 27, 31]. Finally, there are also data to support the role of aerobic training in ameliorating body composition, either by decreasing waist circumference [32] or by increasing bone density [33].

There are very few resistance training intervention studies involving individuals with type 1 diabetes, and those that do exist tend to involve very small sample sizes. From the limited evidence available, we know that resistance exercise increases muscle strength [34, 35] in individuals with type 1 diabetes. Where body composition is concerned, one study showed a decrease in fat mass along with an increase in lean mass after 10 weeks of resistance training [34]. There is also evidence from a very small study to indicate that resistance exercise may be beneficial in terms of reducing A1c and improving triglycerides [35]. Training programs that combined both aerobic (or high-intensity interval training) and resistance exercises have resulted in increased aerobic fitness [36, 37], greater muscle strength [36, 37], improved lipid profiles [36, 37], lower A1c [34, 37], and reduction in insulin needs [34, 36].

Intervention studies of HIIE in individuals with type 1 diabetes are currently just as rare as studies of resistance exercise and also involve small sample sizes. One of the consistent findings is that this type of training increases aerobic capacity [29, 34, 38, 39]. There is also evidence to indicate that HIIE may decrease aortic stiffness (as measured by pulse wave velocity) [38], improve endothelial function [29, 38], reduce fat mass [34, 39], increase lean mass [34, 39], and lower fasting glucose levels [39] in individuals with type 1 diabetes. Whether or not the improvements in aerobic fitness and endothelial function are greater with HIIE than with aerobic training are unclear, with one study finding HIIE to be superior [29], while another found that gains in these areas were similar to aerobic training [38]. As the two studies differed with respect to the length of the intervention, matching (or not) of participants within groups, duration/intensity/frequency of the intervals in the HIIE, and aerobic exercise protocols, the data are difficult to interpret.

In spite of the many known benefits of various types of exercise and physical activity for individuals with type 1 diabetes, a large proportion of adults with type 1 diabetes fail to meet the weekly recommendations of 150 minutes of moderate to vigorous physical activity (MVPA) [16, 40]. Women with type 1 diabetes tend to have lower activity levels than men with type 1 diabetes [2], and adolescents with type 1 diabetes are less active than their nondiabetic counterparts [41]. In addition to the regular barriers that exist where exercise and physical activity are concerned (lack of time, lack of money, lack of resources, etc.), fear of hypoglycemia and fear of losing control over diabetes management are major barriers to becoming more active in this population [42]. As such, a great deal of research has gone into determining the acute effects of different types, timings, durations, and intensities of exercise on blood glucose levels in individuals with type 1 diabetes in order to better understand the risk of hypoglycemia both during and after exercise. To date, a great amount of variability has been found, which may, to a certain extent, be due to individual characteristics such as age, sex, and fitness level [43] in addition to the exercise characteristics (type, intensity, duration) themselves.

The Right Treatment: Acute Glycemic Effects of Exercise in Individuals with Type 1 Diabetes

While exercise and physical activity are highly recommended for individuals with type 1 diabetes [44, 45], being physically active also complicates blood glucose management, resulting in an increased risk for both hypoglycemia and hyperglycemia. Where endogenously produced insulin has a half-life of approximately 5 minutes, even the fastest-acting synthetic insulins used for blood glucose management among individuals with type 1 diabetes take over an hour to hit their peak and several hours to be cleared from the system [46]. As a result, most people with type 1 diabetes undertake exercise in a hyperinsulinemic state. Depending on the type, intensity, or duration of exercise performed, excess insulin can increase the risk of hypoglycemia either during or after activity. In order to individualize exercise recommendations, a clear understanding of the acute effects of each type of exercise on blood glucose and any factors that might mediate these effects is essential.

Lipids are the primary source of fuel for low-intensity *aerobic exercise* [47], with its relative contribution to the fuel mix decreasing as exercise intensity increases. The secondary source of fuel at low intensity is glucose, but more specifically blood glucose, with the reliance on muscle glycogen as a fuel source increasing in proportion to exercise intensity. In people without diabetes, a delicate balance between insulin and its functional antagonist, glucagon, is maintained in order to ensure adequate blood glucose levels. As a result, both sympathetic nervous system signaling [48] and a small decline in blood glucose [49] are among the signals that lead to a decrease in insulin secretion from the pancreatic beta cells once activity has started. The naturally short half-life of endogenous insulin ensures a decrease in circulating insulin, with a concomitant increase in glucagon release by the alpha cells in the pancreas. Glucagon is then able to exert its effects on the liver to ensure release of glucose from storage and maintain blood glucose levels in a tight range for up to 2 hours of activity, even in the absence of carbohydrate intake.

In individuals with type 1 diabetes, the amount of insulin in circulation is dependent on the most recent bolus (either by injection or by infusion) along with the basal insulin that has been administered to manage blood glucose levels. To have appreciably lower insulin in circulation, preparation *at least* 90 minutes to 2 hours before exercise is necessary (discussed in section "Insulin Management"). As a result, most individuals with type 1 diabetes will start exercise in a hyperinsulinemic state, which is often exacerbated by the fact that the accompanying elevation in blood flow can also increase the absorption of insulin (particularly short- and intermediate-acting) from subcutaneous depots [50–53], resulting in even higher levels of insulin during activity. Consequently, it is common for large declines in blood glucose to be experienced during aerobic exercise [54, 55], unless an effort to decrease circulating insulin has been made in advance or unless exercise is performed in the fasting state (see section "Timing of Exercise: Fasting Versus Fed Exercise"). To complicate the situation further, these declines in blood glucose during exercise are often followed by a resurgence in blood glucose levels to the point of hyperglycemia in the hours postexercise [54], followed by an elevated risk of late-onset hypoglycemia [56], particularly if exercise is performed later in the day. It is often suggested that individuals with type 1 diabetes either decrease their basal insulin overnight, eat a low-glycemic index snack before bedtime, or combine both of these strategies to decrease the risk of nocturnal hypoglycemia after performing physical activity/exercise late in the day.

Studies to date would indicate that increasing exercise intensity is associated with smaller declines and potentially even increases in blood glucose during anaerobic activity in individuals with type 1 diabetes [57–59]. Activities, such as resistance exercise [54, 60], HIIE [55, 61–63], and subsequently several team sports, often result in smaller changes in blood glucose during exercise, thereby carrying a lower risk of hypoglycemia during activity and often necessitating smaller insulin adjustments (if any) prior to exercise. In addition to these types of exercise using muscle glycogen as a fuel source (which is used less during aerobic exercise), the smaller declines and/or increases in blood glucose in individuals with type 1 diabetes are often attributed to higher circulating levels of catecholamines, and in particular epinephrine, stimulating hepatic glycogenolysis [58, 62, 64]. While there is some disagreement among studies to date, it is likely that anaerobic activities carry a greater risk of late-onset postexercise hypoglycemia [54, 65, 66], due to the need to replenish glycogen stores used to fuel the activity. Similar to aerobic activities, this risk is likely higher if exercise takes place later in the day (see section "Timing of Exercise: Late Afternoon/Evening Exercise") and may be prevented by decreasing pre-bedtime insulin doses or eating a bedtime snack.

The knowledge that high-intensity activities can have a glucose-stabilizing effect has led to the suggestion that these types of activities can be included before, during, or after aerobic exercise to decrease the acute risk of hypoglycemia during exercise. One small study involving 12 individuals with type 1 diabetes demonstrated that performing resistance exercise (3 sets of 8 repetitions of 7 different exercises, involving all major muscle groups) can delay the declines in blood glucose during subsequent aerobic exercise [67]. Similarly, other studies have shown that 4-second maximal sprints performed every 2 minutes during a low-intensity aerobic exercise session [62] or even a single 10-second sprint at the end of 20 minutes of low-intensity aerobic exercise [68] can lead to smaller exercise-induced declines in blood glucose during activity compared to aerobic exercise on its own.

The Right Patient

While several generalities about exercise in individuals with type 1 diabetes have been listed in section "The Right Treatment: Acute Glycemic Effects of Exercise in Individuals with Type 1 Diabetes", it is important to consider individual characteristics when providing exercise and physical activity advice. Insulin regimens, physiological/physical characteristics, and patient goals will all be relevant with respect to the type, timing, and intensity of activities selected. They may also play a role in the risk of hypoglycemia during and after exercise.

Insulin Management

There are currently three main ways that individuals with type 1 diabetes administer their insulin to manage blood glucose levels, albeit a great deal of variability exists within each category [69]. The first of these is multiple daily injections of insulin

(MDI). This type of regimen generally involves one daily injection of long-lasting (basal) insulin, plus several injections of short-acting (bolus) insulin to manage blood glucose around meals and snacks or to correct for blood glucose levels in a hyperglycemic range. The second type of treatment involves continuous subcutaneous insulin infusion (CSII) of fast-acting insulin via an insulin pump. Rates of basal infusion can be programmed to vary throughout the day to manage diurnal variations in blood glucose. The user also has the ability to administer a bolus of insulin to account for carbohydrate intake in meals and snacks (or to correct for high blood glucose levels). The final and more recent type of system is referred to as a closed-loop system, where insulin is administered via an insulin pump, with information from a continuous glucose monitoring (CGM) sensor providing the data for an algorithm to adjust insulin infusion based on interstitial glucose levels [70]. Adjusting insulin dosages for exercise will vary depending on the type, timing, and intensity of exercise but also on the type of insulin regimen being followed.

For individuals administering insulin via MDI, there are two main options for adjusting insulin dosage prior to exercise. Where a weekly pattern of exercise days is well established, decreasing the basal insulin injection by ~20% the night before (or morning of depending on insulin management routines) the activity is recommended [45]. Where exercise and physical activity are less predictable, individuals with type 1 diabetes using MDI also have the option to decrease the size of their meal bolus if exercise is to take place within a few hours after a meal [63]. Should the activity be spontaneous and advance adjustments to insulin were not possible, fast-acting carbohydrates can be consumed before, during, and after exercise to maintain blood glucose levels in a euglycemic range. The size of the insulin adjustment and/or the amount of carbohydrate intake will depend on the type, timing, intensity, and duration of exercise, along with pre-exercise blood glucose levels [45]. The 2017 consensus statement by Riddell et al. [45] provides a detailed and comprehensive overview of exercise-related insulin adjustments and carbohydrate intake for individuals using an MDI insulin regimen.

Insulin pumps are often preferred by physically active individuals with type 1 diabetes as using only fast-acting insulin and being able to alter basal insulin infusion rates allow more flexibility for adjusting insulin before, during, and after exercise. While one observational study comparing MDI and CSII users showed comparable changes in blood glucose during exercise in both groups, those using CSII were better able to prevent postexercise hyperglycemia with small correction boluses, without increasing the occurrence of nocturnal hypoglycemia [71]. Current recommendations call, once again, for one of two strategies to be used in adjusting insulin delivery: either a decrease in basal rate (from 50% to 100%) at least 90 minutes before exercise or a reduced bolus with a meal or a snack prior to exercise (in particular for aerobic exercise) [45]. Studies have recently shown that adjusting basal rates closer to the start of exercise (either 40 or 20 minutes in advance) [72] and suspending insulin completely at the start of exercise [55] are less effective at preventing hypoglycemia during exercise than planning 90 minutes ahead. Where insulin has not been adjusted in advance, once again, carbohydrates will probably be required in order to maintain blood glucose levels in a euglycemic range during exercise, especially if that exercise is aerobic in nature. A further advantage of CSII is the ability to lower basal rates overnight postexercise (especially if exercise is performed late in the day) without causing next-day hyperglycemia. The consensus statement by Riddell et al. [45] provides a great deal more details about the size of insulin adjustments recommended for different types, intensities, and durations of exercise for individuals using CSII.

A recent randomized crossover trial also showed that using a combination of CSII and MDI (referred to as the "untethered" approach) can be effective for managing blood glucose levels around both aerobic and HIIE sessions [73]. The hybrid approach consisted of a single daily injection of long-acting insulin (basal dose) while using an insulin pump to deliver bolus insulin throughout the day. The comparator was usual CSII treatment. Insulin infusion was suspended 60 minutes prior to exercise. Compared to standard CSII therapy, the hybrid regimen was associated with more time in a euglycemic range during and after lab-based aerobic exercise and HIIE sessions, along with more time in euglycemia and less time in hyperglycemia during and after four high-intensity and two moderate-intensity home-based exercise sessions [73]. The authors argue that this particular approach to insulin management may offer more flexibility while still effectively managing blood glucose levels in physically active individuals with type 1 diabetes [73].

Recently developed closed-loop systems are very effective at managing blood glucose levels both overnight and for most day-to-day activities in individuals with type 1 diabetes of all ages [70, 74]. Exercise and physical activity, however, are still a challenge for closed-loop systems where blood glucose management is concerned. These single hormone systems [available in both commercial and do-it-yourself (also known as "looping") forms] use interstitial glucose data sent from a CGM system to adjust insulin infusion via an insulin pump with minimal input from the user. As mentioned above, however, simply having insulin infusion shut off at the beginning of exercise (if the system were able to detect the activity) often fails to prevent large declines in blood glucose during exercise [55, 72]. Companies producing commercial closed-loop, single hormone systems will thus recommend setting a higher blood glucose target (which subsequently reduces insulin infusion) 90 to 120 minutes before exercise, which should be maintained until the end of exercise [75]. Bihormonal systems (using both insulin and glucagon) are predicted to have greater success with respect to glucose management during exercise, with studies to date showing successful prevention of almost all hypoglycemic episodes [76–79]. The progress of these systems, which have not met with commercial approval to date, continues to be hampered by the lack of a stable glucagon solution and relatively little safety data surrounding the effects of the long-term use of injected glucagon.

Pancreatic islet transplantation is a less often used means of recovering endogenous insulin secretion in individuals with type 1 diabetes. One small study found that those who had undergone transplantation and were independent of exogenous insulin were still likely to experience greater declines in blood glucose and overall lower blood glucose levels during exercise compared to control participants without diabetes matched for height, weight, age, sex, and physical activity level [80]. Hypoglycemia, however, was no more common in the transplant recipients than it was in the control participants, indicating that transplanted islets are generally able to cope with the demands of exercise. More widespread use of this procedure is still being limited by the need for lifelong immune suppression therapy posttransplant. While methods to circumvent the need for this medication are being explored, many experts are still leaning toward fully automated insulin delivery as the preferred means of decreasing the burden of insulin management in individuals with type 1 diabetes [81].

Continuous Glucose Monitoring/Intermittently Scanned Continuous Glucose Monitoring (CGM/isCGM)

Many individuals with type 1 diabetes whether using MDI or CSII will also use CGM or intermittently scanned CGM (isCGM) to help monitor and manage blood glucose levels throughout the day. As these monitors provide not only information about current interstitial glucose levels but also about the rate of change of glucose (in the form of trend arrows), they can be used to assist in making decisions around insulin adjustments and carbohydrate intake before, during, and after exercise. Recent studies of CGM [82–85] and isCGM [86, 87] show that there is a tendency for most, but not all [88], of these systems to decrease in accuracy during exercise, due to the time lag for plasma glucose and interstitial glucose levels to equilibrate [89]. Users are therefore advised to consider trend arrows in addition to CGM glucose values in making decisions during exercise. A recent consensus statement has been published with recommendations on insulin adjustment and carbohydrate intake before and during exercise based on the type, timing, and intensity of exercise, along with starting CGM glucose values and trend arrows [90]. These recommendations are not meant to be a set of rules, but rather a starting point for developing individual management strategies.

Individual Characteristics

A majority of the studies of exercise responses in individuals with type 1 diabetes were performed with younger individuals who were habitually physically active and, for the most part, male. As such, very little is known about the impact of age, sex, or physical fitness on blood glucose responses to exercise and related hypoglycemia risk in this population [43]. What little we know comes from observational studies or secondary analyses of data that were collected for different purposes.

Among individuals with type 1 diabetes, one large observational study ($n = 18{,}028$) found that the frequency of self-reported exercise decreased with age [16]. In the youngest patients (aged 18 to <30 years), 25.8% reported exercising at least twice per week, compared to only 10.0% of individuals ($p < 0.0001$) in the oldest age group (45 to <80 years). Older individuals who were more physically active, however, also reported higher rates of severe hypoglycemia than younger individuals with similar activity levels. Those who were most active were also likely to have the lowest A1c and the smallest insulin dosage (IU/kg/day), along with a tendency to be less obese/overweight, with a healthier lipid profile and a lower frequency of diabetes complications such as retinopathy and nephropathy.

The same observational study found that women with type 1 diabetes were more likely to be inactive than men with type 1 diabetes: 66% of women reported no weekly physical activity, compared to 60.5% of men ($p < 0.0001$) [16]. This higher level of inactivity may be related to the fact that women who were active in the study also reported higher rates of severe hypoglycemia than those who were inactive, whereas the opposite was found among men up to the age of 45 years.

These data conflict to a certain extent with the only study to date examining sex-related differences in acute blood glucose responses to exercise. This secondary analysis of resistance exercise found that male participants had a greater decline in blood glucose during resistance exercise and a higher risk of postexercise hypoglycemia compared to female participants [91]. Another secondary analysis examining the effects of aerobic fitness found that blood glucose levels decreased more during aerobic exercise in individuals of higher aerobic fitness, compared to those of lower aerobic fitness [92]. In both instances, the greater changes in glucose may have been due to a greater amount of work performed or a higher lean body mass in the group that experienced greater changes. The latter argument is supported by yet another secondary analysis, showing that declines in blood glucose during exercise were greater in those with a higher amount of lean body mass [93].

In addition to knowing little about the blood glucose response to physical activity and exercise in women with type 1 diabetes in general, less is known about how the menstrual cycle (or the use of hormonal contraception) may affect blood glucose outcomes. In women with type 1 diabetes, cyclic changes in blood glucose levels have been observed throughout the menstrual cycle with higher blood glucose levels reported in many women during the luteal phase [94–98]. While one case study indicated that oral contraception decreased luteal hyperglycemia [99], another study of self-reported blood glucose in 124 women observed that perimenstrual fluctuations in glucose were still present in 67% of the sample that were using a fixed dose combined oral contraceptive pill [100]. To date, no studies have examined how the menstrual cycle and the use of hormonal contraception affect blood glucose responses to exercise and the resulting risk of postexercise hypoglycemia. Overall, more research is necessary involving studies designed specifically to examine the impact of age, sex, and physical fitness.

A recently described confounding factor explaining some of the variability in blood glucose responses during and after exercise is residual beta-cell function [12]. Recent studies have found that a relatively substantial proportion of individuals with type 1 diabetes still maintain some residual beta-cell function (as measured by c-peptide levels) long after their diagnosis [7, 8]. While many of these individuals would be considered "micro-secretors" [8], some individuals will maintain an amount of endogenous insulin secretion that is clinically relevant [8]. One small study to date examining the impact of residual beta-cell function on blood glucose responses to exercise found that individuals with the highest levels of c-peptide spent roughly 70% more time in a euglycemic range following exercise than those with low or undetectable levels of c-peptide [12]. The authors conclude that quantifying c-peptide could be useful in explaining individual responses to exercise and in personalizing exercise programs to individual patients [12].

A consideration of patient goals is essential to providing the right exercise and physical activity advice, especially where carbohydrate intake is concerned. Where a person is training to compete, finding the right combination of insulin adjustments and carbohydrate intake for optimal athletic performance [45, 101] is necessary. Where weight maintenance/weight loss is goals, finding ways to reduce the risk of hypoglycemia through insulin adjustments in order to prevent the need for additional carbohydrate intake will be essential. For detailed reviews of insulin adjustments for different intensities of exercise, the reader is referred to Riddell et al. [45].

The Right Time

In discussing the "right time" for exercise, it is important to consider benefits of regular exercise throughout disease progression and the life span, in addition to the acute effects of exercise timing throughout the day. With much of the focus in the area of exercise and type 1 diabetes being on acute hypoglycemia prevention, the effects of exercise timing throughout the day and with respect to food intake have been the focus of a great deal more research. There are, however, some important points to be made about exercise through different stages of life and diabetes progression.

The "Honeymoon" Phase

In the initial stages of type 1 diabetes, there are often a significant number of beta cells that continue to function [102], which tend to decline in number and in their ability to secrete insulin over time. This time after diagnosis is often referred to as the "honeymoon" phase; however, as mentioned earlier, some individuals maintain some residual function for an extended period of time post-diagnosis [7, 8]. Higher levels of meal-stimulated c-peptide ($\geq$200 pmol/l) have been associated with lower A1c, less frequent hypoglycemia, and reduced risk of nephropathy and retinopathy [103]. Consequently, several studies have attempted to maintain beta-cell function and extend the "honeymoon" phase in recently diagnosed individuals. Studies involving various pharmaceuticals have not been successful [104], but one case-control study suggested that those who exercise regularly are able to substantially extend their honeymoon phase [105]. These data, however, conflict with the results of a randomized controlled trial of exercise in newly diagnosed individuals with type 1 diabetes [106]. Narendran et al. found improvements in physical fitness and insulin sensitivity in the study participants after performing a minimum of

150 minutes/week of MVPA for 12 months, but there did not seem to be any impact on the rate of beta-cell loss [106]. Newly diagnosed individuals with type 1 diabetes are, nonetheless, encouraged to exercise for all of the other benefits that can be gained. There may, however, be a requirement for additional support in this particular subgroup of individuals, as there may be a tendency to avoid physical activity in those who are recently diagnosed [107], for fear of hypoglycemia.

Children and Adolescents with Type 1 Diabetes

It is generally recommended that children and adolescents acquire at least twice as much weekly physical activity as adults (60–90 minutes/day for toddlers, 90–120 minutes/day for preschoolers, and 60 minutes/day for school-aged children and adolescents) [108]. A meta-analysis of exercise studies involving children and youth with type 1 diabetes found that potential benefits of exercise included lower A1c [109, 110], decreased BMI [109], and improved triglyceride levels [109]. While the benefits of physical activity with respect to mental health are well-documented in children and adolescents without diabetes [111, 112], these benefits have not been well-researched in youth with diabetes. There is observational evidence from studies using CGM that physical activity, particularly if it is performed in the afternoon, is associated with an increase in hypoglycemia for youth with T1D [113, 114]. Conversely, intervention studies promoting an increase in physical activity have generally not found an increase in hypoglycemic events with increasing activity levels [109].

The risk of cardiovascular disease is much higher in individuals with type 1 diabetes than in people without diabetes and is higher for those who are diagnosed with type 1 diabetes at a younger age [115]. There is also evidence that children and youth with type 1 diabetes may already possess cardiovascular risk factors [116]. As the cardiovascular benefits of physical activity and exercise are well-established in individuals with type 1 diabetes [13, 16, 17, 117] and physical activity patterns from youth tend to track into adulthood [118], developing regular physical activity habits in children and youth with type 1 diabetes will be essential to their long-term health.

Pregnancy

Data on the risks and benefits of exercise during pregnancy in women with type 1 diabetes are very sparse. Compared to nondiabetic women, pregnant women with type 1 diabetes are at a higher risk of preeclampsia, miscarriage, congenital anomalies, preterm birth, and large for gestational age babies [119–121]. Several of these risks are associated with higher levels of A1c [119]. One nonrandomized intervention with a small sample size (n = 10) found a decrease in average daily glucose levels, less time spent in hyperglycemia, and less glucose variability (measured by CGM) on a day where participants performed three 20-min self-paced walks and two 50-min sessions of brisk walking compared to their regular routine [122]. Unfortunately, these changes were also associated with an increased risk of symptomatic hypoglycemia, and frequent/prolonged hypoglycemia has been associated with adverse fetal outcomes [123]. Further research is required in order to determine appropriate levels of exercise for this population in order to maximize health benefits while also minimizing risks.

Older Adults

Due to improvements in diabetes care, individuals with type 1 diabetes are living longer than they have in the past [124]. Older adults with type 1 diabetes are at a higher risk of frailty than adults with type 1 diabetes due to a faster loss of muscle mass with aging [125]. There is evidence to indicate that individuals with type 1 diabetes also have an accelerated loss of bone quality [126]. Combined, these factors produce a higher risk of falls and fall-related injuries, including fractures, in older adults with type 1 diabetes compared to those without diabetes [127]. While exercise is known to counteract all of these functional declines, type 1 diabetes-specific data related to exercise for older adults are currently lacking. Data related to hypoglycemia frequency in this population indicate that they are at a high risk of hypoglycemia in general [128] and therefore probably have a higher risk of hypoglycemia with exercise than younger individuals. This premise is consistent with the findings from a large observational study, where rates of hypoglycemia in physically active adults with type 1 diabetes aged 45 to <80 years were higher than their counterparts under the age of 45 with similar physical activity frequency [16]. As the benefits of exercise on functional mobility [129, 130] and quality of life [129, 131] in older adults have been clearly demonstrated, older adults with type 1 diabetes should make an effort to remain active while also remaining vigilant of their blood glucose levels during and after activity.

Timing of Exercise: Fasting Versus Fed Exercise

While most studies comparing fasted to fed exercise involve small sample sizes, there seems to be consensus that blood glucose responses to acute exercise, regardless of modality, are different when exercise is performed in a fasting state. In general, there tends to be little change or even an increase in blood glucose during fasted morning exercise, compared to the decrease that is generally observed with postprandial exercise [132–135]. The strength of existing studies is in their crossover design, where all participants were asked to perform a standard exercise protocol in both a fed (postprandial state) and fasted (postabsorptive) state on separate days, in a randomized order, with a washout period between the sessions. These divergent blood glucose responses to an identical exercise protocol performed by the same participants have been found with aerobic exercise [132, 133], resistance exercise [135], and HIIE [134] of short to moderate (i.e., 30 to 45 minutes) duration. While the mechanism behind these trends has yet to be elucidated, it is possible that they are simply the result of lower circulating insulin when participants exercise in a fasting state. It has also been surmised that variations in cortisol and growth hormone throughout the day could affect insulin sensitivity and fuel selection during exercise [136–138]. Thus, fasted morning exercise may be more appropriate for those who struggle with hypoglycemia during their activities, while those who experience frequent hyperglycemia may wish to exercise postprandially.

Timing of Exercise: Late Afternoon/Evening Exercise

It is generally accepted that when individuals with type 1 diabetes perform exercise later in the day, the risk of nocturnal hypoglycemia is increased [45]. This phenomenon is generally attributed to the fact that there will be fewer meals from which glycogen reserves can be replenished prior to bedtime, when exercise takes place later in the day. One observational study of adolescents and young adults with type 1 diabetes showed that late-day MVPA (as measured by accelerometry) increased the risk of overnight hypoglycemia (measured by CGM) independent of sex, fitness, and concurrent MVPA [114]. These findings are consistent with two crossover studies comparing morning versus afternoon exercise, where afternoon exercise was associated with a greater frequency of nocturnal hypoglycemia [135, 139]. One very tightly controlled study involving 45 minutes of moderate aerobic exercise in individuals with type 1 diabetes using glucose infusion overnight postexercise to maintain euglycemia showed that glucose needs increased in the early morning (between 1 and 3 am) after a late-day (4 pm) exercise session [56]. As such, a low-glycemic index bedtime snack [140] or a reduction in nocturnal basal insulin [141] is highly recommended after late-day activities.

Timing of Exercise Relative to Meals/Snacks

As previously mentioned, the timing of exercise with respect to previous meals and snacks is an important consideration where exercise is concerned. It is generally recommended to avoid exercise when circulating insulin will be at its peak (usually within 1 to 3 hours of a bolus, depending on the type of insulin administered). If exercise is taking place during this window and adjustments have not been made to basal insulin in advance, carbohydrate consumption will likely be required to prevent hypoglycemia during exercise, regardless of exercise intensity. As mentioned above, another option for maintaining blood glucose levels during the postprandial period is to consume a pre-exercise snack with a reduced insulin bolus. The size of this reduction will depend on how close to exercise the snack is being consumed and what type of activity the individual is about to undertake [142]. A more comprehensive discussion on this topic is provided by Riddell et al. [45].

Type 2 Diabetes

Type 2 diabetes has long been known to be a heterogeneous disease, and there have been many approaches to characterize the diverse phenotype. As the change from previous nomenclature suggested (i.e., the terms adult-onset diabetes or non-insulin-dependent diabetes are no longer in use), type 2 diabetes can develop at different ages and different levels of endogenous insulin secretion. More recent efforts to characterize type 2 diabetes have led to the identification of four subgroups by Ahlqvist et al. [143]:

- SIDD = severe insulin-deficient diabetes.
- SIRD = severe insulin-resistant diabetes.
- MOD = mild obesity-related diabetes.
- MARD = mild age-related diabetes.

The main commonality among the subgroups is the presence of hyperglycemia. Many exercise studies in this population have, therefore, focused on decreasing average blood glucose levels.

The Right Treatment

General Considerations

Compared to type 1 diabetes, the acute risk of hypoglycemia or hyperglycemia during or following exercise is typically less of a concern in type 2 diabetes. In the latter, a much larger number of exercise trials have been conducted from the perspective of improving longer-term indicators of glycemic management (e.g., A1c) [144, 145] and cardiovascular risk factors [146, 147]. Different forms of exercise training (e.g., aerobic, resistance, HIIE) have often been found to have relatively similar effects on A1c [145, 148]; however, other considerations may make one form of exercise preferable over others.

Aerobic Training

Aerobic training, such as brisk walking, is the most commonly prescribed exercise for people with diabetes. This is in part due to low cost, low risk, and ease of accessibility for many. It is also one of the preferred types of physical activity by the largest proportion of people with type 2 diabetes [149]. However, walking may not always be appropriate. For example, some people may have lower body limitations to walking, and other factors such as neighborhood safety or environmental conditions (e.g., extreme heat or icy sidewalks) may render walking unpleasant or unfeasible. There is no evidence, to our knowledge, that other forms of aerobic exercise are less effective (e.g., [150]). Cycling, including stationary cycling, or water-based activities could therefore be used to achieve a wide range of health benefits from glycemic management to lowering of blood pressure and improving lipid/lipoprotein profiles. That said, it is also important to have realistic expectations in regard to changes in body composition or fitness with most aerobic training programs, in part due to the moderate volumes and intensities of activity achieved with most interventions in people with type 2 diabetes. In many trials, meaningful improvements in A1c occur in the absence of major changes in body composition or body weight [144, 151].

Resistance Training

Resistance training is also firmly established as part of most guidelines and consensus statements for people with type 2 diabetes (e.g., [44, 152]). Improvements in mean blood glucose levels (as measured by reductions in A1c) are often comparable between aerobic and resistance training, and the benefits of aerobic and resistance training are likely additive [151]. However, many of the adaptations that are targeted by resistance training are different to aerobic training. In the general population, resistance training is normally performed with the goal of increasing muscle strength, power, and/or size. Such changes could be particularly desirable in some people with type 2 diabetes, such as older adults, and those with low muscle mass/function (i.e., sarcopenia) who may have poorer metabolic health to begin with [153]. From a behavioral perspective, resistance training may be considered in those who have access to resistance training equipment or for whom there are more barriers to aerobic training. Other forms of resistance training, which include less expensive and more accessible equipment, do exist. These alternatives, such as using resistance bands, may be good for beginning resistance training or maintenance, but a beneficial effect on A1c has not been consistently demonstrated [154, 155].

High-Intensity Interval Exercise (HIIE)

In recent years, HIIE has received growing attention in people with and without diabetes. It can result in similar, and perhaps slightly better, reductions in insulin resistance and A1c compared to more traditional forms of aerobic training [148, 156, 157]. One of the proposed advantages of HIIE training is that with some forms the benefits can be achieved with less time or exercise volume than continuous exercise of more moderate intensities. On the other hand, higher-intensity activities can be intimidating to some participants, as self-efficacy for higher-intensity exercise is lower [158]. However, it is important to keep in mind that in the context of HIIE, the term "high intensity" is most often a relative term which is set as a proportion of the participants' maximal aerobic fitness level and is not a fixed absolute workload that might be unattainable by those with lower fitness. Nonetheless, higher-intensity exercise may come with additional barriers, and there may be associated risks for some people. Most organizations recommend additional screening for cardiovascular risk before performing such activities [44, 152]. In terms of benefits, it is clear that HIIE training can result in greater improvements in aerobic fitness [156]. Aerobic fitness is often low in people with type 2 diabetes and can be important to facilitate activities of daily living. Aerobic fitness is also one of the strongest independent predictors of all-cause mortality [159, 160].

Breaking Sedentary Time

We are not aware of any long-term intervention study focusing on the effect of breaking sedentary time (e.g., breaks in sitting) in people with type 2 diabetes. There are several short-term studies in people with and without diabetes (as reviewed by Loh et al. [161]). Meta-analyses show relatively consistent reduction in cardiometabolic risk factors such as glucose and triglycerides with breaking of sedentary time [161]. Some studies emphasize standing to break up period of sitting, whereas others add brief exercise periods [161]. Interestingly, when the short-term efficacy of breaks in sedentary time is compared to continuous aerobic exercise, studies have shown mixed results. For example, Duvivier et al. [162] found that breaking sitting with a mix of standing and light-intensity walking improved 24-hour glucose concentrations to a greater extent than structured exercise. On the other hand, in the study by Blankenship et al. [163], continuous walking was more effective than short walking breaks in lowering daily hyperglycemia. Differences among studies may be due to the total number and duration of breaks.

Although there are no longer-term intervention studies, cohort studies have identified associations between the amount of sedentary behavior and the prevalence of type 2 diabetes [164]. Others have noted that more frequent breaks in sedentary time are associated with better glycemic management or insulin sensitivity in adults with type 2 diabetes [165].

The Right Patient

General Considerations

We are not aware of any studies comparing the effectiveness of different exercise interventions within the subgroups of type 2 diabetes described by Ahlqvist et al. [143] and described in section "Type 2 Diabetes". However, in secondary analyses of the Look AHEAD trial, 5145 participants with type 2 diabetes were categorized as "younger onset," "older onset," "severe obesity," and "poor glucose control" [166]. The Look AHEAD trial compared an intensive lifestyle intervention to standard education. The lifestyle intervention aimed to increase physical activity to 175 minutes per week and achieve/maintain a weight loss of 10%. A composite outcome of cardiovascular events/complications was collected over a median follow-up of 9.4 years. There was a significant interaction among the four subgroups and the cardiovascular protectiveness of the combined diet and physical activity intervention. Only the "poor glucose control" group was associated with increased risk for adverse cardiovascular outcomes [166]. Other analyses suggested that previous cardiovascular diseases may also have contributed to negative cardiovascular outcomes from the lifestyle intervention, but the association did not reach statistical significance ($p = 0.06$) [167].

Another approach to studying the heterogeneity of type 2 diabetes is to consider the pathological role of various organ systems. Defronzo had characterized the triumvirate (i.e., insulin resistance in muscle, insulin resistance in the liver, and impaired insulin secretion from beta cells) and later increased this to the ominous octet which added other defects (i.e., increased fatty acid release in adipose tissue, increased glucagon secretion from alpha cells, decreased incretin effect from the gastrointestinal tract, increased glucose reabsorption in kidneys, and neurotransmitter dysfunction in the brain) [168]. It remains to be seen if different exercise interventions can preferentially target some specific organ systems. Clearly, regular aerobic or resistance training can target improvements in insulin resistance at the level of the skeletal muscle (likely in part through different mechanisms); however, less is known about the impact on other organ systems (e.g., incretins).

Age and/or Duration of Diabetes

Although age is associated with an increased risk of developing type 2 diabetes, this disease can present at younger ages. The risk and benefits of physical activity would also be expected to change with aging or duration of diabetes. Both the categorization from Ahlqvist et al. [143] and a recent meta-analysis [169] suggest that diagnosis of diabetes at an older age can be associated with reduced risk of complications. Few exercise studies have been large enough to compare the effects of exercise in people with type 2 diabetes of different age or duration of the condition. Both older age and longer duration of diabetes are associated with a greater risk of cardiovascular disease, which may affect the choice of exercise (e.g., see previous discussion on exercise intensity). Greater duration of diabetes is also associated with a progressive decline in pancreatic volume and insulin secretory capacity [170, 171]. This decline may indirectly, through medications such as insulin, increase the risk of hypoglycemia during exercise [172].

From a behavioral perspective, it is also likely that aging is associated with different barriers to physical activity. For example, retirement from employment may be accompanied with more time for recreational activities. This may, in part, explain why the Diabetes Prevention Program (DPP) found that a lifestyle intervention composed of an energy-reduced diet and physical activity led to greater increases in physical activity and greater reductions in the risk of developing type 2 diabetes compared to placebo or metformin in older adults [173, 174]. More specifically, in participants between 25 and 44 years of age, the incidence of diabetes was reduced by a similar extent in the lifestyle and metformin groups compared to the placebo group (6.2 vs. 6.7 vs 11.6 cases/100 person-years) [175]. However, in the participants between 60 and 85 years of age, the lifestyle intervention reduced the incidence of diabetes more than both the metformin and placebo groups (3.1 vs. 9.6 vs. 11.8 cases/100 person-years) [175].

Sex

Although the prevalence of diabetes is similar in men and women [176] or perhaps slightly greater in men [177], the relative importance of the underlying pathophysiology can be different. For example, men tend to have greater insulin resistance but also greater insulin secretion [178]. In addition, men tend to meet the criteria for fasting hyperglycemia more frequently, whereas women meet the criteria for postprandial hyperglycemia more often (as previously reviewed [179]). Some of these discrepancies may be due to differences in body fat distribution (e.g., men tend to have more visceral and hepatic fat) but also other less appreciated differences such as more pronounced counterregulatory responses in men and greater reliance on fat as fuel in women.

Given the small size of most exercise trials involving people with type 2 diabetes, most have been underpowered to examine if men and women respond differently to the interventions. Again, turning to the DPP, which had a combined dietary and physical activity intervention, it was observed that a greater proportion of men met the objectives of 7% weight loss and 150 minutes/week of physical activity [180]. Despite these gender differences, the progression to diabetes was similar in both men and women, perhaps due to the fact that men had slightly more elevated cardiometabolic risk factors at baseline (e.g., fasting glucose) [180]. Looking at a large ($n = 596$), rigorously controlled exercise study in previously sedentary adults without diabetes, insulin sensitivity increased to a greater extent following training in men compared to women [178].

Obesity, Body Fat Distribution, and Sarcopenia

It has long been known that type 2 diabetes affects people of different shapes and sizes. Obesity, and in particular abdominal obesity, is a well-established modifiable risk factor of type 2 diabetes. However, it has also been recognized that not all people with type 2 diabetes have excess adiposity. Likewise, the prevalence of sarcopenia is enhanced in type 2 diabetes [181]. Although there is likely a bidirectional relationship between type 2 diabetes and sarcopenia (reviewed by Scott et al. [182]), evidence suggests that both impaired insulin sensitivity and secretion can contribute to sarcopenia [183]. Unfortunately, as for age and sex, there is no strong body of evidence to recommend one form of exercise over another in people with type 2 diabetes who have more/less adiposity or muscle mass. In the DPP, reductions in the incidence of type 2 diabetes in the lifestyle intervention group were significant in all three BMI categories compared to placebo (BMI from 22 to <30 kg/m^2 = 65%; BMI from 30 to <35 kg/m^2 = 61%; BMI ≥35 kg/m^2 = 51% reduction in the incidence of diabetes). Reductions in the incidence of diabetes were also superior to metformin except in participants with BMI ≥35 kg/m^2 in whom metformin had similar efficacy compared to those randomized to the lifestyle intervention [175].

From an adiposity perspective, aerobic training of moderate or higher intensity can result in reductions in fat mass, including visceral fat [184]. The effect of resistance training may not be as large [185]. However, reductions would typically be considered small and not largely different from one type of exercise intervention to another. While small amounts of weight loss are typically observed in overweight/obese individuals without diabetes with regular exercise training, it may not be as consistently observed in adults with type 2 diabetes [144]. Changes in visceral fat or health outcomes can, however, occur in the absence of weight loss [186]. As a result, changes in total body weight or body fat should not be used to judge the success of an exercise intervention in type 2 diabetes.

It might seem logical to target sarcopenia with resistance training interventions designed to target increases in muscle size or function [151, 187]. However, there is no clear evidence that resistance training is more effective at improving glycemic management in people with type 2 diabetes and sarcopenia versus those without sarcopenia [153].

Other Treatments (e.g., Medications or Nutrition)

Even though regular exercise or physical activity is considered a frontline therapy for the management of type 2 diabetes, it is rarely prescribed in isolation. When combining multiple therapies, it is possible that their effects are simply additive, that they have synergistic interactions (i.e., the benefits of combined treatment are superior to the additive effect of each treatment), or that one interferes or complicates another (i.e., negative interaction). Given the great number of options in regard to interventions such as glucose-lowering medications, dietary approaches, and bariatric surgeries, it would not be feasible to discuss all potential interactions with exercise (and, in many cases, these have not been studied). Consequently, we will discuss one example each of a likely additive, synergistic, and interference effect from combining other therapies with exercise.

Example 1: Additive Effect – Benefits of Combining Aerobic and Resistance Training In the Diabetes Aerobic and Resistance Exercise (DARE) trial, participants with type 2 diabetes were randomly assigned to a control group, resistance training, aerobic training, or fourth group that completed both the aerobic and resistance training protocols [151]. At both 3 months and 6 months, the effects of the combined training group seemed additive when compared to the groups that performed aerobic and resistance training alone. Although speculative, it would seem that only the two groups performing aerobic training (i.e., the aerobic and combined training groups) showed beneficial changes in A1c during the first 3 months, whereas the two groups that completed resistance training (i.e., the resistance and combined training groups) were the only ones who saw beneficial changes from months 3 to 6 [151].

Such additive effects are important to highlight because it is not always the case that doubling the amount of exercise leads to a doubling of the improvements in select outcomes. For example, Church et al. [188] randomly assigned 464 postmenopausal women with a BMI above 25 kg/m^2 and elevated blood pressure to a control group or 3 exercise groups with increasing volume (i.e., energy expenditure of 4 vs. 8 or 12 kcal/kg, per week). There was no difference in weight loss or waist circumference between exercise groups [188]. In another study by Church et al. [189], 262 people with type 2 diabetes were randomly assigned to a control group, resistance training, aerobic training, or combined resistance plus aerobic training. However, as opposed to the previously described DARE study, the amount of exercise in the combined training group was similar to the other two training groups, and only the combined training protocol was associated with improvements in A1c [189].

Example 2: Potential Synergistic Interaction – High-Protein Diet and Exercise Reductions in muscle mass are common with aging, particularly in those with type 2 diabetes. Exercise can contribute to increasing lean body mass or muscle mass, and there is evidence that this effect can be improved with the consumption of higher amounts of dietary protein. Evidence to support this premise has been at times correlative in nature, such as in one study where greater habitual protein intake was associated with greater improvements in strength and skeletal muscle mass following only 8 weeks of resistance training in elderly women [190]. However, when participants with type 2 diabetes are randomly assigned to different protein intakes, the results have not been fully consistent. In a recent study by Memelink et al. [191], an enriched protein drink, which included leucine and vitamin D, or isocaloric control drink was provided in the morning and immediately following combined HIIE and resistance exercise sessions performed 3 times per week over 13 weeks. Total lean mass and insulin sensitivity increased to a greater extent in the group that received the protein-enriched drink [191].

Wycherley et al. [192] used a factorial design in which an energy-restricted diet included random assignment of participants with type 2 diabetes to resistance training or no exercise with and without a high-protein diet. Reductions in body weight and total fat mass were largest in the combined resistance training and high-protein group. However, contrary to Memelink et al. [191], this group did not experience the most favorable changes in fat-free mass. Differences among studies may be due to factors such as the amount of energy restriction or the timing of protein intake. Indeed, larger improvements in lean body mass and in strength have been shown in older adults assigned to consume a protein supplement immediately after, as opposed to 2 hours after, resistance training sessions [193].

Example 3: Negative Interaction – Metformin and Exercise Unlike type 1 diabetes where the interactions between exercise and insulin treatments are often studied, little is known regarding the effect of glucose-lowering medications on responses to exercise in type 2 diabetes. For example, in the previously discussed DPP, participants were randomly assigned to placebo, an intensive lifestyle intervention, or metformin, but there wasn't a combined lifestyle intervention plus metformin group

[175]. However, the Indian Diabetes Prevention Program (IDPP) trial used a similar design as the DPP with the addition of a combined metformin and lifestyle modification group [194]. Surprisingly, the combined effect was similar to either metformin or lifestyle modification alone (ranging from 26.4% to 28.5% reductions in the risk of developing diabetes).

In people with type 2 diabetes, there is also evidence to suggest that combinations of metformin and exercise can at times lead to surprising, if not to say disappointing, results. Recently, a study of 6447 people with type 2 diabetes from the NHANES survey (1999–2018) found that increasing physical activity was associated with improved A1c in those who were not treated with metformin but not in those who were. We are not aware of longer-term randomized trials in which participants with type 2 diabetes were assigned to exercise and/or metformin, but several short-term studies have confirmed these potential negative interactions [195, 196]. Most of these studies have focused on aerobic exercise. However, in older adults without diabetes, metformin interfered with resistance training-induced increases in muscle mass [197]. These findings do not necessarily mean that exercise should not be prescribed in those treated with metformin or that metformin should not be prescribed to those who exercise. There may be other benefits of combined treatment, and further studies are needed. However, people treated with metformin should not be surprised if some of the effects of exercise are less pronounced than anticipated.

The Right Time

General Considerations

Unlike some glucose-lowering medications, increasing physical activity, including participation in structured exercise, is indicated at all stages (healthy, prediabetes, new-onset diabetes, and long-duration diabetes) of disease progression. Consequently, most people receive advice at all stages, and we are not aware of any studies, comparing exercise to delayed exercise prescription in people with type 2 diabetes. Some such studies exist in other chronic conditions such as severe obesity, which did not suggest advantages of delaying the addition of physical activity to an energy-restricted diet [198]. On the other hand, there are recent trials addressing issues pertaining to the timing of individual bouts of exercise in relation to the time of day or other factors such as meal or medication intake.

Speculations on When Delaying Exercise Interventions (or Co-Interventions) Could Be Considered

As we highlighted in the previous studies in prediabetes (e.g., the DPP and IDPP), lifestyle interventions that include exercise can play an important role in delaying diabetes and improving many cardiometabolic risk factors. The evidence on combining exercise and metformin is not definitive, but the potential negative interaction between the two lends support to the idea that it may be worthwhile delaying metformin treatment in those who want to attempt to increase physical activity levels. Delaying metformin may be particularly useful in older participants with low muscle mass given the greater efficacy of lifestyle interventions in older participants [175] (and the potential for greater reductions in fat-free mass with metformin [197]). Perhaps once it is determined that increasing physical is difficult to achieve, metformin could be added.

At the diagnosis of prediabetes or type 2 diabetes, there is evidence that some, but not all, people can be very receptive to behavior change [199, 200]. However, this time is characterized by many potential other changes such as diet and medications. Some patients may prefer making one behavior change at a time to avoid being overwhelmed. That said, there is also evidence that the barriers to physical activity can be very different to the barriers to diet changes [201, 202]. Consequently, there may be times when people with type 2 diabetes are more receptive to some lifestyle interventions than others.

Exercise Timing (e.g., Time of Day)

The questions of the timing of specific bouts of exercise have not received much attention in type 2 diabetes. In general, it would seem that when circulating glucose and insulin are elevated, the rate of decline in glucose during exercise can be more pronounced. For example, exercise performed ~1 hour after a meal leads to a greater decline in glucose during the exercise bout itself, whereas exercise in the fasted state would lead to little change [203, 204]. Of note, glucose may have declined in the former situation even in the absence of exercise as postprandial glucose eventually declines due to glucoregulatory processes. In addition, differences in the change in glucose during exercise may not reflect glucose changes over a 24-hour period [205, 206]. For example, in the study by Munan et al. [206], exercise after an overnight fast led to a lesser acute reduction in glucose compared to afternoon exercise (−0.4 vs −1.5 mmol/L, $p = 0.02$), but there was no difference over 24 hours (7.5 vs 7.3 mmol/L, $p = 0.57$). Interestingly, fasting glucose was lower the day after fasting exercise only (6.8 vs 7.3 mmol/L, $p = 0.003$) suggesting that the timing of exercise is an important consideration as it can affect some glycemic outcomes but not others.

On the other hand, Savikj et al. [207] compared HIIE performed either in the morning or the afternoon in participants with type 2 diabetes and concluded that afternoon HIIE was more efficacious than morning HIIE at improving blood glucose. Differences between this study and the one by Munan et al. [206] include the fact that Munan prescribed morning exercise after an overnight fast, whereas Savikj prescribed exercise after a light breakfast and provided a postexercise snack in the morning condition only. Indeed, a complete understanding of the effects of exercise timing is not available and includes the timing in the day, the timing in relation to meals or medications, as well as the type of exercise or characteristics of participants.

Several recent studies, commentaries, and reviews have suggested that exercise should be performed shortly after meals to cause greater immediate improvements in mean blood glucose levels [208–215]. In spite of this attention, clear recommendations for post-meal (i.e., postprandial) exercise are not yet endorsed by Canadian [216] or American [44] physical activity guidelines. However, as we and others have argued [215, 217], the emphasis on post-meal exercise may come at a cost. There is growing evidence supporting more favorable long-term adaptations when exercise is performed after an overnight fast, which results in greater depletion of endogenous energy reserves. For example, a study by Van Proeyen et al. showed that regular exercise training increased muscle glycogen and improved mitochondrial function when performed in the fasted state but not when exercise was performed with carbohydrate supplementation [218]. This is noteworthy because impairments in glycogen storage [219–221] and mitochondrial mass or function [222–224] are linked to insulin resistance and type 2 diabetes.

We have studied exercise in the fasted state in several contexts [157, 203, 225, 226]. For example, we compared the effects of 4 weeks of the same exercise prescription performed after an overnight fast versus after breakfast in recreational cyclists. We observed greater improvements in aerobic fitness, as well as lower glucagon and glucose levels when exercise was performed after fasting overnight [157]. These findings are in line with another study by Van Proeyen et al. [227] who studied active young men (mean physical activity of ~3.5 hours per week at baseline) and found improvements in oral glucose tolerance after 6 weeks of training in the fasted state but not when similar training was performed after breakfast [227]. However, to date, only two studies have compared training adaptations to several weeks of training in the fasted state (pre breakfast) versus postprandial exercise training in type 2 diabetes [228, 229]. The studies were relatively small and did not show consistently superior benefits of fasted training, in comparison to training in postprandial state.

Summary

There are many health outcomes that are improved (on average) with regular physical activity in both type 1 and type 2 diabetes. While most activities can be performed safely with gradual progression and appropriate adjustments, a great deal of variability exists in the physiological responses to exercise and physical activity. There is also a great deal of variability in exercise and physical activity preferences among individuals with diabetes. An effort should be made to tailor recommendations to individual needs (Fig. 13.1) in order to optimize the use of this "treatment" to improve the health and quality of life of individuals with diabetes.

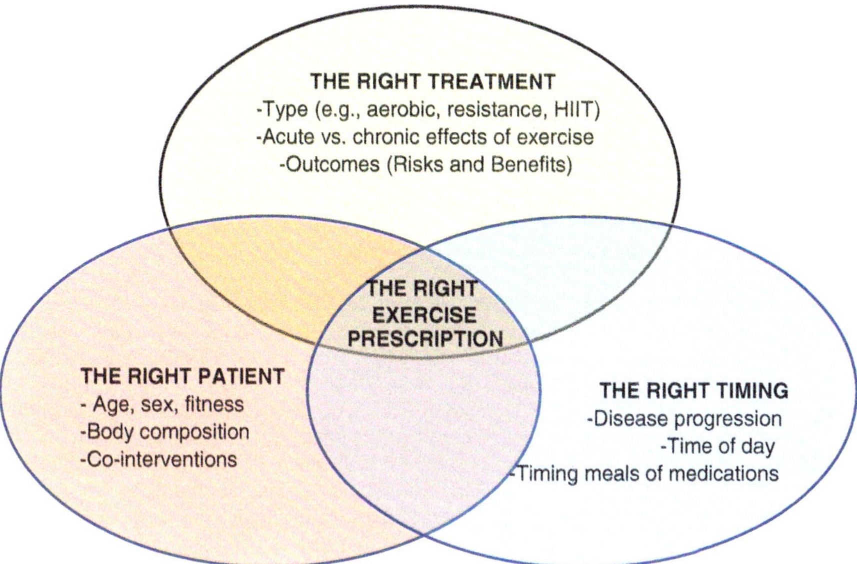

Fig. 13.1 Precision medicine considerations for exercise/physical activity in diabetes mellitus

References

1. Katz S. Assessing self-maintenance: activities of daily living, mobility, and instrumental activities of daily living. J Am Geriatr Soc. 1983;31(12):721–7.
2. Physical Activity Guidelines Advisory Committee. Physical activity guidelines advisory committee report. Washington, DC: U.S. Department of Health and Human Services; 2008.
3. Garber CE, Blissmer B, Deschenes MR, Franklin BA, Lamonte MJ, Lee IM, et al. American College of Sports Medicine position stand. Quantity and quality of exercise for developing and maintaining cardiorespiratory, musculoskeletal, and neuromotor fitness in apparently healthy adults: guidance for prescribing exercise. Med Sci Sports Exerc. 2011;43(7):1334–59.
4. Behm DG, Faigenbaum AD, Falk B, Klentrou P. Canadian Society for Exercise Physiology position paper: resistance training in children and adolescents. Appl Physiol Nutr Metab. 2008;33(3):547–61.
5. Cassidy S, Thoma C, Houghton D, Trenell MI. High-intensity interval training: a review of its impact on glucose control and cardiometabolic health. Diabetologia. 2017;60(1):7–23.
6. Chung WK, Erion K, Florez JC, Hattersley AT, Hivert MF, Lee CG, et al. Precision medicine in diabetes: a consensus report from the American Diabetes Association (ADA) and the European Association for the Study of Diabetes (EASD). Diabetes Care. 2020;43(7):1617–35.
7. Williams GM, Long AE, Wilson IV, Aitken RJ, Wyatt RC, McDonald TJ, et al. Beta cell function and ongoing autoimmunity in long-standing, childhood onset type 1 diabetes. Diabetologia. 2016;59(12):2722–6.
8. Oram RA, McDonald TJ, Shields BM, Hudson MM, Shepherd MH, Hammersley S, et al. Most people with long-duration type 1 diabetes in a large population-based study are insulin microsecretors. Diabetes Care. 2015;38(2):323–8.

9. Fadiga L, Saraiva J, Catarino D, Frade J, Melo M, Paiva I. Adult-onset autoimmune diabetes: comparative analysis of classical and latent presentation. Diabetol Metab Syndr. 2020;12(1):107.
10. Popovic DS, Papanas N. Double diabetes: a growing problem requiring solutions. Exp Clin Endocrinol Diabetes. 2021. https://doi.org/10.1055/a-1392-0590.
11. Simoniene D, Platukiene A, Prakapiene E, Radzeviciene L, Velickiene D. Insulin resistance in type 1 diabetes mellitus and its association with Patient's micro- and macrovascular complications, sex hormones, and other clinical data. Diabetes Ther. 2020;11(1):161–74.
12. Taylor GS, Smith K, Capper TE, Scragg JH, Bashir A, Flatt A, et al. Postexercise Glycemic control in type 1 diabetes is associated with residual beta-cell function. Diabetes Care. 2020;43(10):2362–70.
13. Tielemans SM, Soedamah-Muthu SS, De Neve M, Toeller M, Chaturvedi N, Fuller JH, et al. Association of physical activity with all-cause mortality and incident and prevalent cardiovascular disease among patients with type 1 diabetes: the EURODIAB Prospective Complications Study. Diabetologia. 2013;56(1):82–91.
14. Moy CS, Songer TJ, LaPorte RE, Dorman JS, Kriska AM, Orchard TJ, et al. Insulin-dependent diabetes mellitus, physical activity, and death. Am J Epidemiol. 1993;137(1):74–81.
15. Kriska AM, LaPorte RE, Patrick SL, Kuller LH, Orchard TJ. The association of physical activity and diabetic complications in individuals with insulin-dependent diabetes mellitus: the Epidemiology of Diabetes Complications Study–VII. J Clin Epidemiol. 1991;44(11):1207–14.
16. Bohn B, Herbst A, Pfeifer M, Krakow D, Zimny S, Kopp F, et al. Impact of physical activity on glycemic control and prevalence of cardiovascular risk factors in adults with type 1 diabetes: a cross-sectional multicenter study of 18,028 patients. Diabetes Care. 2015;38(8):1536–43.
17. Tikkanen-Dolenc H, Waden J, Forsblom C, Harjutsalo V, Thorn LM, Saraheimo M, et al. Frequent and intensive physical activity reduces risk of cardiovascular events in type 1 diabetes. Diabetologia. 2017;60(3):574–80.
18. Waden J, Tikkanen HK, Forsblom C, Harjutsalo V, Thorn LM, Saraheimo M, et al. Leisure-time physical activity and development and progression of diabetic nephropathy in type 1 diabetes: the FinnDiane study. Diabetologia. 2015;58(5):929–36.
19. Tikkanen-Dolenc H, Waden J, Forsblom C, Harjutsalo V, Thorn LM, Saraheimo M, et al. Frequent physical activity is associated with reduced risk of severe diabetic retinopathy in type 1 diabetes. Acta Diabetol. 2020;57(5):527–34.
20. Yardley JE, Sigal RJ, Perkins BA, Riddell MC, Kenny GP. Resistance exercise in type 1 diabetes. Can J Diabetes. 2013;37(6):420–6.
21. Yardley JE, Hay J, Abou-Setta AM, Marks SD, McGavock J. A systematic review and meta-analysis of exercise interventions in adults with type 1 diabetes. Diabetes Res Clin Pract. 2014;106(3):393–400.
22. Laaksonen DE, Atalay M, Niskanen LK, Mustonen J, Sen CK, Lakka TA, et al. Aerobic exercise and the lipid profile in type 1 diabetic men: a randomized controlled trial. Med Sci Sports Exerc. 2000;32(9):1541–8.
23. Wallberg-Henriksson H, Gunnarsson R, Rossner S, Wahren J. Long-term physical training in female type 1 (insulin-dependent) diabetic patients: absence of significant effect on glycaemic control and lipoprotein levels. Diabetologia. 1986;29(1):53–7.
24. Yki-Jarvinen H, DeFronzo RA, Koivisto VA. Normalization of insulin sensitivity in type I diabetic subjects by physical training during insulin pump therapy. Diabetes Care. 1984;7(6):520–7.
25. Fuchsjager-Mayrl G, Pleiner J, Wiesinger GF, Sieder AE, Quittan M, Nuhr MJ, et al. Exercise training improves vascular endothelial function in patients with type 1 diabetes. Diabetes Care. 2002;25(10):1795–801.
26. Landt KW, Campaigne BN, James FW, Sperling MA. Effects of exercise training on insulin sensitivity in adolescents with type I diabetes. Diabetes Care. 1985;8(5):461–5.

27. Rigla M, Sanchez-Quesada JL, Ordonez-Llanos J, Prat T, Caixas A, Jorba O, et al. Effect of physical exercise on lipoprotein(a) and low-density lipoprotein modifications in type 1 and type 2 diabetic patients. Metabolism. 2000;49(5):640–7.
28. de Moraes R, Van Bavel D, Gomes MB, Tibirica E. Effects of non-supervised low intensity aerobic excise training on the microvascular endothelial function of patients with type 1 diabetes: a non-pharmacological interventional study. BMC Cardiovasc Disord. 2016;16:23.
29. Boff W, da Silva AM, Farinha JB, Rodrigues-Krause J, Reischak-Oliveira A, Tschiedel B, et al. Superior effects of high-intensity interval vs. moderate-intensity continuous training on endothelial function and cardiorespiratory fitness in patients with type 1 diabetes: a randomized controlled trial. Front Physiol. 2019;10:450.
30. Wrobel M, Rokicka D, Czuba M, Golas A, Pyka L, Greif M, et al. Aerobic as well as resistance exercises are good for patients with type 1 diabetes. Diabetes Res Clin Pract. 2018;144:93–101.
31. Wallberg-Henriksson H, Gunnarsson R, Henriksson J, DeFronzo R, Felig P, Ostman J, et al. Increased peripheral insulin sensitivity and muscle mitochondrial enzymes but unchanged blood glucose control in type I diabetics after physical training. Diabetes. 1982;31(12):1044–50.
32. Ramalho AC, de Lourdes Lima M, Nunes F, Cambui Z, Barbosa C, Andrade A, et al. The effect of resistance versus aerobic training on metabolic control in patients with type-1 diabetes mellitus. Diabetes Res Clin Pract. 2006;72(3):271–6.
33. Maggio AB, Rizzoli RR, Marchand LM, Ferrari S, Beghetti M, Farpour-Lambert NJ. Physical activity increases bone mineral density in children with type 1 diabetes. Med Sci Sports Exerc. 2012;44(7):1206–11.
34. Farinha JB, Ramis TR, Vieira AF, Macedo RCO, Rodrigues-Krause J, Boeno FP, et al. Glycemic, inflammatory and oxidative stress responses to different high-intensity training protocols in type 1 diabetes: a randomized clinical trial. J Diabetes Complicat. 2018;32(12):1124–32.
35. Durak EP, Jovanovic-Peterson L, Peterson CM. Randomized crossover study of effect of resistance training on glycemic control, muscular strength, and cholesterol in type I diabetic men. Diabetes Care. 1990;13(10):1039–43.
36. D'Hooge R, Hellinckx T, Van Laethem C, Stegen S, De Schepper J, Van Aken S, et al. Influence of combined aerobic and resistance training on metabolic control, cardiovascular fitness and quality of life in adolescents with type 1 diabetes: a randomized controlled trial. Clin Rehabil. 2011;25(4):349–59.
37. Mosher PE, Nash MS, Perry AC, LaPerriere AR, Goldberg RB. Aerobic circuit exercise training: effect on adolescents with well-controlled insulin dependent diabetes mellitus. Arch Phys Med Rehabil. 1998;79(6):652–7.
38. Scott SN, Cocks M, Andrews RC, Narendran P, Purewal TS, Cuthbertson DJ, et al. High-intensity interval training improves aerobic capacity without a detrimental decline in blood glucose in people with type 1 diabetes. J Clin Endocrinol Metab. 2019;104(2):604–12.
39. Alarcon-Gomez J, Calatayud J, Chulvi-Medrano I, Martin-Rivera F. Effects of a HIIT protocol on cardiovascular risk factors in a type 1 diabetes mellitus population. Int J Environ Res Public Health. 2021;18(3):1262.
40. Plotnikoff RC, Taylor LM, Wilson PM, Courneya KS, Sigal RJ, Birkett N, et al. Factors associated with physical activity in Canadian adults with diabetes. Med Sci Sports Exerc. 2006;38(8):1526–34.
41. Valerio G, Spagnuolo MI, Lombardi F, Spadaro R, Siano M, Franzese A. Physical activity and sports participation in children and adolescents with type 1 diabetes mellitus. Nutr Metab Cardiovasc Dis. 2007;17(5):376–82.
42. Brazeau AS, Rabasa-Lhoret R, Strychar I, Mircescu H. Barriers to physical activity among patients with type 1 diabetes. Diabetes Care. 2008;31(11):2108–9.
43. Yardley JE, Brockman NK, Bracken RM. Could age, sex and physical fitness affect blood glucose responses to exercise in type 1 diabetes? Front Endocrinol (Lausanne). 2018;9:674.

44. Colberg SR, Sigal RJ, Yardley JE, Riddell MC, Dunstan DW, Dempsey PC, et al. Physical activity/exercise and diabetes: a position statement of the American Diabetes Association. Diabetes Care. 2016;39(11):2065–79.
45. Riddell MC, Gallen IW, Smart CE, Taplin CE, Adolfsson P, Lumb AN, et al. Exercise management in type 1 diabetes: a consensus statement. Lancet Diabetes Endocrinol. 2017;5(5):377–90.
46. Rodbard HW, Rodbard D. Biosynthetic human insulin and insulin analogs. Am J Ther. 2020;27(1):e42–51.
47. Romijn JA, Coyle EF, Sidossis LS, Gastaldelli A, Horowitz JF, Endert E, et al. Regulation of endogenous fat and carbohydrate metabolism in relation to exercise intensity and duration. Am J Phys. 1993;265(3 Pt 1):E380–91.
48. Jarhult J, Holst J. The role of the adrenergic innervation to the pancreatic islets in the control of insulin release during exercise in man. Pflugers Arch. 1979;383(1):41–5.
49. Hedeskov CJ. Mechanism of glucose-induced insulin secretion. Physiol Rev. 1980;60(2):442–509.
50. Ferrannini E, Linde B, Faber O. Effect of bicycle exercise on insulin absorption and subcutaneous blood flow in the normal subject. Clin Physiol. 1982;2(1):59–70.
51. McAuley SA, Horsburgh JC, Ward GM, La Gerche A, Gooley JL, Jenkins AJ, et al. Insulin pump basal adjustment for exercise in type 1 diabetes: a randomised crossover study. Diabetologia. 2016;59(8):1636–44.
52. Ronnemaa T, Koivisto VA. Combined effect of exercise and ambient temperature on insulin absorption and postprandial glycemia in type I patients. Diabetes Care. 1988;11(10):769–73.
53. Thow JC, Johnson AB, Antsiferov M, Home PD. Exercise augments the absorption of isophane (NPH) insulin. Diabet Med. 1989;6(4):342–5.
54. Yardley JE, Kenny GP, Perkins BA, Riddell MC, Balaa N, Malcolm J, et al. Resistance versus aerobic exercise: acute effects on glycemia in type 1 diabetes. Diabetes Care. 2013;36(3):537–42.
55. Zaharieva D, Yavelberg L, Jamnik V, Cinar A, Turksoy K, Riddell MC. The effects of basal insulin suspension at the start of exercise on blood glucose levels during continuous versus circuit-based exercise in individuals with type 1 diabetes on continuous subcutaneous insulin infusion. Diabetes Technol Ther. 2017;19(6):370–8.
56. McMahon SK, Ferreira LD, Ratnam N, Davey RJ, Youngs LM, Davis EA, et al. Glucose requirements to maintain euglycemia after moderate-intensity afternoon exercise in adolescents with type 1 diabetes are increased in a biphasic manner. J Clin Endocrinol Metab. 2007;92(3):963–8.
57. Mitchell TH, Abraham G, Schiffrin A, Leiter LA, Marliss EB. Hyperglycemia after intense exercise in IDDM subjects during continuous subcutaneous insulin infusion. Diabetes Care. 1988;11(4):311–7.
58. Purdon C, Brousson M, Nyveen SL, Miles PD, Halter JB, Vranic M, et al. The roles of insulin and catecholamines in the glucoregulatory response during intense exercise and early recovery in insulin-dependent diabetic and control subjects. J Clin Endocrinol Metab. 1993;76(3):566–73.
59. Sigal RJ, Purdon C, Fisher SJ, Halter JB, Vranic M, Marliss EB. Hyperinsulinemia prevents prolonged hyperglycemia after intense exercise in insulin-dependent diabetic subjects. J Clin Endocrinol Metab. 1994;79(4):1049–57.
60. Turner D, Gray BJ, Luzio S, Dunseath G, Bain SC, Hanley S, et al. Similar magnitude of post-exercise hyperglycemia despite manipulating resistance exercise intensity in type 1 diabetes individuals. Scand J Med Sci Sports. 2016;26(4):404–12.
61. Campbell MD, West DJ, Bain SC, Kingsley MI, Foley P, Kilduff L, et al. Simulated games activity vs continuous running exercise: a novel comparison of the glycemic and metabolic responses in T1DM patients. Scand J Med Sci Sports. 2015;25(2):216–22.

62. Guelfi KJ, Jones TW, Fournier PA. The decline in blood glucose levels is less with intermittent high-intensity compared with moderate exercise in individuals with type 1 diabetes. Diabetes Care. 2005;28(6):1289–94.
63. Moser O, Tschakert G, Mueller A, Groeschl W, Pieber TR, Obermayer-Pietsch B, et al. Effects of high-intensity interval exercise versus moderate continuous exercise on glucose homeostasis and hormone response in patients with type 1 diabetes mellitus using novel ultra-Long-acting insulin. PLoS One. 2015;10(8):e0136489.
64. Sigal RJ, Fisher SJ, Halter JB, Vranic M, Marliss EB. Glucoregulation during and after intense exercise: effects of beta-adrenergic blockade in subjects with type 1 diabetes mellitus. J Clin Endocrinol Metab. 1999;84(11):3961–71.
65. Maran A, Pavan P, Bonsembiante B, Brugin E, Ermolao A, Avogaro A, et al. Continuous glucose monitoring reveals delayed nocturnal hypoglycemia after intermittent high-intensity exercise in nontrained patients with type 1 diabetes. Diabetes Technol Ther. 2010;12(10):763–8.
66. Rempel M, Yardley JE, MacIntosh A, Hay JL, Bouchard D, Cornish S, et al. Vigorous intervals and hypoglycemia in type 1 diabetes: a randomized cross over trial. Sci Rep. 2018;8(1):15879.
67. Yardley JE, Kenny GP, Perkins BA, Riddell MC, Malcolm J, Boulay P, et al. Effects of performing resistance exercise before versus after aerobic exercise on glycemia in type 1 diabetes. Diabetes Care. 2012;35(4):669–75.
68. Bussau VA, Ferreira LD, Jones TW, Fournier PA. The 10-s maximal sprint: a novel approach to counter an exercise-mediated fall in glycemia in individuals with type 1 diabetes. Diabetes Care. 2006;29(3):601–6.
69. Kesavadev J, Saboo B, Krishna MB, Krishnan G. Evolution of insulin delivery devices: from syringes, pens, and pumps to DIY artificial pancreas. Diabetes Ther. 2020;11(6):1251–69.
70. Cengiz E. Automated insulin delivery in children with type 1 diabetes. Endocrinol Metab Clin N Am. 2020;49(1):157–66.
71. Yardley JE, Iscoe KE, Sigal RJ, Kenny GP, Perkins BA, Riddell MC. Insulin pump therapy is associated with less post-exercise hyperglycemia than multiple daily injections: an observational study of physically active type 1 diabetes patients. Diabetes Technol Ther. 2013;15(1):84–8.
72. Roy-Fleming A, Taleb N, Messier V, Suppere C, Cameli C, Elbekri S, et al. Timing of insulin basal rate reduction to reduce hypoglycemia during late post-prandial exercise in adults with type 1 diabetes using insulin pump therapy: a randomized crossover trial. Diabetes Metab. 2019;45(3):294–300.
73. Aronson R, Li A, Brown RE, McGaugh S, Riddell MC. Flexible insulin therapy with a hybrid regimen of insulin degludec and continuous subcutaneous insulin infusion with pump suspension before exercise in physically active adults with type 1 diabetes (FIT untethered): a single-Centre, open-label, proof-of-concept, randomised crossover trial. Lancet Diabetes Endocrinol. 2020;8(6):511–23.
74. Boughton CK, Hovorka R. Automated insulin delivery in adults. Endocrinol Metab Clin N Am. 2020;49(1):167–78.
75. Zaharieva DP, Messer LH, Paldus B, O'Neal DN, Maahs DM, Riddell MC. Glucose control during physical activity and exercise using closed loop technology in adults and adolescents with type 1 diabetes. Can J Diabetes. 2020;44(8):740–9.
76. Jacobs PG, El Youssef J, Reddy R, Resalat N, Branigan D, Condon J, et al. Randomized trial of a dual-hormone artificial pancreas with dosing adjustment during exercise compared with no adjustment and sensor-augmented pump therapy. Diabetes Obes Metab. 2016;18(11):1110–9.
77. Taleb N, Emami A, Suppere C, Messier V, Legault L, Ladouceur M, et al. Efficacy of single-hormone and dual-hormone artificial pancreas during continuous and interval exercise in adult patients with type 1 diabetes: randomised controlled crossover trial. Diabetologia. 2016;59(12):2561–71.

78. Haidar A, Rabasa-Lhoret R, Legault L, Lovblom LE, Rakheja R, Messier V, et al. Single- and dual-hormone artificial pancreas for overnight glucose control in type 1 diabetes. J Clin Endocrinol Metab. 2016;101(1):214–23.
79. Castle JR, El Youssef J, Wilson LM, Reddy R, Resalat N, Branigan D, et al. Randomized outpatient trial of single- and dual-hormone closed-loop systems that adapt to exercise using wearable sensors. Diabetes Care. 2018;41(7):1471–7.
80. Yardley JE, Rees JL, Funk DR, Toghi-Eshghi SR, Boule NG, Senior PA. Effects of moderate cycling exercise on blood glucose regulation following successful clinical islet transplantation. J Clin Endocrinol Metab. 2019;104(2):493–502.
81. Senior P, Lam A, Farnsworth K, Perkins B, Rabasa-Lhoret R. Assessment of risks and benefits of beta cell replacement versus automated insulin delivery systems for type 1 diabetes. Curr Diab Rep. 2020;20(10):52.
82. Zaharieva DP, Turksoy K, McGaugh SM, Pooni R, Vienneau T, Ly T, et al. Lag time remains with newer real-time continuous glucose monitoring technology during aerobic exercise in adults living with type 1 diabetes. Diabetes Technol Ther. 2019;21(6):313–21.
83. Larose S, Rabasa-Lhoret R, Roy-Fleming A, Suppere C, Tagougui S, Messier V, et al. Changes in accuracy of continuous glucose monitoring using Dexcom G4 platinum over the course of moderate intensity aerobic exercise in type 1 diabetes. Diabetes Technol Ther. 2019;21(6):364–9.
84. Biagi L, Bertachi A, Quiros C, Gimenez M, Conget I, Bondia J, et al. Accuracy of continuous glucose monitoring before, during, and after aerobic and anaerobic exercise in patients with type 1 diabetes mellitus. Biosensors (Basel). 2018;8(1).
85. Taleb N, Emami A, Suppere C, Messier V, Legault L, Chiasson JL, et al. Comparison of two continuous glucose monitoring systems, Dexcom G4 platinum and Medtronic paradigm Veo Enlite system, at rest and during exercise. Diabetes Technol Ther. 2016;18(9):561–7.
86. Moser O, Eckstein ML, McCarthy O, Deere R, Pitt J, Williams DM, et al. Performance of the freestyle libre flash glucose monitoring (flash GM) system in individuals with type 1 diabetes: a secondary outcome analysis of a randomized crossover trial. Diabetes Obes Metab. 2019;21(11):2505–12.
87. Fokkert M, van Dijk PR, Edens MA, Diez Hernandez A, Slingerland R, Gans R, et al. Performance of the Eversense versus the free style libre flash glucose monitor during exercise and normal daily activities in subjects with type 1 diabetes mellitus. BMJ Open Diabetes Res Care. 2020;8(1):e001193.
88. Guillot FH, Jacobs PG, Wilson LM, Youssef JE, Gabo VB, Branigan DL, et al. Accuracy of the Dexcom G6 glucose sensor during aerobic, resistance, and interval exercise in adults with type 1 diabetes. Biosensors (Basel). 2020;10(10):138.
89. Moser O, Yardley JE, Bracken RM. Interstitial glucose and physical exercise in type 1 diabetes: integrative physiology, technology, and the gap in-between. Nutrients. 2018;10(1):93.
90. Moser O, Riddell MC, Eckstein ML, Adolfsson P, Rabasa-Lhoret R, van den Boom L, et al. Glucose management for exercise using continuous glucose monitoring (CGM) and intermittently scanned CGM (isCGM) systems in type 1 diabetes: position statement of the European Association for the Study of Diabetes (EASD) and of the International Society for Pediatric and Adolescent Diabetes (ISPAD) endorsed by JDRF and supported by the American Diabetes Association (ADA). Pediatr Diabetes. 2020;63:2501–20.
91. Brockman NK, Sigal RJ, Kenny GP, Riddell MC, Perkins BA, Yardley JE. Sex-related differences in blood glucose responses to resistance exercise in adults with type 1 diabetes: a secondary data analysis. Can J Diabetes. 2020;44(3):267–73 e1.
92. Al Khalifah RA, Suppere C, Haidar A, Rabasa-Lhoret R, Ladouceur M, Legault L. Association of aerobic fitness level with exercise-induced hypoglycaemia in type 1 diabetes. Diabet Med. 2016;33(12):1686–90.
93. Tagougui S, Goulet-Gelinas L, Taleb N, Messier V, Suppere C, Rabasa-Lhoret R. Association between body composition and blood glucose during exercise and recovery in adolescent and adult patients with type 1 diabetes. Can J Diabetes. 2020;44(2):192–5.

94. Barata DS, Adan LF, Netto EM, Ramalho AC. The effect of the menstrual cycle on glucose control in women with type 1 diabetes evaluated using a continuous glucose monitoring system. Diabetes Care. 2013;36(5):e70.
95. Widom B, Diamond MP, Simonson DC. Alterations in glucose metabolism during menstrual cycle in women with IDDM. Diabetes Care. 1992;15(2):213–20.
96. Trout KK, Rickels MR, Schutta MH, Petrova M, Freeman EW, Tkacs NC, et al. Menstrual cycle effects on insulin sensitivity in women with type 1 diabetes: a pilot study. Diabetes Technol Ther. 2007;9(2):176–82.
97. Goldner WS, Kraus VL, Sivitz WI, Hunter SK, Dillon JS. Cyclic changes in glycemia assessed by continuous glucose monitoring system during multiple complete menstrual cycles in women with type 1 diabetes. Diabetes Technol Ther. 2004;6(4):473–80.
98. Brown SA, Jiang B, McElwee-Malloy M, Wakeman C, Breton MD. Fluctuations of Hyperglycemia and insulin sensitivity are linked to menstrual cycle phases in women with T1D. J Diabetes Sci Technol. 2015;9(6):1192–9.
99. Sacerdote A, Bleicher SJ. Oral contraceptives abolish luteal phase exacerbation of hyperglycemia in type I diabetes. Diabetes Care. 1982;5(6):651–2.
100. Lunt H, Brown LJ. Self-reported changes in capillary glucose and insulin requirements during the menstrual cycle. Diabetic Med. 1996;13(6):525–30.
101. Riddell MC, Scott SN, Fournier PA, Colberg SR, Gallen IW, Moser O, et al. The competitive athlete with type 1 diabetes. Diabetologia. 2020;63(8):1475–90.
102. Campbell-Thompson M, Fu A, Kaddis JS, Wasserfall C, Schatz DA, Pugliese A, et al. Insulitis and beta-cell mass in the natural history of type 1 diabetes. Diabetes. 2016;65(3):719–31.
103. Steffes MW, Sibley S, Jackson M, Thomas W. Beta-cell function and the development of diabetes-related complications in the diabetes control and complications trial. Diabetes Care. 2003;26(3):832–6.
104. Skyler JS. Prevention and reversal of type 1 diabetes–past challenges and future opportunities. Diabetes Care. 2015;38(6):997–1007.
105. Chetan MR, Charlton MH, Thompson C, Dias RP, Andrews RC, Narendran P. The type 1 diabetes 'honeymoon' period is five times longer in men who exercise: a case-control study. Diabet Med. 2019;36(1):127–8.
106. Narendran P, Jackson N, Daley A, Thompson D, Stokes K, Greenfield S, et al. Exercise to preserve beta-cell function in recent-onset type 1 diabetes mellitus (EXTOD) – a randomized controlled pilot trial. Diabet Med. 2017;34(11):1521–31.
107. Matson RIB, Leary SD, Cooper AR, Thompson C, Narendran P, Andrews RC. Objective measurement of physical activity in adults with newly diagnosed type 1 diabetes and healthy individuals. Front Public Health. 2018;6:360.
108. American Academic of Pediatrics, American Public Health Association, Education NRCfHaSiCCaE. Caring for our children: national health and safety performance standards; Guidelines for early care and education programs. 3rd ed. Washington, DC: American Academy of Pediatrics; 2011.
109. Quirk H, Blake H, Tennyson R, Randell TL, Glazebrook C. Physical activity interventions in children and young people with type 1 diabetes mellitus: a systematic review with meta-analysis. Diabet Med. 2014;31(10):1163–73.
110. MacMillan F, Kirk A, Mutrie N, Matthews L, Robertson K, Saunders DH. A systematic review of physical activity and sedentary behavior intervention studies in youth with type 1 diabetes: study characteristics, intervention design, and efficacy. Pediatr Diabetes. 2014;15(3):175–89.
111. Ahn S, Fedewa AL. A meta-analysis of the relationship between children's physical activity and mental health. J Pediatr Psychol. 2011;36(4):385–97.
112. Larun L, Nordheim LV, Ekeland E, Hagen KB, Heian F. Exercise in prevention and treatment of anxiety and depression among children and young people. Cochrane Database Syst Rev. 2006;3:CD004691.

113. Bachmann S, Hess M, Martin-Diener E, Denhaerynck K, Zumsteg U. Nocturnal Hypoglycemia and physical activity in children with diabetes: new insights by continuous glucose monitoring and Accelerometry. Diabetes Care. 2016;39(7):e95–6.
114. Metcalf KM, Singhvi A, Tsalikian E, Tansey MJ, Zimmerman MB, Esliger DW, et al. Effects of moderate-to-vigorous intensity physical activity on overnight and next-day hypoglycemia in active adolescents with type 1 diabetes. Diabetes Care. 2014;37(5):1272–8.
115. Rawshani A, Sattar N, Franzen S, Rawshani A, Hattersley AT, Svensson AM, et al. Excess mortality and cardiovascular disease in young adults with type 1 diabetes in relation to age at onset: a nationwide, register-based cohort study. Lancet. 2018;392(10146):477–86.
116. Snell-Bergeon JK, Nadeau K. Cardiovascular disease risk in young people with type 1 diabetes. J Cardiovasc Transl Res. 2012;5(4):446–62.
117. Herbst A, Kordonouri O, Schwab KO, Schmidt F, Holl RW. Impact of physical activity on cardiovascular risk factors in children with type 1 diabetes: a multicenter study of 23,251 patients. Diabetes Care. 2007;30(8):2098–100.
118. Telama R, Yang X, Leskinen E, Kankaanpaa A, Hirvensalo M, Tammelin T, et al. Tracking of physical activity from early childhood through youth into adulthood. Med Sci Sports Exerc. 2014;46(5):955–62.
119. Suhonen L, Hiilesmaa V, Teramo K. Glycaemic control during early pregnancy and fetal malformations in women with type I diabetes mellitus. Diabetologia. 2000;43(1):79–82.
120. Evers IM, de Valk HW, Visser GH. Risk of complications of pregnancy in women with type 1 diabetes: nationwide prospective study in the Netherlands. BMJ. 2004;328(7445):915.
121. Lin SF, Kuo CF, Chiou MJ, Chang SH. Maternal and fetal outcomes of pregnant women with type 1 diabetes, a national population study. Oncotarget. 2017;8(46):80679–87.
122. Kumareswaran K, Elleri D, Allen JM, Caldwell K, Westgate K, Brage S, et al. Physical activity energy expenditure and glucose control in pregnant women with type 1 diabetes: is 30 minutes of daily exercise enough? Diabetes Care. 2013;36(5):1095–101.
123. Rosenn BM, Miodovnik M, Khoury JC, Siddiqi TA. Deficient counterregulation: a possible risk factor for excessive fetal growth in IDDM pregnancies. Diabetes Care. 1997;20(5):872–4.
124. Lin X, Xu Y, Pan X, Xu J, Ding Y, Sun X, et al. Global, regional, and national burden and trend of diabetes in 195 countries and territories: an analysis from 1990 to 2025. Sci Rep. 2020;10(1):14790.
125. Krause MP, Riddell MC, Hawke TJ. Effects of type 1 diabetes mellitus on skeletal muscle: clinical observations and physiological mechanisms. Pediatr Diabetes. 2011;12(4 Pt 1):345–64.
126. Halper-Stromberg E, Gallo T, Champakanath A, Taki I, Rewers M, Snell-Bergeon J, et al. Bone mineral density across the lifespan in patients with type 1 diabetes. J Clin Endocrinol Metab. 2020;105(3):746–53.
127. Rasmussen NH, Dal J, den Bergh JV, de Vries F, Jensen MH, Vestergaard P. Increased risk of falls, fall-related injuries and fractures in people with type 1 and type 2 diabetes – a Nationwide Cohort Study. Curr Drug Saf. 2021;16(1):52–61.
128. Carlson AL, Kanapka LG, Miller KM, Ahmann AJ, Chaytor NS, Fox S, et al. Hypoglycemia and Glycemic control in older adults with type 1 diabetes: baseline results from the WISDM study. J Diabetes Sci Technol. 2019;15(3):582–92. 1932296819894974
129. Campbell E, Petermann-Rocha F, Welsh P, Celis-Morales C, Pell JP, Ho FK, et al. The effect of exercise on quality of life and activities of daily life in frail older adults: a systematic review of randomised control trials. Exp Gerontol. 2021;147:111287.
130. Ramsey KA, Rojer AGM, D'Andrea L, Otten RHJ, Heymans MW, Trappenburg MC, et al. The association of objectively measured physical activity and sedentary behavior with skeletal muscle strength and muscle power in older adults: a systematic review and meta-analysis. Ageing Res Rev. 2021;67:101266.
131. Cunningham C, O'Sullivan R, Caserotti P, Tully MA. Consequences of physical inactivity in older adults: a systematic review of reviews and meta-analyses. Scand J Med Sci Sports. 2020;30(5):816–27.

132. Ruegemer JJ, Squires RW, Marsh HM, Haymond MW, Cryer PE, Rizza RA, et al. Differences between prebreakfast and late afternoon glycemic responses to exercise in IDDM patients. Diabetes Care. 1990;13(2):104–10.
133. Yamanouchi K, Abe R, Takeda A, Atsumi Y, Shichiri M, Sato Y. The effect of walking before and after breakfast on blood glucose levels in patients with type 1 diabetes treated with intensive insulin therapy. Diabetes Res Clin Pract. 2002;58(1):11–8.
134. Yardley JE. Fasting may alter blood glucose responses to high intensity interval exercise in adults with type 1 diabetes: a randomized acute crossover study. Can J Diabetes. 2020;44(8):727–33.
135. Toghi-Eshghi SR, Yardley JE. Morning (fasting) vs afternoon resistance exercise in individuals with type 1 diabetes: a randomized crossover study. J Clin Endocrinol Metab. 2019;104(11):5217–24.
136. Yardley JE, Sigal RJ, Riddell MC, Perkins BA, Kenny GP. Performing resistance exercise before versus after aerobic exercise influences growth hormone secretion in type 1 diabetes. Appl Physiol Nutr Metab. 2014;39(2):262–5.
137. Vendelbo MH, Christensen B, Gronbaek SB, Hogild M, Madsen M, Pedersen SB, et al. GH signaling in human adipose and muscle tissue during 'feast and famine': amplification of exercise stimulation following fasting compared to glucose administration. Eur J Endocrinol. 2015;173(3):283–90.
138. Vieira AF, Costa RR, Macedo RC, Coconcelli L, Kruel LF. Effects of aerobic exercise performed in fasted v. fed state on fat and carbohydrate metabolism in adults: a systematic review and meta-analysis. Br J Nutr. 2016;116(7):1153–64.
139. Gomez AM, Gomez C, Aschner P, Veloza A, Munoz O, Rubio C, et al. Effects of performing morning versus afternoon exercise on glycemic control and hypoglycemia frequency in type 1 diabetes patients on sensor-augmented insulin pump therapy. J Diabetes Sci Technol. 2015;9(3):619–24.
140. Campbell MD, Walker M, Trenell MI, Stevenson EJ, Turner D, Bracken RM, et al. A low-glycemic index meal and bedtime snack prevents postprandial hyperglycemia and associated rises in inflammatory markers, providing protection from early but not late nocturnal hypoglycemia following evening exercise in type 1 diabetes. Diabetes Care. 2014;37(7):1845–53.
141. Campbell MD, Walker M, Bracken RM, Turner D, Stevenson EJ, Gonzalez JT, et al. Insulin therapy and dietary adjustments to normalize glycemia and prevent nocturnal hypoglycemia after evening exercise in type 1 diabetes: a randomized controlled trial. BMJ Open Diabetes Res Care. 2015;3(1):e000085.
142. West DJ, Stephens JW, Bain SC, Kilduff LP, Luzio S, Still R, et al. A combined insulin reduction and carbohydrate feeding strategy 30 min before running best preserves blood glucose concentration after exercise through improved fuel oxidation in type 1 diabetes mellitus. J Sports Sci. 2011;29(3):279–89.
143. Ahlqvist E, Storm P, Karajamaki A, Martinell M, Dorkhan M, Carlsson A, et al. Novel subgroups of adult-onset diabetes and their association with outcomes: a data-driven cluster analysis of six variables. Lancet Diabetes Endocrinol. 2018;6(5):361–9.
144. Boule NG, Haddad E, Kenny GP, Wells GA, Sigal RJ. Effects of exercise on glycemic control and body mass in type 2 diabetes mellitus: a meta-analysis of controlled clinical trials. JAMA. 2001;286(10):1218–27.
145. Umpierre D, Ribeiro PA, Kramer CK, Leitao CB, Zucatti AT, Azevedo MJ, et al. Physical activity advice only or structured exercise training and association with HbA1c levels in type 2 diabetes: a systematic review and meta-analysis. JAMA. 2011;305(17):1790–9.
146. Snowling NJ, Hopkins WG. Effects of different modes of exercise training on glucose control and risk factors for complications in type 2 diabetic patients: a meta-analysis. Diabetes Care. 2006;29(11):2518–27.
147. Pan B, Ge L, Xun YQ, Chen YJ, Gao CY, Han X, et al. Exercise training modalities in patients with type 2 diabetes mellitus: a systematic review and network meta-analysis. Int J Behav Nutr Phys Act. 2018;15(1):72.

148. Liubaoerjijin Y, Terada T, Fletcher K, Boule NG. Effect of aerobic exercise intensity on glycemic control in type 2 diabetes: a meta-analysis of head-to-head randomized trials. Acta Diabetol. 2016;53(5):769–81.
149. Forbes CC, Plotnikoff RC, Courneya KS, Boule NG. Physical activity preferences and type 2 diabetes: exploring demographic, cognitive, and behavioral differences. Diabetes Educ. 2010;36(5):801–15.
150. Rees JL, Johnson ST, Boule NG. Aquatic exercise for adults with type 2 diabetes: a meta-analysis. Acta Diabetol. 2017;54(10):895–904.
151. Sigal RJ, Kenny GP, Boule NG, Wells GA, Prud'homme D, Fortier M, et al. Effects of aerobic training, resistance training, or both on glycemic control in type 2 diabetes: a randomized trial. Ann Intern Med. 2007;147(6):357–69.
152. Sigal RJ, Armstrong MJ, Bacon SL, Boule NG, Dasgupta K, Kenny GP, et al. Physical activity and diabetes. Can J Diabetes. 2018;42(Suppl 1):S54–63.
153. Terada T, Boule NG, Forhan M, Prado CM, Kenny GP, Prud'homme D, et al. Cardiometabolic risk factors in type 2 diabetes with high fat and low muscle mass: at baseline and in response to exercise. Obesity (Silver Spring). 2017;25(5):881–91.
154. Sigal RJ, Armstrong JA, Fowles JR, Kenny GP, McGinley SK, Dineen T, et al. Resistance bands training improved strength and glycemic control: the DARE-bands trial. Can J Diabetes. 2018;42(5 Suppl):S11.
155. McGinley SK, Armstrong MJ, Boule NG, Sigal RJ. Effects of exercise training using resistance bands on glycaemic control and strength in type 2 diabetes mellitus: a meta-analysis of randomised controlled trials. Acta Diabetol. 2015;52(2):221–30.
156. Jelleyman C, Yates T, O'Donovan G, Gray LJ, King JA, Khunti K, et al. The effects of high-intensity interval training on glucose regulation and insulin resistance: a meta-analysis. Obes Rev. 2015;16(11):942–61.
157. Terada T, Toghi Eshghi SR, Liubaoerjijin Y, Kennedy M, Myette-Cote E, Fletcher K, et al. Overnight fasting compromises exercise intensity and volume during sprint interval training but improves high-intensity aerobic endurance. J Sports Med Phys Fitness. 2019;59(3):357–65.
158. Rodgers WM, Blanchard CM, Sullivan MJ, Bell GJ, Wilson PM, Gesell JG. The motivational implications of characteristics of exercise bouts. J Health Psychol. 2002;7(1):73–83.
159. Wei M, Gibbons LW, Kampert JB, Nichaman MZ, Blair SN. Low cardiorespiratory fitness and physical inactivity as predictors of mortality in men with type 2 diabetes. Ann Intern Med. 2000;132(8):605–11.
160. Myers J, Prakash M, Froelicher V, Do D, Partington S, Atwood JE. Exercise capacity and mortality among men referred for exercise testing. N Engl J Med. 2002;346(11):793–801.
161. Loh R, Stamatakis E, Folkerts D, Allgrove JE, Moir HJ. Effects of interrupting prolonged sitting with physical activity breaks on blood glucose, insulin and triacylglycerol measures: a systematic review and meta-analysis. Sports Med. 2020;50(2):295–330.
162. Duvivier BM, Schaper NC, Hesselink MK, van Kan L, Stienen N, Winkens B, et al. Breaking sitting with light activities vs structured exercise: a randomised crossover study demonstrating benefits for glycaemic control and insulin sensitivity in type 2 diabetes. Diabetologia. 2017;60(3):490–8.
163. Blankenship JM, Chipkin SR, Freedson PS, Staudenmayer J, Lyden K, Braun B. Managing free-living hyperglycemia with exercise or interrupted sitting in type 2 diabetes. J Appl Physiol (1985). 2019;126(3):616–25.
164. van der Berg JD, Stehouwer CD, Bosma H, van der Velde JH, Willems PJ, Savelberg HH, et al. Associations of total amount and patterns of sedentary behaviour with type 2 diabetes and the metabolic syndrome: the Maastricht study. Diabetologia. 2016;59(4):709–18.
165. Sardinha LB, Magalhaes JP, Santos DA, Judice PB. Sedentary patterns, physical activity, and cardiorespiratory fitness in association to Glycemic control in type 2 diabetes patients. Front Physiol. 2017;8:262.

166. Bancks MP, Chen H, Balasubramanyam A, Bertoni AG, Espeland MA, Kahn SE, et al. Type 2 diabetes subgroups, risk for complications, and differential effects due to an intensive lifestyle intervention. Diabetes Care. 2021;44(5):1203–10.
167. Look AHEAD Research Group, Wing RR, Bolin P, Brancati FL, Bray GA, Clark JM, et al. Cardiovascular effects of intensive lifestyle intervention in type 2 diabetes. N Engl J Med. 2013;369(2):145–54.
168. Defronzo RA. Banting Lecture. From the triumvirate to the ominous octet: a new paradigm for the treatment of type 2 diabetes mellitus. Diabetes. 2009;58(4):773–95.
169. Nanayakkara N, Curtis AJ, Heritier S, Gadowski AM, Pavkov ME, Kenealy T, et al. Impact of age at type 2 diabetes mellitus diagnosis on mortality and vascular complications: systematic review and meta-analyses. Diabetologia. 2021;64(2):275–87.
170. Lu J, Guo M, Wang H, Pan H, Wang L, Yu X, et al. Association between pancreatic atrophy and loss of insulin secretory capacity in patients with type 2 diabetes mellitus. J Diabetes Res. 2019;2019:6371231.
171. Zangeneh F, Arora PS, Dyck PJ, Bekris L, Lernmark A, Achenbach SJ, et al. Effects of duration of type 2 diabetes mellitus on insulin secretion. Endocr Pract. 2006;12(4):388–93.
172. Zammitt NN, Frier BM. Hypoglycemia in type 2 diabetes: pathophysiology, frequency, and effects of different treatment modalities. Diabetes Care. 2005;28(12):2948–61.
173. Wing RR, Hamman RF, Bray GA, Delahanty L, Edelstein SL, Hill JO, et al. Achieving weight and activity goals among diabetes prevention program lifestyle participants. Obes Res. 2004;12(9):1426–34.
174. Diabetes Prevention Program Research Group, Crandall J, Schade D, Ma Y, Fujimoto WY, Barrett-Connor E, et al. The influence of age on the effects of lifestyle modification and metformin in prevention of diabetes. J Gerontol A Biol Sci Med Sci. 2006;61(10):1075–81.
175. Knowler WC, Barrett-Connor E, Fowler SE, Hamman RF, Lachin JM, Walker EA, et al. Reduction in the incidence of type 2 diabetes with lifestyle intervention or metformin. N Engl J Med. 2002;346(6):393–403.
176. Bullard KM, Cowie CC, Lessem SE, Saydah SH, Menke A, Geiss LS, et al. Prevalence of diagnosed diabetes in adults by diabetes type – United States, 2016. MMWR Morb Mortal Wkly Rep. 2018;67(12):359–61.
177. Cowie CC, Casagrande SS, Geiss LS. Prevalence and incidence of type 2 diabetes and prediabetes. In: Cowie CC, Casagrande SS, Menke A, Cissell MA, Eberhardt MS, et al. editors. Diabetes in america. Bethesda: national institute of diabetes and digestive and kidney diseases (US). 2018.
178. Boule NG, Weisnagel SJ, Lakka TA, Tremblay A, Bergman RN, Rankinen T, et al. Effects of exercise training on glucose homeostasis: the HERITAGE Family Study. Diabetes Care. 2005;28(1):108–14.
179. Tramunt B, Smati S, Grandgeorge N, Lenfant F, Arnal JF, Montagner A, et al. Sex differences in metabolic regulation and diabetes susceptibility. Diabetologia. 2020;63(3):453–61.
180. Perreault L, Ma Y, Dagogo-Jack S, Horton E, Marrero D, Crandall J, et al. Sex differences in diabetes risk and the effect of intensive lifestyle modification in the Diabetes Prevention Program. Diabetes Care. 2008;31(7):1416–21.
181. Kim TN, Park MS, Yang SJ, Yoo HJ, Kang HJ, Song W, et al. Prevalence and determinant factors of sarcopenia in patients with type 2 diabetes: the Korean Sarcopenic Obesity Study (KSOS). Diabetes Care. 2010;33(7):1497–9.
182. Scott D, de Courten B, Ebeling PR. Sarcopenia: a potential cause and consequence of type 2 diabetes in Australia's ageing population? Med J Aust. 2016;205(7):329–33.
183. Tanaka K, Kanazawa I, Sugimoto T. Reduction in endogenous insulin secretion is a risk factor of sarcopenia in men with type 2 diabetes mellitus. Calcif Tissue Int. 2015;97(4):385–90.
184. Vissers D, Hens W, Taeymans J, Baeyens JP, Poortmans J, Van Gaal L. The effect of exercise on visceral adipose tissue in overweight adults: a systematic review and meta-analysis. PLoS One. 2013;8(2):e56415.

185. Ismail I, Keating SE, Baker MK, Johnson NA. A systematic review and meta-analysis of the effect of aerobic vs. resistance exercise training on visceral fat. Obes Rev. 2012;13(1):68–91.
186. Kay SJ, Fiatarone Singh MA. The influence of physical activity on abdominal fat: a systematic review of the literature. Obes Rev. 2006;7(2):183–200.
187. Davidson LE, Hudson R, Kilpatrick K, Kuk JL, McMillan K, Janiszewski PM, et al. Effects of exercise modality on insulin resistance and functional limitation in older adults: a randomized controlled trial. Arch Intern Med. 2009;169(2):122–31.
188. Church TS, Earnest CP, Skinner JS, Blair SN. Effects of different doses of physical activity on cardiorespiratory fitness among sedentary, overweight or obese postmenopausal women with elevated blood pressure: a randomized controlled trial. JAMA. 2007;297(19):2081–91.
189. Church TS, Blair SN, Cocreham S, Johannsen N, Johnson W, Kramer K, et al. Effects of aerobic and resistance training on hemoglobin A1c levels in patients with type 2 diabetes: a randomized controlled trial. JAMA. 2010;304(20):2253–62.
190. Nabuco HC, Tomeleri CM, Junior PS, Fernandes RR, Cavalcante EF, Nunes JP, et al. Effects of higher habitual protein intake on resistance-training-induced changes in body composition and muscular strength in untrained older women: a clinical trial study. Nutr Health. 2019;25(2):103–12.
191. Memelink RG, Pasman WJ, Bongers A, Tump A, van Ginkel A, Tromp W, et al. Effect of an enriched protein drink on muscle mass and Glycemic control during combined lifestyle intervention in older adults with obesity and type 2 diabetes: a double-blind RCT. Nutrients. 2020;13(1):64.
192. Wycherley TP, Noakes M, Clifton PM, Cleanthous X, Keogh JB, Brinkworth GD. A high-protein diet with resistance exercise training improves weight loss and body composition in overweight and obese patients with type 2 diabetes. Diabetes Care. 2010;33(5):969–76.
193. Esmarck B, Andersen JL, Olsen S, Richter EA, Mizuno M, Kjaer M. Timing of postexercise protein intake is important for muscle hypertrophy with resistance training in elderly humans. J Physiol. 2001;535(Pt 1):301–11.
194. Ramachandran A, Snehalatha C, Mary S, Mukesh B, Bhaskar AD, Vijay V, et al. The Indian Diabetes Prevention programme shows that lifestyle modification and metformin prevent type 2 diabetes in Asian Indian subjects with impaired glucose tolerance (IDPP-1). Diabetologia. 2006;49(2):289–97.
195. Boule NG, Robert C, Bell GJ, Johnson ST, Bell RC, Lewanczuk RZ, et al. Metformin and exercise in type 2 diabetes: examining treatment modality interactions. Diabetes Care. 2011;34(7):1469–74.
196. Sharoff CG, Hagobian TA, Malin SK, Chipkin SR, Yu H, Hirshman MF, et al. Combining short-term metformin treatment and one bout of exercise does not increase insulin action in insulin-resistant individuals. Am J Physiol Endocrinol Metab. 2010;298(4):E815–23.
197. Walton RG, Dungan CM, Long DE, Tuggle SC, Kosmac K, Peck BD, et al. Metformin blunts muscle hypertrophy in response to progressive resistance exercise training in older adults: a randomized, double-blind, placebo-controlled, multicenter trial: the MASTERS trial. Aging Cell. 2019;18(6):e13039.
198. Goodpaster BH, Delany JP, Otto AD, Kuller L, Vockley J, South-Paul JE, et al. Effects of diet and physical activity interventions on weight loss and cardiometabolic risk factors in severely obese adults: a randomized trial. JAMA. 2010;304(16):1795–802.
199. Kuznetsov L, Simmons RK, Sutton S, Kinmonth AL, Griffin SJ, Hardeman W, et al. Predictors of change in objectively measured and self-reported health behaviours among individuals with recently diagnosed type 2 diabetes: longitudinal results from the ADDITION-Plus trial cohort. Int J Behav Nutr Phys Act. 2013;10:118.
200. Youngs W, Gillibrand WP, Phillips S. The impact of pre-diabetes diagnosis on behaviour change: an integrative literature review. Pract Diabetes. 2016;33(5):171–5.
201. Ali HI, Baynouna LM, Bernsen RM. Barriers and facilitators of weight management: perspectives of Arab women at risk for type 2 diabetes. Health Soc Care Community. 2010;18(2):219–28.

202. Sohal T, Sohal P, King-Shier KM, Khan NA. Barriers and facilitators for Type-2 diabetes management in South Asians: a systematic review. PLoS One. 2015;10(9):e0136202.
203. Terada T, Friesen A, Chahal BS, Bell GJ, McCargar LJ, Boule NG. Exploring the variability in acute glycemic responses to exercise in type 2 diabetes. J Diabetes Res. 2013;2013:591574.
204. Poirier P, Tremblay A, Catellier C, Tancrede G, Garneau C, Nadeau A. Impact of time interval from the last meal on glucose response to exercise in subjects with type 2 diabetes. J Clin Endocrinol Metab. 2000;85(8):2860–4.
205. Terada T, Wilson BJ, Myette-Cote E, Kuzik N, Bell GJ, McCargar LJ, et al. Targeting specific interstitial glycemic parameters with high-intensity interval exercise and fasted-state exercise in type 2 diabetes. Metabolism. 2016;65(5):599–608.
206. Munan M, Dyck RA, Houlder S, Yardley JE, Prado CM, Snydmiller G, et al. Does exercise timing affect 24-hour glucose concentrations in adults with type 2 diabetes? A follow up to the exercise-physical activity and diabetes glucose monitoring study. Can J Diabetes. 2020;44(8):711–8.e1.
207. Savikj M, Gabriel BM, Alm PS, Smith J, Caidahl K, Bjornholm M, et al. Afternoon exercise is more efficacious than morning exercise at improving blood glucose levels in individuals with type 2 diabetes: a randomised crossover trial. Diabetologia. 2019;62(2):233–7.
208. Nygaard H, Ronnestad BR, Hammarstrom D, Holmboe-Ottesen G, Hostmark AT. Effects of exercise in the fasted and postprandial state on interstitial glucose in Hyperglycemic individuals. J Sports Sci Med. 2017;16(2):254–63.
209. Heden TD, Winn NC, Mari A, Booth FW, Rector RS, Thyfault JP, et al. Postdinner resistance exercise improves postprandial risk factors more effectively than predinner resistance exercise in patients with type 2 diabetes. J Appl Physiol (1985). 2015;118(5):624–34.
210. Colberg SR, Zarrabi L, Bennington L, Nakave A, Thomas Somma C, Swain DP, et al. Postprandial walking is better for lowering the glycemic effect of dinner than pre-dinner exercise in type 2 diabetic individuals. J Am Med Dir Assoc. 2009;10(6):394–7.
211. Chacko E. Timing and intensity of exercise for glucose control. Diabetologia. 2014;57(11):2425–6.
212. Chacko E. Timing, intensity and frequency of exercise for glucose control. Acta Diabetol. 2016;54(1):103–4.
213. Chacko E. A time for exercise: the exercise window. J Appl Physiol (1985). 2017;122(1):206–9.
214. Erickson ML, Jenkins NT, McCully KK. Exercise after you eat: hitting the postprandial glucose target. Front Endocrinol. 2017;8:228.
215. Haxhi J, Scotto di Palumbo A, Sacchetti M. Exercising for metabolic control: is timing important? Ann Nutr Metab. 2013;62(1):14–25.
216. Diabetes Canada Clinical Practice Guidelines Expert C, Sigal RJ, Armstrong MJ, Bacon SL, Boule NG, Dasgupta K, et al. Physical activity and diabetes. Can J Diabetes. 2018;42(Suppl 1):S54–63.
217. Boule NG, Terada T, Francois ME, Hawley JA, Cotter JD, Kruse NT, et al. Commentaries on viewpoint: a time for exercise: the exercise window. J Appl Physiol (1985). 2017;122(1):210–3.
218. Van Proeyen K, Szlufcik K, Nielens H, Ramaekers M, Hespel P. Beneficial metabolic adaptations due to endurance exercise training in the fasted state. J Appl Physiol (1985). 2011;110(1):236–45.
219. Shulman GI, Rothman DL, Jue T, Stein P, DeFronzo RA, Shulman RG. Quantitation of muscle glycogen synthesis in normal subjects and subjects with non-insulin-dependent diabetes by 13C nuclear magnetic resonance spectroscopy. N Engl J Med. 1990;322(4):223–8.
220. Perseghin G, Price TB, Petersen KF, Roden M, Cline GW, Gerow K, et al. Increased glucose transport-phosphorylation and muscle glycogen synthesis after exercise training in insulin-resistant subjects. N Engl J Med. 1996;335(18):1357–62.
221. Macauley M, Smith FE, Thelwall PE, Hollingsworth KG, Taylor R. Diurnal variation in skeletal muscle and liver glycogen in humans with normal health and type 2 diabetes. Clin Sci. 2015;128(10):707–13.

222. Goodpaster BH, Brown NF. Skeletal muscle lipid and its association with insulin resistance: what is the role for exercise? Exerc Sport Sci Rev. 2005;33(3):150–4.
223. Boushel R, Gnaiger E, Schjerling P, Skovbro M, Kraunsoe R, Dela F. Patients with type 2 diabetes have normal mitochondrial function in skeletal muscle. Diabetologia. 2007;50(4):790–6.
224. Ritov VB, Menshikova EV, Azuma K, Wood R, Toledo FG, Goodpaster BH, et al. Deficiency of electron transport chain in human skeletal muscle mitochondria in type 2 diabetes mellitus and obesity. Am J Physiol Endocrinol Metab. 2010;298(1):E49–58.
225. Terada T, Wilson BJ, Myette-Cote E, Kuzik N, Bell GJ, McCargar LJ, et al. Targeting specific interstitial glycemic parameters with high-intensity interval exercise and fasted-state exercise in type 2 diabetes. Metab Clin Exp. 2016;65(5):599–608.
226. Eshghi SR, Fletcher K, Myette-Cote E, Durrer C, Gabr RQ, Little JP, et al. Glycemic and metabolic effects of two long bouts of moderate-intensity exercise in men with normal glucose tolerance or type 2 diabetes. Front Endocrinol. 2017;8:154.
227. Van Proeyen K, Szlufcik K, Nielens H, Pelgrim K, Deldicque L, Hesselink M, et al. Training in the fasted state improves glucose tolerance during fat-rich diet. J Physiol. 2010;588(Pt 21):4289–302.
228. Brinkmann C, Weh-Gray O, Brixius K, Bloch W, Predel HG, Kreutz T. Effects of exercising before breakfast on the health of T2DM patients-a randomized controlled trial. Scand J Med Sci Sports. 2019;29(12):1930–6.
229. Verboven K, Wens I, Vandenabeele F, Stevens AN, Celie B, Lapauw B, et al. Impact of exercise-nutritional state interactions in patients with type 2 diabetes. Med Sci Sports Exerc. 2020;52(3):720–8.

Chapter 14
Diabetes Technology for Precision Therapy in Children, Adults, and Pregnancy

Roger S. Mazze, Alice Pik Shan Kong, Goran Petrovski, and Rita Basu

Introduction

In their comprehensive review of precision medicine, Mering and Florez conclude that "Clinical decision-making is, by necessity, dichotomous: on the basis of complex and often continuous information, the practitioner needs to decide whether to act or not to act, to intervene or to merely observe. One course must be taken among several possible options, and the key question is whether modern omics technologies will be able to capture enough biological variation to enable the construction of sensible discrete categories to facilitate rational decision analysis, or this will remain the province of 'boutique' rare forms of diabetes" [1]. They, of course, were writing about the contributions of genomics, proteomics, metabolomics, and glycomics as a means of characterizing individuals with diabetes in order to identify effective treatments. They conclude that "Treatment personalisation requires initial identification of key characteristics of the patient with diabetes" [2]. Gloyn and Drucker, in their review of type 2 diabetes, agree, arguing that genetics helps to distinguish between subtypes and thereby provides more precision in diagnosis and treatment [3]. An alternative view advanced by Dennis and associates suggests that "The known heterogeneity in type 2 diabetes, together with the differences we have observed in clinical outcomes, raises the possibility of a practical clinical application of

R. S. Mazze (✉)
AGP Clinical Academy, Portsmouth, UK

A. P. S. Kong
Chinese University of Hong Kong, Hong Kong, PRC, China

G. Petrovski
Cornell University/Sidra Medicine, Doha, Qatar

R. Basu
Division of Endocrinology, University of Virginia, Charlottesville, VA, USA
e-mail: basu.rita@virginia.edu

R. Basu (ed.), *Precision Medicine in Diabetes*,
https://doi.org/10.1007/978-3-030-98927-9_14

precision medicine in type 2 diabetes in the near future. Our study supports the suggestion that the optimal approach to tailor management on the basis of risk of progression and therapeutic response will be to use phenotypic measures to predict specific outcomes for individuals using multivariable models… In particular, specific clinical characteristics have been shown to have robust associations with response to specific type 2 diabetes drug options [which raises] the possibility that the relative glucose-lowering benefit of the different drugs might be identifiable by combining *simple clinical measures* in a model for treatment selection" [4].

Changing the Precision Medicine Paradigm

Clearly, while advancing "omics," credence must be given to clinical observations. Two of the most promising and far-reaching technologies in clinical practice which enable the collection and application of accurate, reliable, and verifiable data are often overlooked in terms of their contributions to precision medicine, specifically continuous glucose monitoring (CGM) and continuous subcutaneous insulin infusion (pump). These technologies have the potential of revolutionizing precision medicine if the paradigm underlying their use shifts. If these technologies are employed for the "… comprehensive capture of multiple data points across orthogonal axes of information [to develop] … analytical methods that permit the interpretation of complex data [this will] … enable the construction of more refined categories, and concomitant advances in targeted therapeutics" [1].

The question is whether glucose sensing and insulin delivery systems have an expanded role in precision medicine. Can the use of CGM for the management of diabetes be extended to encompass improving diagnostic and treatment precision by identifying with greater specificity the underlying metabolic abnormalities that characterize diabetes? Currently, CGM is employed to measure glucose in an effort to guide and assess treatment. When optimized, CGM provides a diurnal profile of glucose perturbations which may uncover defects that otherwise go undetected. Similarly, can the insulin pump functionality go beyond attempting to mimic physiologic insulin delivery in type 1 diabetes? These traditional practices of CGM and pump technologies have stifled the myriad purposes both technologies may serve in precision medicine. This chapter addresses three areas: (1) how these technologies function, (2) optimization of their current roles in clinical practice, and (3) their potential contributions to precision medicine.

A change in the paradigms that have guided the use of CGM and pump technologies since their introduction is needed if their roles in precision medicine are to be maximized. Both technologies were originally introduced without a clear understanding of their purpose. As with many technological advances in diabetes, the focus was on how these technologies functioned and their accuracy and reliability. In general, their purpose in clinical practice was left to the physician's and/or patient's prerogative. Consequently, for many years, the implementation of these technologies in clinical practice has been stilted. Accordingly, for both technologies, it is important to understand their purpose, so that their potential usage in terms of precision medicine can be explored. What is the purpose of continuous glucose monitoring (CGM)? CGM is used to provide a means of *accurate* and *verifiable* glucose data in order to make clinical decisions that improve the *diurnal glucose profile* with the goal of mimicking normal glucose metabolism [5]. Insulin pumps are employed to *mimic normal glucose metabolism* by infusing insulin in response to diurnal glucose patterns.

CGM Technology

There are two types of CGM systems: external and implantable [6]. External systems are further divided into real-time (rtCGM) and intermittently scanned (isCGM). They consist of a sensor/transmitter and receiver. The transmitter rests on the surface of the skin with the attached sensor component (filament) inserted 5 mm under the skin resting in the interstitium. There it reacts with interstitial glucose molecules which liberate electrons. The electrons are then transferred to the electrode where electric current proportionate to the glucose concentration is generated. The transmitter relays data to a wireless receiver (either a free-standing reader or a smart phone). The receiver uses an algorithm to convert the interstitial glucose reading into a blood glucose equivalent value. Data are transmitted and recorded in 1-, 2-, 5-, 10-, and 15-minute intervals, depending upon the manufacturer. Additionally, the length of time the sensor remains in place is manufacturer-dependent—from 3 to 14 days. There is currently one implantable CGM device. It consists of an under-the-skin sensor that remains in place for 90 days, an external rechargeable smart transmitter, and a smart phone application for real-time glucose data. The reader-stored data for all devices can be uploaded to a computer where proprietary software produces a variety of reports.

The fundamental difference between the rtCGM and isCGM is the availability of glucose readings. The rtCGM system data can be accessed anytime by turning on the display, while the isCGM requires scanning the sensor with the receiver. Both systems provide alarms and alerts at preset glucose levels [7]. Most CGM systems have the option of blinding the data to the user. CGM displays include the current glucose value, the trend (shown using an arrow), and the previous 8 hours represented by a curve [8].

External real-time and intermittent CGM glucose sensors use electrochemical- and enzymatic-based methods (i.e., glucose oxidase and glucose dehydrogenase) to measure interstitial glucose. There are three generations of glucose sensors [9]. First-generation sensors rely on oxygen (cofactors of glucose oxidase compete with oxygen), and therefore, conditions leading to tissue hypoxia can result in overestimation of glucose concentration. Second-generation sensors are not affected by hypoxemia because nonphysiological electron acceptors are used to shuttle electrons. Third-generation sensors adopt oxygen-independent cofactor to accept electrons liberated from glucose in interstitial tissues and are without toxicity. All sensors use an adhesive to hold the sensor/transmitter to the skin.

Measurement of interstitial glucose (ISG) presents some important challenges that impact its accuracy and reliability. Glucose is transported into the interstitium via passive diffusion when the volume of glucose in the capillary system is greater than in the interstitial fluid. From there, glucose passes into insulin-sensitive tissue with the aid of insulin. However, prior to CGM, clinical decision-making relied on glucose measurement in blood either by laboratory assay or by SMBG. The introduction of ISG raises an important question: Is ISG an accurate and reliable reflection of blood glucose? The solution was to convert ISG to blood glucose using simultaneous SMBG calibrations. However, when glucose rapidly changes, the difference between blood glucose and ISG can be as large as 20% [10]. In terms of precision medicine, this is a significant error if real-time glucose levels are guiding clinical decisions. First-generation receivers had to employ multiple calibrations to readjust the current CGM reading. For patients dependent upon real-time blood glucose levels, the time lag is a problem if they rely on alarms when glucose levels reach low thresholds [11]. Consequently, multiple SMBG calibrations are needed. In 2015, factory calibration was introduced employing the glucose oxidase mechanism for glucose measurement updated with a wired enzyme sensor incorporating osmium [12]. Because this sensor technology does not produce as much "drift" as earlier CGM sensors and has a more stable response over time in glucose measurements, it can be calibrated at the time of manufacturing and *does not require recalibration by the patient*. In a study in which two CGM devices (with and without factory calibration) were worn by the same subject, the difference in glucose values was negligible [13].

As with all newer technologies, generalized use helps identify their limitations. It has been found that exogenous and endogenous substances can potentially interfere with CGM sensors leading to inaccurate readings. These include ascorbic acid (vitamin C), acetaminophen, albuterol, atenolol, dopamine, maltose, xylose, mannitol, red wine, and uric acid [14, 15]. It has been reported that some CGM systems, which use an abiotic (nonenzyme-based), fluorescent glucose-indicating polymer to measure interstitial glucose levels, are not affected by ascorbic acid and acetaminophen, but the readings may be interfered by tetracycline and mannitol [12]. Therefore, specific drug interference profile of different CGM systems should be noted, especially when there are discrepancies between CGM readings and capillary blood or plasma glucose levels.

CGM Clinical Outcomes

CGM's primary contribution to precision medicine is the provision of verifiable and unbiased continuous data. CGM can generate between 96 and 288 measurements per day (dependent upon the system). It has been shown that CGM helps to improve diabetes care in terms of reduction of hypoglycemic episodes and glycated hemoglobin (HbA_{1c}), lessen glycemic variability, and improve quality of life in people with type 1 and type 2 diabetes receiving different treatment regimens [16]. The use of CGM also helps to reduce diabetes-related complications [17].

As a component of precision medicine, CGM is complementary to HbA_{1c}. As a general marker of glycemic control and prognostic indicator of incident diabetes-related complications, HbA_{1c} cannot address an individual's glycemic excursions and does not provide insights regarding the adjustment of the treatment regimen on a personalized basis; whereas, CGM provides a means of assessing diurnal glucose patterns under conditions of daily living to guide clinicians and patients in making decisions related to treatment. With the standardization of the reporting format and inclusion of key metrics from CGM data through international consensus and clinical targets specific for CGM from international experts, the interpretation of CGM data has become more straightforward [13, 18, 19].

CGM and the Ambulatory Glucose Profile (AGP)

The myriad uses of CGM rely on an understanding of the innovative approaches CGM employs to display glucose data. Figure 14.1 illustrates the scope of information provided by CGM. It contains two ambulatory glucose profiles (AGPs), each based on 2 weeks of continuous monitoring of the same individual with type 1 DM. AGP graphics are a means of representing continuous glucose data as a "typical" diurnal glucose pattern using five frequency distribution curves [20–22]. Figure 14.1 displays two consecutive time periods during which time estimated A1c and mean glucose are stable. In this instance, the contribution to precision medicine

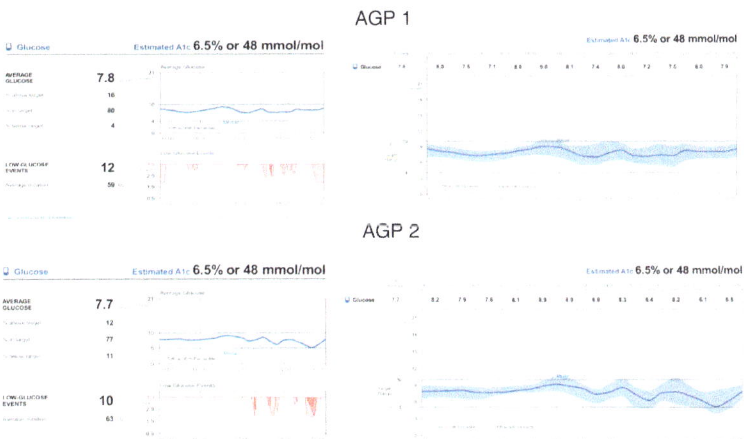

Fig. 14.1 Consecutive AGPs with Analytics. The AGP is comprised of the 10th, 25th 50th 75th and 90 frequency percentile curves produced by using all CGM values collected between 8 and 14 days and plotted by time without regards to date. Glucose exposure is measured by area under the median (50th percentile) curve, variability by inter-quartile range (dark gray area) and stability by change in the median. The report includes specific information related to time in range which is pre-set by the health care professional and hypoglycemia, in terms of its incidence, duration, magnitude and frequency

lies in the discovery of the frequency, duration, magnitude, and distribution of hypoglycemic events. Depsite a stable average glucose (7.7–7.8 mmol/L), the incidence of hypoglycemia increased threefold from 4 to 11%. In AGP 1, hypoglycemia occurs between 16:00 and 19:00 hours and is mild, while in AGP 2, it begins at noon and continues until near midnight. Furthermore, variability (interquartile range) averages 7 mmol/L in AGP 1 and 11 mmol/L in the later AGP 2.

This level of specificity is only possible using CGM technology. It identifies underlying dysglycemia that would otherwise have gone undetected. Since both variability and stability have been identified as potential contributors to long-term complications, their discovery and amelioration are critical. In this case, neither the average glucose nor the eA1c would have detected these anomalies. Furthermore, only through CGM can they be specified as to their magnitude, frequency, distribution, and duration.

Expanding the Role of CGM: Real-Life Applications

Application of AGP analytics has already expanded the role of CGM in terms of precision medicine. As shown, CGM can function to identify metabolic defects under real-life conditions. Can the same technology be used as a diagnostic tool? Figure 14.2 contains the AGP and daily profiles of a 34-year-old pregnant individual (BMI 34) whose diagnosis of gestational diabetes during her 26th gestational week was inconclusive. Consequently, 12 days of blinded CGM (to minimize bias) was initiated to identify underlying metabolic defects and determine a course of treatment. Based on the AGP and daily profiles, it was possible to confirm that on at least three occasions glucose values reached just below 10 mmol/L, which would be considered diagnostic for diabetes in pregnancy. Since the AGP identified a slightly elevated fasting glucose and meal-related excursions, 500-mg metformin plus a routine of multiple small meals to reduce glucose excursions was initiated. The patient was given an open CGM system allowing her to see in real time the impact of diet on glucose levels. The results are displayed on the right panel of Fig. 14.3. If the treatment was efficacious, the overnight and fasting glucose levels should decrease, and postprandial excursions should be reduced.

As shown in Fig. 14.3, the AGP allows precise identification of the *underlying defect* at the time of diagnosis (left panel) and provides a means of *pinpointing the impact of the treatment* (right panel). The CGM provides the evidence of a change in the daytime glucose pattern revealing lower glucose exposure and narrower variability; consequently, it can be reported that both exposure and variability were addressed by the combination of metformin and meal planning. In this case, CGM served multiple purposes: it confirmed the diagnosis and specified the metabolic abnormalities which allowed for a more precise treatment regiment, resulting in improved glycemic control.

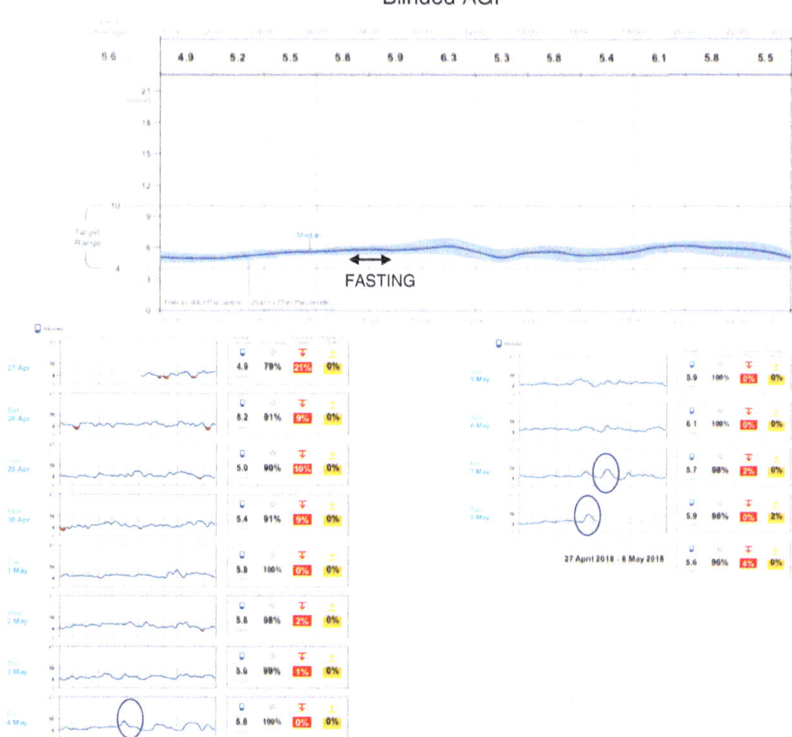

Fig. 14.2 CGM in Pregnancy. The top panel is the AGP of an individual diagnosed with GDM by 100g OGTT (fasting 6.3 mmol/L and 2 hours 8.5 mmol/L). The subsequent 12 days showed fasting glucose (08:30-09:30) ranging between 5 and 7.5 mmol/L; and three postprandial incidents (solid oval) of glucose reaching just below 10 mmol/L

Background and Rationale for Pump Therapy

The paradigm shift for CGM allowed for expanded diagnostic and treatment functionality in terms of precision medicine: Is there a parallel in terms of the insulin pump? With the advent of CGM came the possibility of connecting the two technologies and expanding their purpose. For the most part, the pump is reserved for individuals with type 1 diabetes whose glucose control using more conservative multiple daily injections (MDI) is not adequate in terms of achieving three overall goals: an improved diurnal glucose profile, lessening hypoglycemia, and enhanced quality of life [23]. Recently, pumps have been employed in individuals with type 2 diabetes and women with GDM or pre-GDM requiring intensive insulin therapy. How has the automated insulin delivery by advanced algorithms guided by CGM contributed to precision medicine?

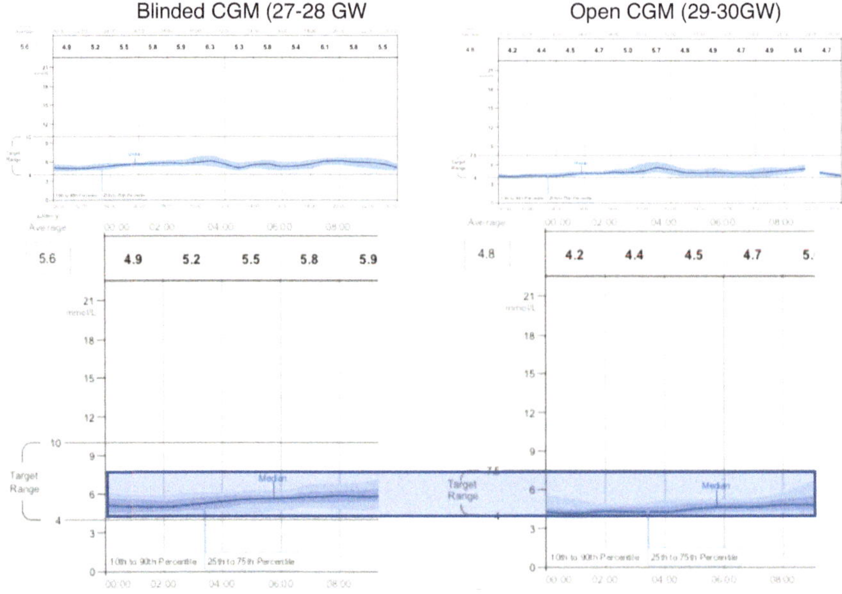

Fig. 14.3 CGM in Pregnancy. Comparing the blinded CGM with the open GDM the average glucose exposure has decreased by 0.6 mmol/L. The bottom panels show for the period mid-night to 09:30 hrs glucose exposure declined from 54.6 mmol/L/9.5 hours to 45.6 mmol/L/9.5 hours). Daytime exposure (top panels) reduced from 79.8 mmol/L/14.5 hours to 64.8 mmol/L/14.5 hours

The insulin pump is a portable device attached to the skin surface that continuously delivers short-acting insulin via a catheter placed under the skin. There are two types of devices. A traditional pump which employs a fine tube to connect the pump to the cannula inserted under the skin. A second type is the patch pump which is directly linked to a cannula inserted under the skin. Both devices are guided by algorithms which direct the insulin infusion rate. Insulin pumps provide basal and bolus infusions. Basal insulin is continuous insulin delivery based on preprogramed basal rates (open loop system) or insulin dose adjusted based on real-time CGM sensor glucose levels (hybrid closed-loop system). The basal insulin attempts to mimic physiologic insulin delivery. Bolus insulin is episodically delivered using either a bolus advisor (or wizard) or an onboard algorithm. The meal-related bolus dose is dependent upon carbohydrate data entered by the user. The correction bolus is based on a pre-programed glucose targets.

Pumps with Integrated CGM

Fundamentally, there are two ways in which the pump and CGM can be integrated: open-loop and hybrid closed loop. For open-loop systems, the CGM data is entered by the user. Hybrid systems (HCL) provide a direct connection between the pump and the CGM device allowing both devices to directly interact. The most advanced development in this area are the automated insulin delivery systems that use real-time glucose readings from a CGM device and a specific algorithm to adjust insulin delivery via the pump. There are a number of different versions of the HCL. The more advanced HCL systems contain both automatic basal insulin delivery and correction boluses when CGM readings are high. Some of these systems utilize a smart phone which receives data from a CGM sensor and uses a cloud-based adaptive predictive control algorithm to direct insulin delivery. In this manner, the smart phone acts as a CGM receiver and includes a basal and bolus calculator. It sends the calculations to the pump which then adjusts the timing and insulin infusion rates. Data are transmitted approximately every 5–15 minutes from the sensor. The control algorithm residing on the smart phone calculates the insulin infusion rate that is communicated wirelessly to the pump via a Bluetooth communication's protocol. The algorithms are initialized using patient-specific data, such as weight, caloric intake, activity level, and previous insulin regimen. To meet the dual goals of reduced hypoglycemia and hyperglycemia, a glucose range is set and adjusted over time. Advanced HCL systems are designed to continually alter the algorithm to optimize control. The user is vital in this construct. While glucose and insulin data are accurate and verifiable, the HCL also depends upon dietary and activity information which must be entered by the user.

Hybrid Closed Loop in Clinical Practice: Following the Principles of Precision Medicine

In terms of precision medicine, it has become axiomatic that "[…] insulin delivery via CSII pump is more consistent and precise in providing patient's individual insulin requirements with low risk of severe hypoglycaemia than conventional delivery devices" [24]. How has this need for "precision insulin delivery" been translated into clinical practice? The following case report details the myriad functions HCL therapy may perform.

A 13-year-old female with a 4-year history of type 1 diabetes treated with MDI and 8.9% HbA_{1c} was presented for consideration of pump therapy. Both the patient and parents requested initiation of pump therapy. Under most circumstances, this would be sufficient to start a process of training on the pump's use with CGM. However, applying the principles of precision medicine suggests the need for greater specificity regarding characterizing her current metabolic status and selecting a starting insulin regimen. This was accomplished by having the patient wear a CGM sensor for 7 days while maintaining her current insulin regimen (16 units of long-acting insulin at bedtime, 12 units of rapid-acting insulin before breakfast, and 13 units before dinner). As can be seen in Fig. 14.4 panel a, there is significant hyperglycemia beginning at 13:00 hours and lasting throughout the remainder of the day. During this same period, there is noteworthy glucose variability (11.1 mmol/L average interquartile range). Overnight (10 PM–8 AM), glucose values are more variable, ranging from 10 to 16.7 mmol/L. Three episodes of hypoglycemia and three of hyperglycemia are also present.

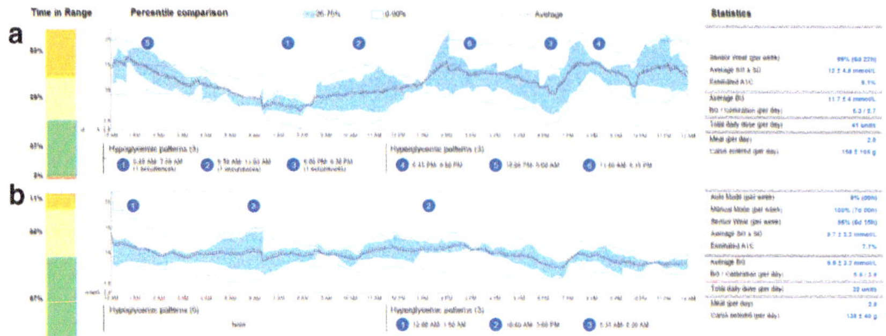

Fig. 14.4 AGP for MDI Period (**a**) and Initiation of HCL (**b**). Time in range uses fixed values: <3.9, 3.9–10, 10–13.9 >13.9 mmol/L. Hypoglycemic (<3.9 mmol/L) and hyperglycemic (>13.9 mmol/L)"patterns" are indicated by numbers. The center curve is the average, the shaded area represents the inter-quartile range (25th to 75th percentile curves) and the outer range is bordered by the 0 and 90th percentile curves. The Statistics reports data sufficiency, glucose exposure by estimated A1c and average, as well as, self-reported insulin dose (top panel), automated insulin dose (lower panel), and self-reported estimated total carbohydrates

Three issues were identifiable: (1) near hypoglycemic levels upon awakening, (2) significant variability throughout the day, and (3) overnight persistent hyperglycemia. It was determined that based on the overall glycemic profile, the patient was a candidate for pump initiation. The baseline period had multiple purpose: (1) to obtain a diurnal glucose profile to identify the magnitude, duration, distribution and frequency of excess glucose exposure reported by the HbA_{1c}, (2) to identify any underlying hypoglycemia to avoid exacerbation during initiation of the pump, (3) to determine the starting dose and timing of insulin infusion, and (4) to enable the patient to experience CGM technology, which is vital to HCL functioning.

Fundamental to initiation of combined pump and CGM technologies is to clearly state the purpose of these technologies so that their efficacy can be assessed. At its initiation, the patient was informed that "success" would be measured by glycemic improvements and patient satisfaction. The baseline AGP serves as an unbiased assessment of the clinical efficacy of MDI therapy; consequently, the use of the pump must be evaluated against the MDI AGP, essentially answering the question: To what degree did the new technology improve glucose exposure, variability, stability, and the incidence of hypoglycemic and hyperglycemic episodes? Patient satisfaction is less quantitative and can be assessed by the following questions: Was the patient able to use the technology? Did the technology measurably improve the quality of life?

Prepump and carbohydrate counting assessment was performed at a clinic visit; once successfully completed, the patient was scheduled for regular pump training. The patient attended practical sessions for pump connection and sensor insertion; pump operations; auto mode feature; auto basal/safe basal; alarms/alerts; troubleshooting and pump failure; temporary disconnection and converting back to MDI; management of hypoglycemia, hyperglycemia, and sick days; DKA; exit to manual mode and temporary basal; diet; and exercise.

Initiation of HCL system was performed in manual mode (requiring patient input) based on evaluation of the AGP produced while using MDI (Fig. 14.4 panel a). It was noted that there was a risk of hypoglycemia; consequently, the total daily insulin was reduced by 10%. Due to the wide variability overnight and during the daytime, five basal rates were set. Based on the previous report during MDI, the insulin to carbohydrate ratio was established as 10 g, and the correction factor of 3 mmol/L was set. Active insulin time was set at 4 hours and the glucose target range was established as 5–7.5 mmol/L to avoid both hypoglycemia and hyperglycemia.

Displayed in Fig. 14.4 panel b is the AGP during the initial pump use when the manual mode with suspend before low feature (3.5 mmol/L) allows the algorithm to establish personalized auto mode initiation parameters. Time in range increased to 58%. Auto mode uses the CGM and insulin infusion data as well as the target settings to determine the optimum infusion rate and timing for both basal and bolus periods. The next period was fully controlled by the auto mode (see Fig. 14.5 panel c). Time in range continued to increase reaching 69% in the first week of auto mode initiation, where postmeal hyperglycemia was noted.

By the third week, the patient reached a steady state. Comparing the baseline AGP (Fig. 14.4 panel a) to the final AGP (Fig. 14.5 panel d), time in range reached 86%, with no hypoglycemic episodes, reduction in hyperglycemia episodes to one, and overall glucose exposure reduced from 11.7 to 7.7 mmol/L with a concomitant decrease in eA1C. Glucose variability (as shown by the shaded area) decreased to 2 mmol/L. There was no significant difference in sensor wear, calibrations, set/reservoir change, meals, and carbohydrates per day during this period.

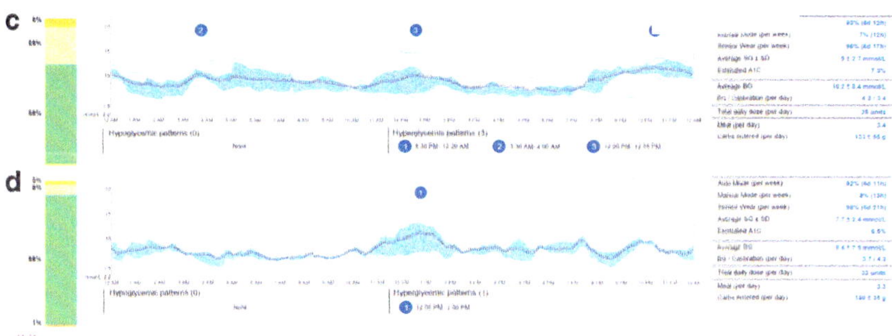

Fig. 14.5 AGP for Pump Adjustments (**c**) and Stabilization (**d**). Comparing the adjustment (**c**) with the stabilization phase, the magnitude, duration, frequency and distribution of glucose exposure improved. It appears as if the entire AGP narrowed and lowered. This is consistent with a structured approach in which narrowing the variability and stabilizing the average glucose throughout the day precede lowering the glucose f = values. Note that this was accomplished without an increase in total daily insulin. The algorithm maintains glycemic control by using the CGM data to "teach" the algorithm. As with all technology human behavior can counter the algorithm as shown by the wide inter-quartile range and outlier range at noon. This is indicative of alterations in diet each day, interfering with the ability of the algorithm to detect a predictable pattern

The use of the HCL system following principles of precision medicine resulted in a logical process of clinical decision-making relying on accurate and verifiable data. The onboard algorithm followed a rational series of steps that targeted reduced variability and increased stability ahead of glucose exposure. This approach lessened the risk of hypoglycemia and suggests a model that can be applied to MDI therapies as well. In this case, CGM corroborated the need for pump therapy and served to identify the underlying dysglycemia with sufficient specificity to allow a more rapid initiation of pump therapy.

Expanding the Role of Pumps

This chapter began with the proposition that the current paradigm for precision medicine needs to be altered. The role of glucose sensing and pump technologies in the diagnosis and treatment of diabetes can be expanded and become central to the notion of precision medicine. Close examination of the heterogeneity within diabetes classifications suggests new roles for insulin delivery technologies. At diagnosis, individuals with type 1 diabetes present with varying degrees of β-cell function. This leads to a variety of glucose patterns that suggest the need for highly individualized treatment. Two specific benefits of initiation of pump therapy combined with CGM at diagnosis are prolonging β-cell function and characterizing insulin requirements. Both benefits require restoration of near euglycemia. It is argued that for newly diagnosed children with type 1 diabetes, "Sensor-augmented pump therapy starting from the diagnosis of type 1 diabetes can be associated with less decline in fasting C-peptide…" [25]. In a study in adolescents, pumps were initiated between one day and one month after diagnosis. The 28 subjects experienced a decline in HbA_{1c} from 10.5 +/− 2.4% to between 6.5% and 7.4% over the next 18 months [26]. Endogenous insulin secretion, measured by C-peptide values, remained stable during the first 12 months after diagnosis. The researchers concluded that "The study provided a positive experience with CSII as the initial insulin replacement therapy in newly diagnosed patients with T1DM with excellent clinical outcomes and apparent prolongations of the honeymoon period" [26].

Compared to type 1 diabetes, type 2 diabetes is highly heterogeneous. The underlying defects that characterize type 2 diabetes range from impaired β-cell function to reduced incretin production. They can be mechanistic, chemical, behavioral, or a combination. The contributions of insulin resistance and β-cell dysfunction differ to such an extent that it has been hypothesized that there are a number of subgroups within the classification. It has been noted that at diagnosis even with comparable HbA_{1c}, diurnal glucose profiles differ extensively. While measurement of insulin level and insulin resistance may provide evidence of reduced or impaired β-cell function, they are limited. What is missing at diagnosis is an understanding of how much supplemental insulin, if any, is needed. Consequently, the selection of treatment is often "hit or miss," primarily because the diagnostic criteria and initial treatments rely on very limited data. This is especially problematic as diagnosis of type 2 diabetes is often delayed until it becomes symptomatic.

In a study of individuals newly diagnosed with type 2 DM, subjects were hospitalized for 3 weeks during which time they underwent episodic pump therapy using CGM before, during, and after pump therapy to "define the features of patients" in order to determine whether long-term insulin therapy was required [27]. Hypothetically, if near euglycemia could be maintained using the pump, the precise insulin regimen could be identified, and the decision could be made as to whether to continue with pump therapy or MDI and, more importantly, whether insulin therapy could be discarded if, for instance, a negligible amount of insulin were required to achieve near euglycemia. At diagnosis, using pump therapy with CGM may foster a "better understanding of the underlying mechanisms responsible for elevated fasting versus postprandial glucose concentration, as well as knowledge about the expected responsiveness to treatment in individuals with different clinical characteristics at diagnosis, may contribute to optimising strategies for management of hyperglycaemia in both pre-diabetes and type 2 diabetes" [28].

If glucose sensing technologies are to make a lasting contribution to precision medicine, then we must understand: (1). *how* the current technology is related to the underlying pathophysiology of diabetes, and (2). *how* this relationship can improve clinical practice. The classifications, type 1 and type 2 diabetes, as well as diabetes in pregnancy are placeholders suggesting that "one term fits all." Genomics has identified numerous subtypes, suggesting that all diabetes within the same classification are not the same. Metabolic profiling can take precision medicine one step further. Using CGM can identify the distinguishing features within diabetes subgroups that contribute to greater diagnostic specificity and consequently, improved therapeutics. For example, informed treatment selection requires an understanding of glucose exposure, variability, and stability, as well as the incidence of hypoglycemia and how these characteristics reflect the underlying pathophysiology of diabetes.

The purpose of CGM is manifold. First, it characterizes patients in new and innovative ways using recognized data patterns related to the disease pathophysiology. Second, it assists in the interpretation of these patterns (AGPs) to better identify and manage patients with diabetes. Third, because CGM provides a means of collecting accurate, verifiable, and reliable glucose data under conditions of daily living that cannot otherwise be obtained, it facilitates insights into the inter-relationships between behavior and pathophysiology. Fourth, by providing diurnal and nocturnal glycemic patterns vital to the detection of dysglycemic patterns, it aids in the selection and adjustment of therapies. Essentially, CGM technologies bring the goal of achieving normal metabolic patterns closer.

The role of CGM in precision management of diabetes was recently enhanced by the recommendation of the American Diabetes Association that CGM reports with AGP graphic displays should be used to detect dysglycemic patterns and associate these patterns with their underlying pathophysiology [29]. CGM allows greater specificity in selecting the appropriate therapy to correct the underlying defect. Essentially, when used in type 2 diabetes to detect fasting, postprandial and overnight dysglycemia, CGM analytics provide clues related to their underlying causes.

For example, overnight glucose utilization is lower and glucose production higher in individuals with type 2 diabetes than their nondiabetic counterparts [30]. Reflected in CGM overnight hyperglycemic patterns, this is due to the central role the liver plays in regulating carbohydrate tolerance. Furthermore, it is likely that the diabetic state per se determines the severity of extrahepatic and hepatic insulin resistance [31]. CGM patterns that show fasting hyperglycemia may be the direct result of defects in beta cell function which lead to reduced insulin secretion overnight. In a similar manner, CGM postprandial hyperglycemic patterns may also be the result of defects in beta cell function [32]. Overnight CGM patterns that show significant variability, with glucose levels ranging from normal to hyperglycemia, may be indicative of early type 2 diabetes due to disturbances in nocturnal regulation of glycemia which are affected by varying degrees of overnight hepatic insulin resistance. This leads to increase in glucose production in type 2 diabetes during the night [33]. Thus, the underlying cause for abnormal nocturnal glucose production as revealed in CGM patterns appears to be mild physiological hyperglucagonemia rather than increase in cortisol [34].

Detecting underlying pathophysiology by employing CGM-based glucose patterns is equally effective in type 1 diabetes by characterizing dysglycemic patterns that aid in the decision to initiate pump therapy, select the starting basal and bolus regimen, and guide adjustments. Similarly, CGM may be used to detect dysglycemic patterns in pregnancy caused by human placental lactogen-induced insulin resistance. Even subtle rises in overnight and postprandial glucose during the first and second trimesters may be indicators of impending gestational diabetes.

Pump therapy plays a different role in precision medicine, as its purpose is to mimic the normal physiology of insulin secretion. While CGM aids this by corroborating normal insulin action, it is pump technology that achieves this by integrating glycemic patterns reflected in CGM analytics with infusion algorithms. Precision medicine demands that the goal of pump therapy no longer be defined by HbA_{1c}, rather by specific characteristics of diurnal glucose exposure, variability, stability, and hypoglycemia derived from CGM. These characteristics of normal glucose metabolism under conditions of daily living, in turn, are associated with normal physiology, which in turn is correlated with prevention of diabetes-related complications.

The integration of new technologies is a vital element of precision medicine. It is an essential step if these technologies are to be optimized and if precision medicine is to meet the goal of individualizing care by identifying the nature of the underlying defects related to diabetes specific to the individual and designing interventions that target the defect. CGM does this by characterizing the glucose patterns of a single individual, not a classification of diabetes; the pump does this by developing an infusion regimen particular to the individual based on both physiology and behavior.

References

1. Mering J, Florez J. Precision medicine in diabetes: an opportunity for clinical translation. Ann N Y Acad Sci. 2018;1411(1):140–52.

2. Del Prato S. Heterogeneity of diabetes: heralding an era of precision medicine. Lancet. 2019;7(9):659–61.
3. Gloyn AL, Drucker DJ. Precision medicine in the management of type 2 diabetes. Lancet Diabetes Endocrinol. 2018;6:891–900.
4. Dennis JM, Shields BM, Henley W, et al. Disease progression and treatment response in data-driven subgroups of type 2 diabetes compared with models based on simple clinical features: an analysis using clinical trial data. Lancet. 2019;7(6):442–51.
5. American Diabetes Association. Guidelines for the use of Continuous Glucose Monitors (CGM) and Sensors in the School Setting. ADA; 2020.
6. The rtCGM devices: MiniMed Guardian Connect® (Medtronic, Northridge CA), Dexcom G7® (Dexcom, San Diego, CA)) and implantable Eversense® (Senseonics, Germantown MD). The isCGM devices: FreeStyle Libre for personal use and FreeStyle Libre professional (Abbott Diabetes Care, Alameda, CA).
7. American Diabetes Association. Diabetes technology: standards of medical Care in Diabetes-2020. Diabetes Care. 2020;43(Suppl 1):S77–88.
8. Danne T, Nimri R, Battelino T, Bergenstal RM, Close KL, DeVries JH, Garg S, Heinemann L, Hirsch I, Amiel SA, Beck R, Bosi E, Buckingham B, Cobelli C, Dassau E, Doyle FJ 3rd, Heller S, Hovorka R, Jia W, Jones T, Kordonouri O, Kovatchev B, Kowalski A, Laffel L, Maahs D, Murphy HR, Nørgaard K, Parkin CG, Renard E, Saboo B, Scharf M, Tamborlane WV, Weinzimer SA, Phillip M. International consensus on use of continuous glucose monitoring. Diabetes Care. 2017;40(12):1631–40.
9. Klonoff DC, Ahn D, Drincic A. Continuous glucose monitoring: a review of the technology and clinical use. Diabetes Res Clin Pract. 2017;133:178–92.
10. Kulcu E, Tamada J, Reach G, et. al. Physiological differences between interstitial glucose and blood glucose measured in human subjects. Diabetes Care 2003; 26:2405–2409.
11. Cappon G, Vettoretti M, Sparacino G, Facchinetti A. Continuous glucose monitoring sensors for diabetes management: a review of technologies and applications. Diabetes Metab J. 2019;43(4):383–97.
12. Hoss U, Budiman E, Liu H, Christiansen H. Continuous glucose monitoring in the subcutaneous tissue over a 14-day sensor wear period. Diabetes Sci Technol. 2013;7(5):1210–9.
13. Danne T, Nimri R, Battelino T, et al. International consensus on use of continuous glucose monitoring. Diabetes Care. 2017;40:1631–40.
14. Basu A, Slama MQ, Nicholson WT, Langman L, Peyser T, Carter R, Basu R. Continuous glucose monitor interference with commonly prescribed medications: a pilot study. J Diabetes Sci Technol. 2017;11(5):936–41.
15. Lorenz C, Sandoval W, Mortellaro M. Interference assessment of various endogenous and exogenous substances on the performance of the Eversense long-term implantable continuous glucose monitoring system. Diabetes Technol Ther. 2018;20(5):344–52.
16. Rodbard D. Continuous glucose monitoring: a review of recent studies demonstrating improved glycemic outcomes. Diabetes Technol Ther. 2017;19(S3):S25–s37.
17. Huang ES, O'Grady M, Basu A, Winn A, John P, Lee J, Meltzer D, Kollman C, Laffel L, Tamborlane W, Weinzimer S, Wysocki T. The cost-effectiveness of continuous glucose monitoring in type 1 diabetes. Diabetes Care. 2010;33(6):1269–74.
18. Bergenstal RM, Ahmann AJ, Bailey T, et al. Recommendations for standardizing glucose reporting and analysis to optimize clinical decision making in diabetes: the ambulatory glucose profile (agp). Diabetes Technol Ther. 2013;15:198–211.
19. Matthaei S, Dealaiz RA, Bosp E, et al. Consensus recommendations for the use of ambulatory glucose profile in clinical practice. Br J Diabetes Vas Dis. 2014;14:153–7.
20. Mazze RS, Lucido D, Langer O, Hartmann K, Rodbard D. Ambulatory glucose profile: representation of verified self-monitored blood glucose data. Diabetes Care. 1987;10(1):111–7.
21. Mazze RS, Strock E, Wesley D, Borgman S, Morgan B, Bergenstal R, Cuddihy R. Characterizing glucose exposure for individuals with normal glucose tolerance using continuous glucose monitoring and ambulatory glucose profile analysis. Diabetes Technol Ther. 2008;10(3):149–59.
22. Mazze R, Strock E, Cuddihy R, Wesley D. Ambulatory glucose profile (AGP) development of a common, web-based application to record and report continuous glucose monitoring data. Can J Diabetes. 2009;33(3):215.

23. DiMeglio LA, Acerini CL, Codner E, et al. ISPAD clinical practice consensus guidelines 2018: glycemic control targets and glucose monitoring for children, adolescents, and young adults with diabetes. Pediatr Diabetes. 2018;19(S27):105–14.
24. Kesavadev J, Jaim SM, Muruganathan A, Das AK. Consensus evidence-based guidelines for use of insulin pump therapy in the management of diabetes as per indian clinical practice supplement. J Assoc Physicians India. 2014;62.
25. Kordonouri O, Pankowska E, Rami B, et al. Sensor-augmented pump therapy from the diagnosis of childhood type 1 diabetes: results of the Paediatric Onset Study (ONSET) after 12 months of treatment Diabetologia. 2010;53(12):2487–95.
26. Ramchandani N, Ten S, Anhalt H, et al. Insulin pump therapy from the time of diagnosis of type 1 diabetes. Diabetes Technol Ther. 2006;8(6):663–70.
27. Li F-F, Liu B-L, Zhu H-H, et al. Continuous glucose monitoring in newly diagnosed type 2 diabetes patients reveals a potential risk of hypoglycemia in older men. J Diabetes Res. 2017:2740372.
28. Faerch K, Hulman A, Solomon T. Heterogeneity of pre-diabetes and type 2 diabetes: implications for prediction, prevention and treatment responsiveness. Curr Diabetes Rev. 2015;12(1):30–41.
29. American Diabetes Association. Standards of medical care in diabetes-2022. Diab Care. 2022;45(Suppl. 1):S85–7.
30. Basu A, Basu R, Shah P, Vella A, Johnson CM, Nair KS, Jensen MD, Schwenk WF, Rizza RA. Effects of type 2 diabetes on the ability of insulin and glucose to regulate splanchnic and muscle glucose metabolism: evidence for a defect in hepatic glucokinase activity. Diabetes. 2000;49(2):272–83.
31. Basu R, Schwenk WF, Rizza RA. Both fasting glucose production and disappearance are abnormal in people with "mild" and "severe" type 2 diabetes. Am J Physiol Endocrinol Metab. 2004;287(1):E55–62.
32. Basu A, Dalla Man C, Basu R, Toffolo G, Cobelli C, Rizza RA. Effects of type 2 diabetes on insulin secretion, insulin action, glucose effectiveness, and postprandial glucose metabolism. Diab Care. 2009;32(5):866–72. PMCID: PMC2671126
33. Basu A, Joshi N, Miles J, Carter RE, Rizza RA, Basu R. Paradigm Shifts in Nocturnal Glucose Control in Type 2 Diabetes. J Clin Endocrinol Metab. 2018;103(10):3801–9. PMCID: PMC6179178
34. Basu A, Yadav Y, Carter RE, Basu R. Novel insights into effects of cortisol and glucagon on nocturnal glucose production in Type 2 diabetes. J Clin Endocrinol Metab. 2020;105(7) PMCID: PMC7274493

Chapter 15
Adaptive and Individualized Artificial Pancreas for Precision Management of Type 1 Diabetes

Chiara Toffanin, Claudio Cobelli, and Lalo Magni

Introduction

Automated devices for glycaemic control, the so-called artificial pancreas (AP), are revolutioning diabetes management by reducing patient burden and allowing more effective control. This has been made possible by incredible progresses in subcutaneous (sc) glucose sensing (continuous glucose monitoring (CGM)), by improved technology of sc insulin pumps and by important development in control algorithms, the core of AP technology. A large spectrum of control techniques has been explored including proportional integral derivative (PID) equipped in [1] with insulin feedback to mitigate insulin absorption delays, medical doctor reasoning [2] and model predictive control (MPC) [3–5]. MPC appears to be particularly suited for glucose control in view of its capability to handle constraints (insulin delivery is bounded to be positive) and to mitigate insulin absorption delays employing predictive; it has also been employed in dual-hormone AP, infusing glucagon in addition to insulin [6], and for handling ancillary physical activity measurements [7]. The sc insulin delivery has important limitations, and recently an AP employing the intraperitoneal (ip) insulin delivery has been investigated showing that, at variance with the sc, the ip does not require meal announcements, thanks to much faster insulin kinetics [8, 9].

C. Toffanin
Department of Electrical, Computer and Biomedical Engineering, University of Pavia, Pavia, Italy

C. Cobelli (✉)
Department of Woman and Child's Health, University of Padova, Padova, Italy
e-mail: cobelli@dei.unipd.it

L. Magni
Department of Civil and Architecture Engineering, University of Pavia, Pavia, Italy

R. Basu (ed.), *Precision Medicine in Diabetes*,
https://doi.org/10.1007/978-3-030-98927-9_15

In the last 10 years, an intense clinical research effort has been performed to test AP prototypes, resulting in numerous trials conducted on kid, adolescent, and adult subjects affected by T1D. The first clinical experiments were conducted on hospitalized subjects (inpatient) to test safety and efficacy of this technology, then experiments in semi-controlled outpatient setting were conducted to safely emulate the AP unsupervised use by the patient in real life, and finally various AP prototypes entered the last validation phase, i.e. the sustained independent use of the device in real life (see, for example, [10–24]). Today, there are three commercial devices on the market [25].

In this chapter, we focus on two problems related to the control algorithm which still deserve novel research, i.e. individualization and adaptivity. Individuals are different; thus, strategies to tune the control algorithm to a specific person are needed. In addition, individuals change in time; thus, strategies to adapt the controller configuration to a changing metabolic status of a person are key to improve AP long-term glucose control.

Individualization

The individualization topic has been faced in the last years by several research groups (for a comprehensive literature review, refer to [26, 27]). For example, a well-established approach [28, 29] involved simple black box models with fixed time constants and the possibility to adapt the system gain on the base of well-known clinical parameters such as TDI.

In this section, the techniques studied by the authors will be summarized: CR-based [30], impulse response (IR) [31], constrained optimization (CO) [32], nonparametric (NP) [32] and neural network (NN) approaches. In particular, the main goal of the works was the improvement in terms of performance of the MPC algorithm synthesized by the authors on a population model [5] and to design patient-tailored alarm systems able to prevent hypoglycaemia [33].

CR-Based Models

The first and simpler way to individualize a population model is to divide the population in clusters of patients (classes) with similar characteristics and then to use the average model of the specific cluster the patient belongs to.

The model customization approach [30] is based on subdividing the entire virtual population in subgroups depending on the insulin-to-carbohydrate ratio (CR) parameter. The CR represents the nominal quantity of carbohydrate compensated by 1 U of insulin. Note that the CR is a parameter defined by the physician and customized for each patient, so this grouping considers the individual characteristics of each patient to react to insulin and meals. The subdivision applied in silico [30] involves four classes of the adult population of the UVA/Padova Simulator (UPS), each of which is composed of patients having low, medium-low, medium-high and high insulin sensitivity on the base of the integer approximations of the 25th, 50th, and 75th percentiles associated with the CR distribution of the adult virtual population. For each class, an average model is computed and then linearized around the basal equilibrium.

Impulse Response (IR) Models

The second technique is based on impulse signals, the most exciting inputs, so it is called impulse response (IR). It has been developed in silico [31] and extended on in vivo data in [33, 34].

The subsystems from insulin to glucose and from meal carbohydrates to glucose can be described by two continuous-time transfer functions (TFs). Their structure and complexity are determined by impulse response experiments on the 100 in silico subjects of UPS. The use of the UPS is motivated by the impossibility of performing extensive and possibly unsafe experiments on real subjects: insulin boluses without meal intake and uncontrolled meals (meals without insulin boluses). The identification technique is divided into two steps: the first one is entirely developed on the "average" in silico patient (Av) of the UPS to obtain the TFs, and then a patient-tailored model is identified using patient real-life data collected in closed loop.

Seen the good results obtained in silico, this technique was applied to in vivo data [33] coming from 1-month trial in free-living condition [35]. The technique was adapted to deal with the characteristics of the trial: the system was discretized, and a residual error e(k) was added to consider the effect of unmeasured factors like physical exercise, stress, illness, etc. and other unmodelled dynamics.

Constrained Optimization (CO) Models

The third technique that consists in the identification of a linear model having a fixed parametric structure is a grey-box identification approach based on a constrained optimization (CO) [32]. In particular, the linearization of the metabolic model included in the UPS around the basal equilibrium is considered, and its matrices are identified through the solution of a CO problem. Several elements have been fixed equal to zero according to the structure of the in silico model; in this way, a priori information are included, and the computational burden of the optimization is reduced. The identification is performed by relying on historical input-output data associated with the patient. The CGM subcutaneous glucose measurements need to be prefiltered to be considered for identification; in this case, a moving average filter showed good performances [32]; other techniques, like the retrofitting process [36], could be considered. A substantial advantage of the CO approach is represented by the fixed parametric structure of the identified model, which results in a fixed implementation complexity of the control algorithm for any patient. It has been shown in [32] that the CO approach is able to capture the glucose-insulin dynamics of the patient by relying on shorter identification datasets, which are more easily realizable in a real-life scenario where the patient would be enrolled in a clinical study to produce historical input-output data for identification purposes.

Nonparametric (NP) Models

The nonparametric (NP) approach described in [32] belongs to the class of black box identification techniques and can be used to identify patient-specific glucose-insulin models by relying on historical insulin administrations and meal intakes and CGM measurements. Given a set of historical input-output data associated with a specific patient, the NP approach identifies a one-step ahead predictor that is subsequently converted in a state-space model obtained through a minimal realization of a given dimension. The identification process is performed through a kernel-based regression in which the stable spline kernel introduced in [37] is considered. The final result is a linear time-invariant model involving a white Gaussian noise signal to represent the uncertainties affecting the model. The impulse responses and the Gaussian noise are identified through kernel-based regression processes described in [32].

Neural Network (NN) Models

In the last decade, machine learning approaches have been applied to glucose control problem with promising results. These approaches have been investigated to perform glucose forecasting [38] for in silico adult subjects. In particular, a deep learning approach based on a novel, two-headed long short-term memory implementation is proposed which takes in input the previous values obtained through continue glucose monitoring, the carbohydrate intake, the suggested insulin therapy and that forecasts the interstitial glucose level of the patient. With a large dataset available, these techniques could be directly applied on the in vivo data. In [38], the population model obtained in silico was adapted to a real patient with promising results. These approaches are currently under study for both control and hypo-avoidance purposes.

Adaptivity

One of the main problems related to the glucose control together with the inter-patient variability is the intra-patient variability that calls for time-variant models or adaptation techniques. The significant level of subject-specific glycaemic variability requires continuously adapting the control policy to successfully face daily changes in patient's metabolism and lifestyle. In the last year, several research groups tried to face this problem exploring different techniques. For example, in [39], the authors designed a dual-layer control scheme: the lower layer is composed of multiple controllers that deal with short-term disturbances, while the upper one is responsible for long-term (e.g. weeks) parameter adaptation of lower layer control algorithms. The purpose of this layer is to handle chronic changes in the patient's glucose metabolic process and lifestyle through a long-term data-driven multivariate parameter learning framework based on historical performance. In [40], an online selective reinforcement learning algorithm for a real-time adaptation based on ongoing interactions with the patient is used to tailor the artificial pancreas. Adaptation includes two online procedures: online sparsification and parameter updating of the Gaussian process used to approximate the control policy by detecting novel information from the arriving data stream. The adaptation can also be applied indirectly to advanced techniques such as the MPC [41] through the update of the nominal basal insulin around which the MPC instantaneously varies the basal insulin. In this approach also, the meal bolus is adapted on the base of the correction made by the MPC the previous day. The MPC can be also made adaptive through change of the control penalty in the cost function of the controller as in [42]. This adaptive controller resulted able to actively perform insulin infusion when blood glucose is rapidly increasing but cautiously reduces/suspends insulin infusion when glucose rate of change is positively small or negative. In [43], a run-to-run (R2R) approach adapts the parameters of the model used in the MPC for the prediction, adjusting the insulin sensitivity and postprandial insulin.

The adaptation techniques explored by the authors involve mainly R2R approaches used to daily adapt the aggressiveness of the controller and/or the conventional basal-bolus therapy on the base of the performances achieved the previous day. A very promising approach has been also tested in vivo with interesting results [44]. In particular, in [45], the aggressiveness of the MPC controller proposed by the author was updated considering the patient position on the CVGA [31]: this grid considers the maximum and the minimum BG level reached by the patient in the observation period, and the R2R algorithm tries to lead it to the optimal bottom left corner where no hypoglycaemia/hyperglycaemia events occurred.

An innovative R2R approach to improve the glucose control was presented in [46, 47]. This approach exploits a switching updating law in order to adapt the basal-bolus therapy to avoid at first the hypoglycaemia events and then to improve the time in target, avoiding hyperglycaemia and leading the average glucose to the target. Previous R2R approaches were based on a few blood glucose measurements, while the authors used a subcutaneous continuous glucose monitoring in order to obtain more relevant clinical performance indices, such as the percentage of time spent below 70 mg/dl, above 180 mg/dl, and the average glucose. The convergence of the proposed R2R approach is proved by resorting to the Lyapunov theory for piecewise affine systems [46]. While in [46] only the basal amount along all day is updated, in [47] both, the nocturnal basal and the diurnal CR are changed in order to improve the control obtained via an adaptive MPC approach [5]. The adaptation of the MPC is obtained through the update of the aggressiveness of the controller, thanks to the updating of the CR which the aggressiveness is based on. In silico simulations were performed by using the UPS enriched by incorporating three novel features: intraday and interday variability of insulin sensitivity; different distributions of CR at breakfast, lunch, and dinner; and dawn phenomenon. After about 2 months, using the R2R approach with a scenario characterized by a random ±30% variation of the nominal insulin sensitivity, the time in range and the time in tight range are increased by 11.39% and 44.87%, respectively, and the time spent above 180 mg/dl is reduced by 48.74%. Making an AP adaptive is key for long-term real-life outpatient studies and seen the good in silico results; an in vivo testing was performed on 18 subjects involved in a 1-month trial [44] under free-living conditions. Time in target with adaptive MPC (R2R-AP) was higher than with the non-adaptive one (NA-AP), although the increase was not significant: mean 66.90% (standard deviation: 13.34) versus 61.82% (11.12), $P = 0.10$. The increase was significant during the night, 74.01% (14.61) versus 64.31% (15.71), $P = 0.03$, and at wake-up time, median 92.43% (25th; 75th percentiles: 78.22; 99.53) versus 84.54% (57.14; 88.52), $P = 0.02$. Time above target (>10 mmol/L) during the whole day was 30.98% (13.22) versus 36.17% (11.53), $P = 0.10$. The decrease was significant during the night, 24.23% (15.03) versus 34.49% (16.25), $P = 0.03$, and at wake-up time, 7.57% (0.00; 14.29) versus 14.29% (8.25; 42.86), $P = 0.05$. Time spent below target (<3.9 mmol/L) was low and similar to the two treatments. The R2R-AP improves glucose control over NA-AP during the night, and it maintains equivalent control performance during the day.

New approaches explored by the authors in terms of adaptivity involve the use of a multiple model predictor (MMP) [48] in order to improve the glucose prediction taking into account the intraday variability of the patients. A correlation between postprandial glucose profiles and different day periods (DPs) was found analysing experimental data [35]. The data-driven MMP based on real-data analysis uses three basic models specific of each DP identified through the IR technique. Its prediction capabilities compared to the ones of a daily model predictor, built using a single model identified on a daily subset, showed an improvement in terms of prediction capabilities during breakfast.

Conclusions

In this chapter, we have focused on two important problems related to AP control algorithms which should allow an improved long-term glucose control, i.e. individualization and adaptivity. Both issues are very relevant for precision medicine since they would allow to tune glucose control to a specific person or to a subgroup of people.

References

1. Steil GM, Palerm CC, Kurtz N, Voskanyan G, Roy A, Paz S, Kandeel FR. The effect of insulin feedback on closed loop glucose control. J Clin Endocrinol Metabol. 2011;96(5):1402–8.
2. Atlas E, Nimri R, Miller S, Grunberg EA, Phillip M. MD-logic artificial pancreas system: a pilot study in adults with type 1 diabetes. Diabetes Care. 2010;33(5):1072–6.
3. Hovorka R, Canonico V, Chassin LJ, Haueter U, Massi-Benedetti M, Federici MO, Pieber TR, Schaller HC, Schaupp L, Vering TAO. Nonlinear model predictive control of glucose concentration in subjects with type 1 diabetes. Physiolog Measurement. 2004;25(4):905.
4. Grosman B, Dassau E, Zisser HC, Jovanovi L, Doyle FJ III. Zone model predictive control: a strategy to minimize hyper-and hypoglycemic events. J Diabetes Sci Technol. 2010;4(4):961–75.
5. Toffanin C, Messori M, Di Palma F, De Nicolao G, Cobelli C, Magni L. Artificial pancreas: model predictive control design from clinical experience. J Diabetes Sci Technol. 2013;7(6):1470–83.
6. Russell SJ, El-Khatib FH, Nathan DM, Magyar KL, Jiang J, Damiano ER. Blood glucose control in type 1 diabetes with a bihormonal bionic endocrine pancreas. Diabetes Care. 2012;35(11):2148–55.
7. Turksoy K, Bayrak ES, Quinn L, Littlejohn E, Cinar A. Multivariable adaptive closed-loop control of an artificial pancreas without meal and activity announcement. Diabetes Technol Ther. 2013;15(5):386–400.
8. Renard E. Insulin delivery route for the artificial pancreas: subcutaneous, intraperitoneal, or intravenous? Pros and cons. J Diabetes Sci Technol. 2008;2(4):735–8.
9. Dassau E, Renard E, Place J, Farret A, Pelletier M-J, Lee J, Huyett LM, Chakrabarty A, Doyle FJ III, Zisser HC. Intraperitoneal insulin delivery provides superior glycaemic regulation to subcutaneous insulin delivery in model predictive control-based fully-automated artificial pancreas in patients with type 1 diabetes: a pilot study. Diabetes Obes Metab. 2017;19(12):1698–705.
10. Leelarathna L, Dellweg S, Mader JK, Allen JM, Benesch C, Doll W, Ellmerer M, Hartnell S, Heinemann L, Kojzar HAO. Day and night home closed-loop insulin delivery in adults with type 1 diabetes: three-center randomized crossover study. Diabetes Care. 2014;37(7):1931–7.
11. Russell SJ, El-Khatib FH, Sinha M, Magyar KL, McKeon K, Goergen LG, Balliro C, Hillard MA, Nathan DM, Damiano ER. Outpatient glycemic control with a bionic pancreas in type 1 diabetes. N Engl J Med. 2014;371(4):313–25.
12. Nimri R, Muller I, Atlas E, Miller S, Kordonouri O, Bratina N, Tsioli C, Stefanija MA, Danne T, Battelino TAO. Night glucose control with MD-logic artificial pancreas in home setting: a single blind, randomized crossover trial—interim analysis. Pediatr Diabetes. 2014;15(2):91–9.

13. Russell SJ, El-Khatib FH, Sinha M, Magyar KL, McKeon K, Goergen LG, Balliro C, Hillard MA, Nathan DM, Damiano ER. Outpatient glycemic control with a bionic pancreas in type 1 diabetes. N Engl J Med. 2014;371(4):313–25.
14. Del Favero S, Place J, Kropff J, Messori M, Keith-Hynes P, Visentin R, Monaro M, Galasso S, Boscari F, Toffanin CAO. Multicenter outpatient dinner/overnight reduction of hypoglycemia and increased time of glucose in target with a wearable artificial pancreas using modular model predictive control in adults with type 1 diabetes. Diabetes Obes Metab. 2015;17(5):468–76.
15. Kropff J, Del Favero S, Place J, Toffanin C, Visentin R, Monaro M, Messori M, Di Palma F, Lanzola G, Farret AAO. 2 month evening and night closed-loop glucose control in patients with type 1 diabetes under free-living conditions: a randomised crossover trial. The lancet Diabetes & endocrinology. 2015;3(12):939–47.
16. Thabit H, Tauschmann M, Allen JM, Leelarathna L, Hartnell S, Wilinska ME, Acerini CL, Dellweg S, Benesch C, Heinemann LAO. Home use of an artificial beta cell in type 1 diabetes. N Engl J Med. 2015;373(22):2129–40.
17. Del Favero S, Boscari F, Messori M, Rabbone I, Bonfanti R, Sabbion A, Iafusco D, Schiaffini R, Visentin R, Calore RAO. Randomized summer camp crossover trial in 5-to 9-year-old children: outpatient wearable artificial pancreas is feasible and safe. Diabetes Care. 2016;39(7):1180–5.
18. Bergenstal RM, Garg S, Weinzimer SA, Buckingham BA, Bode BW, Tamborlane WV, Kaufman FR. Safety of a hybrid closed-loop insulin delivery system in patients with type 1 diabetes. JAMA. 2016;316(13):1407–8.
19. Russell SJ, Hillard MA, Balliro C, Magyar KL, Selagamsetty R, Sinha M, Grennan K, Mondesir D, Ekhlaspour L, Zheng HAO. Day and night glycaemic control with a bionic pancreas versus conventional insulin pump therapy in preadolescent children with type 1 diabetes: a randomised crossover trial. The lancet Diabetes & endocrinology. 2016;4(3):233–43.
20. Garg SK, Weinzimer SA, Tamborlane WV, Buckingham BA, Bode BW, Bailey TS, Brazg RL, Ilany J, Slover RH, Erson SMAO. Glucose outcomes with the in-home use of a hybrid closed-loop insulin delivery system in adolescents and adults with type 1 diabetes. Diabetes Technol Ther. 2017;19(3):155–63.
21. Tauschmann M, Thabit H, Bally L, Allen JM, Hartnell S, Wilinska ME, Ruan Y, Sibayan J, Kollman C, Cheng PAO. Closed-loop insulin delivery in suboptimally controlled type 1 diabetes: a multicentre, 12-week randomised trial. Lancet. 2018;392(10155):1321–9.
22. Brown SA, Kovatchev BP, Raghinaru D, Lum JW, Buckingham BA, Kudva YC, Laffel LM, Levy CJ, Pinsker JE, Wadwa RPAO. Six-month randomized, multicenter trial of closed-loop control in type 1 diabetes. N Engl J Med. 2019;381(18):1707–17.
23. Sherr JL, Buckingham BA, Forlenza GP, Galderisi A, Ekhlaspour L, Wadwa RP, Carria L, Hsu L, Berget C, Peyser TAAO. Safety and performance of the omnipod hybrid closed-loop system in adults, adolescents, and children with type 1 diabetes over 5 days under free-living conditions. Diabetes Technol Ther. 2020;22(3):174–84.
24. Collyns OJ, Meier RA, Betts ZL, Chan DS, Frampton C, Frewen CM, Hewapathirana NM, Jones SD, Roy A, Grosman BAO. Improved glycemic outcomes with medtronic minimed advanced hybrid closed-loop delivery: results from a randomized crossover trial comparing automated insulin delivery with predictive low glucose suspend in people with type 1 diabetes. Diabetes Care. 2021;44(4):969–75.
25. Boughton CK, Hovorka R. New closed-loop insulin systems. Diabetologia. 2021:1–9.
26. Zarkogianni K, Litsa E, Mitsis K, Wu P-Y, Kaddi CD, Cheng C-W, Wang MD, Nikita KS. A review of emerging technologies for the management of diabetes mellitus. IEEE Trans Biomed Eng. 2015;62(12):2735–49.
27. Oviedo S, Vehì J, Calm R, Armengol J. A review of personalized blood glucose prediction strategies for T1DM patients. Inter J Numer Meth Biomed Eng. 2017;33(6)
28. van Heusden K, Dassau E, Zisser HC, Seborg DE, Doyle FJ III. Control-relevant models for glucose control using a priori patient characteristics. IEEE Trans Biomed Eng. 2011;59(7):1839–49.
29. Lee JB, Dassau E, Seborg DE, Doyle FJ. Model-based personalization scheme of an artificial pancreas for type 1 diabetes applications. In: 2013 American Control Conference. Washington; 2013.

30. Messori M, Ellis M, Cobelli C, Christofides PD, Magni L. Improved postprandial glucose control with a customized model predictive controller. In: 2015 American Control Conference (ACC). Chicago; 2015.
31. Soru P, De Nicolao G, Toffanin C, Dalla Man C, Cobelli C, Magni L, A. H. C. A. Others. MPC based artificial pancreas: strategies for individualization and meal compensation. Annu Rev Control. 2012;36(1):118–28.
32. Messori M, Toffanin C, Del Favero S, De Nicolao G, Cobelli C, Magni L. Model individualization for artificial pancreas. Comput Methods Prog Biomed. 2019;171:133–40.
33. Toffanin C, Del Favero S, Aiello EM, Messori M, Cobelli C, Magni L. Glucose-insulin model identified in free-living conditions for hypoglycaemia prevention. J Process Control. 2018;64:27–36.
34. Toffanin C, Aiello EM, Cobelli C, Magni L. Hypoglycemia prevention via personalized glucose-insulin models identified in free-living conditions. J Diabetes Sci Technol. 2019;13(6):1008–16.
35. Renard E, Farret A, Kropff J, Bruttomesso D, Messori M, Place J, Visentin R, Calore R, Toffanin C, Di Palma FAO. Day-and-night closed-loop glucose control in patients with type 1 diabetes under free-living conditions: results of a single-arm 1-month experience compared with a previously reported feasibility study of evening and night at home. Diabetes Care. 2016;39(7):1151–60.
36. Del Favero S, Facchinetti R, Sparacino G, Cobelli C. Improving accuracy and precision of glucose sensor profiles: retrospective fitting by constrained deconvolution. IEEE Trans Biomed Eng. 2013;61(4):1044–53.
37. Pillonetto G, De Nicolao G. A new kernel-based approach for linear system identification. Automatica. 2010;46(1):81–93.
38. Aiello EM, Lisanti G, Magni L, Musci M, Toffanin C. Therapy-driven deep glucose forecasting. Eng Appl Artif Intell. 2020;87:103255.
39. Shi D, Dassau E, Doyle FJ III. Multivariate learning framework for long-term adaptation in the artificial pancreas. Bioengineering Translat Med. 4(1):61–74; 019.
40. De Paula M, Acosta GG, Martìnez EC. On-line policy learning and adaptation for real-time personalization of an artificial pancreas. Expert Sys Applicat. 42(4):2234–55, 201.
41. El-Khatib FH, Russell SJ, Magyar KL, Sinha M, McKeon K, Nathan DM, Damiano ER. Autonomous and continuous adaptation of a bihormonal bionic pancreas in adults and adolescents with type 1 diabetes. J Clin Endocrinol Metabol. 2014;99(5):1701–11.
42. Shi D, Dassau E, Doyle FJ. Adaptive zone model predictive control of artificial pancreas based on glucose-and velocity-dependent control penalties. IEEE Trans Biomed Eng. 2018;66(4):1045–54.
43. Resalat N, Hilts W, Youssef JE, Tyler N, Castle JR, Jacobs PG. Adaptive control of an artificial pancreas using model identification, adaptive postprandial insulin delivery, and heart rate and accelerometry as control inputs. J Diabetes Sci Technol. 2019;13(6):1044–53.
44. Messori M, Kropff JADFS, Place J, Visentin R, Calore R, Toffanin C, Di Palma F, Lanzola G, Farret AAO. Individually adaptive artificial pancreas in subjects with type 1 diabetes: a one-month proof-of-concept trial in free-living conditions. Diabetes Technol Ther. 2017;19(10):560–71.
45. Magni L, Forgione M, Toffanin C, Dalla Man C, Kovatchev B, De Nicolao G, Cobelli C. Run-to-run tuning of model predictive control for type 1 diabetes subjects: in silico trial. J Diabetes Sci Technol. 2009;3(5):1091–8.
46. Toffanin C, Messori M, Cobelli C, Magni L. Automatic adaptation of basal therapy for type 1 diabetic patients: a run-to-run approach. Biomedical Signal Processing and Control. 2017;31:539–49.
47. Toffanin C, Visentin R, Messori M, Di Palma F, Magni L, Cobelli C. Toward a run-to-run adaptive artificial pancreas: in silico results. IEEE Trans Biomed Eng. 2017;65(3):479–88.
48. Toffanin C, Aiello E, Del Favero S, Cobelli C, Magni L. Multiple models for artificial pancreas predictions identified from free-living condition data: a proof of concept study. J Process Control. 2019;77:29–37.

Chapter 16
Evolving Approaches to Type 1 Diabetes Management

Jay S. Skyler

Ideal therapeutic goals for type 1 diabetes (T1D) include automated insulin delivery (AID); prevention of immune destruction, to preserve beta cell mass or function; and replacement or regeneration of insulin-secreting beta cells. This chapter will discuss progress in each of these approaches.

Automated Insulin Delivery

A true artificial endocrine pancreas (AEP), or a closed-loop automated insulin delivery system, or, more precisely, a glucose-controlled automated insulin delivery system, has been evolving over the past few decades. Initial systems used a bedside apparatus and required intravenous access both for glucose measurement and for insulin delivery [1]. Continuous subcutaneous insulin infusion (CSII) pumps were introduced in the late 1970s [2–3] and used in clinical practice beginning in the 1980s [4–5]. An implantable system, using an intravascular glucose sensor and intraperitoneal insulin delivery, was briefly used in clinical trials in the early 2000s [6]. In the mid-2000s, continuous glucose monitoring (CGM) systems emerged, and as their accuracy improved, they were coupled with CSII pumps [7–8]. With development of sophisticated algorithms to control CSII delivery based on CGM input, first emerged hybrid systems that controlled basal insulin, and subsequently more sophisticated systems for AID that approach being a true AEP [9–13]. Further evolution will likely be based on advanced data science methods to support diabetes decision support, such as deep learning and big data analytics so that the control

J. S. Skyler (✉)
Diabetes Research Institute, University of Miami Miller School of Medicine,
Miami, FL, USA
e-mail: jskyler@miami.edu

R. Basu (ed.), *Precision Medicine in Diabetes*,
https://doi.org/10.1007/978-3-030-98927-9_16

algorithms evolve to the needs of each individual patient [14–15]. Newer systems may well have algorithms that control delivery of additional hormones besides insulin, such as glucagon and/or an amylin analogue [16–18]. Other chapters in this book discuss the detailed development of control algorithms and the use of AID systems as precision medicine tools for adults and children and during pregnancy.

Automated insulin delivery systems have evolved from "low-glucose suspend" in which insulin delivery was interrupted if the CGM value crossed a low threshold [19] to "predictive low-glucose suspend" in which insulin delivery was interrupted when the CGM value was falling and predicted that it would cross a low threshold [20] to "hybrid closed loop" which provided control of basal glucose (principally overnight) but required mealtime initiation of bolus insulin delivery by the patient [21] to full "automated closed loop" which controls both basal insulin delivery and, to some extent, mealtime bolus insulin delivery [9–13]. Currently available commercial systems have achieved 70–75% time in range (TIR) of 70–180 mg/dl [3.9–10 mmol/l] for adults and 67–73% TIR for children or adolescents. As important, these systems have reduced time spent <54 mg/dl [3.0 mmol/l] to less than 0.5%. The systems still need improvement to achieve ideal glycemic control. Besides improving the control algorithms with such things as deep learning and big data analytics, one limitation that currently exists is the slowness of insulin absorption in response to modulation by the control algorithm. There is hope that the development of ultrarapid insulins, or intra-peritoneal insulin delivery, will speed up directed insulin delivery. Unfortunately, the first evaluation of an ultrarapid insulin in an AID system did not result in improved outcome [22]. Meaningful trials of AID with peritoneal insulin delivery have not yet been reported.

Algorithms for AID are evolving so that the patient may merely have to press a button to indicate initiation of a meal, so that the system will respond differently than it would to mere changes in prevailing glucose level [23]. Future systems potentially may also detect physical activity such as by the use of an accelerometer, sleep pattern, and other variables. However, one must remain cautious, since the more systems and devices that are integrated, the greater the complexity, and the increased potential for technical risks. Nonetheless, technology is advancing to the point that we can anticipate that AID systems will provide near normal glucose levels without risk of hypoglycemia.

Prevention of Immune Destruction to Preserve Beta-Cell Mass or Function

In genetically predisposed individuals, an environmental trigger initiates an immune response directed against pancreatic islet beta cells, resulting in cellular damage, impairment of function, and a potential decrease of beta-cell mass. There is a progressive decline in beta-cell function, spanning years [24]. This gives one the opportunity to intervene in an attempt to modify the course of the disease. Such intervention may precede the clinical stage of the disease, in an attempt to halt the progression of the disease, or may occur after the clinical onset of the disease, in an attempt to preserve – or ideally to improve – residual beta-cell function [25, 26].

Beginning in the 1980s, randomized controlled clinical trials have been conducted in an effort either to delay or prevent clinical onset of the disease or to preserve beta-cell function. Prevention studies have begun in stage 1 of the disease, i.e., individuals with two or more diabetes-related autoantibodies, or in stage 2 of the disease, i.e., those with both autoantibodies and dysglycemia as evidence of decline of beta-cell function. In general, the goal of such prevention studies is to delay progression to stage 3, i.e., clinical T1D. To date, none of the multiple trials initiated in stage 1 have had convincing evidence demonstrating a delay in development of clinical T1D [27]. In contrast, in one trial, the anti-CD3 monoclonal antibody teplizumab, initiated in stage 2 T1D, was shown to delay progression to clinical T1D [28, 29].

There have been a number of interventions tested after clinical onset of T1D that have been shown to preserve residual beta-cell function, at least transiently [30–42]. In some cases, the beneficial effect, compared to that of placebo, was sustained for more than 1 year. Unfortunately, often the intervention was discontinued, on the misguided assumption that the intervention would permanently alter the course of the disease, only to see a decline in beta-cell function toward that of the placebo group [40, 41]. Yet, in a few cases, a short course of therapy – as short as 2 days or 6 or 14 days – has resulted in sustained beneficial effect for 2 years or more [33, 34, 39].

It is possible that intervening after the appearance of antibodies, or certainly after the clinical onset of T1D, may be too late to alter the disease course. In an attempt to intervene prior to the immune process taking hold, efforts are underway to conduct population screening for genetic susceptibility at birth or shortly thereafter and attempt primary prevention before appearance of antibodies [43]. Any such intervention initiated for a primary prevention trial would require that the studies be subject-centric and relatively nonintrusive.

An alternative strategy to potentially improve outcomes in preserving beta-cell function in recent onset T1D is to use a combination of agents. These might include agents that arrest background innate immunity and inflammation (e.g., anti-TNFα), stop adaptive immunity (e.g., anti-CD3 or antithymocyte globulin (ATG)), and/or stimulate protective or regulatory immunity (e.g., low-dose interleukin-2 or infusion of regulatory T cells). In addition to immune intervention, one might consider agents that improve beta-cell health or function (e.g., GLP-1 receptor agonists). It remains to be shown whether a combination strategy might improve outcomes of clinical trials [44, 45].

Replacement of Insulin-Secreting Beta Cells

Beta-cell replacement has been accomplished for many years by either whole pancreas transplantation or isolated islet transplantation [46]. Whole pancreas transplantation has usually accompanied simultaneous kidney transplantation in patients with diabetes with end-stage renal disease, since they will require immune suppression to prevent allograft organ rejection. Occasionally, pancreas transplants have been done following kidney transplantation or have been done alone, in the absence of kidney transplantation [47]. Organs are almost invariably obtained from cadaver donors. Isolated islet transplantation has generally been done in individuals with recurrent severe hypoglycemia resulting in seizures, loss of consciousness, emergency room visits, or hospitalization [48]. Again, islets are obtained from cadaver donor pancreases, with the islets isolated and purified [49] before being transplanted, usually via portal vein infusion, but more recently in other locations such as the omentum [50].

There are three issues which have limited both pancreas and islet transplantation. These are (1) the availability and source of cells (there has been an average of only 1200 pancreas donors per year in the United States) [51], (2) the alloimmune response leading to organ rejection, and (3) the recurrence of the autoimmune response which led to T1D in the first place [52, 53].

To provide availability of cells, there are three strategies that have been proposed: (1) xenotransplantation using pig islets [54], particularly using specially bred pigs that are devoid of porcine viruses [55], (2) use of human embryonic stem cells (hESCs) [56, 57], and (3) use of induced pluripotent stem cells (iPSCs) [58–60]. Each of these strategies has the potential of providing an essentially unlimited source of cells.

There are two general strategies for stem cell transplantation: (1) a patient-specific approach using reprogramming or transdifferentiation of cells to create islets, such as by converting liver cells (obtained by biopsy) to insulin-secreting cells in the laboratory [61], and (2) a generic approach using allogeneic cells, e.g., a bank of human embryonic stem cells (hESCs) or induced pluripotent stem cells (iPSCs). The latter approach creates cells that may be used for multiple patients, using cells that are centrally produced and more easily commercialized. Indeed, randomized clinical trials are currently underway with both hESCs [62] and iPSCs [63].

For both hESCs and iPSCs, there needs to be immune protection both against alloimmune rejection and potentially against autoimmune recurrence. This might be accomplished by the use of immunosuppressive or immunomodulatory drugs. Alternatively, one could create a physical barrier protecting the infused cells from the immune system using encapsulation [64, 65]. Ultimately, one might use gene editing for either immune evasion or immune protection [66].

Regeneration of Beta Cells

Beta-cell regeneration might be a way to improve function and potentially reverse T1D. Although approaches to regeneration have been used in animal models, human studies have not yet been successful [67, 68]. Nonetheless, many laboratories are pursuing beta-cell regeneration, and the hope is that progress will be forthcoming.

Conclusions

My hypothesis is that the ideal therapeutic approaches to T1D, automated insulin delivery (AID); prevention of immune destruction, to preserve beta-cell mass or function; and replacement of insulin-secreting beta-cells and/or regeneration of beta cells, are all approaches that will ultimately come to fruition. The time course of success for each of these approaches is unpredictable. Many investigators, their institutions, or their funders often issue press releases heralding their advances. One must be cautious in reading these, as many overpromote the advances [69]. Nonetheless, there has been a great progress in both innovations and the scientific breakthroughs needed to advance these ideas to clinical reality.

References

1. Clemens AH, Chang PH, Myers RW. The development of Biostator, a glucose controlled insulin infusion system (GCIIS). Horm Metab Res Suppl. 1977;7:23–33.
2. Pickup JC, Keen H, Parsons JA, Alberti KGMM. Continuous subcutaneous insulin infusion: an approach to achieving normoglycemia. Br Med J. 1978;1:204–7.
3. Tamborlane WV, Sherwin RS, Genel M, Felig P. Reduction to normal of plasma glucose in juvenile diabetes by subcutaneous administration of insulin with a portable infusion pump. N Engl J Med. 1979;300:573–8.
4. Skyler JS, Seigler DE, Reeves ML. Optimizing pumped insulin delivery. Diabetes Care. 1982;5:135–9.
5. Farkas-Hirsch R, Hirsch I. Continuous subcutaneous insulin infusion: a review of the past and its implementation for the future. Diabetes Spectrum. 1994;7(80-84):136–8.
6. Renard E. Implantable closed-loop glucose-sensing and insulin delivery: the future for insulin pump therapy. Curr Opin Pharmacol. 2002;2:708–16.
7. Hovorka R. Closed-loop insulin delivery: from bench to clinical practice. Nat Rev Endocrinol. 2011;7:385–95.
8. Weinzimer SA, Steil GM, Swan KL, Dziura J, Kurtz N, Tamborlane WV. Fully automated closed-loop insulin delivery versus semiautomated hybrid control in pediatric patients with type 1 diabetes using an artificial pancreas. Diabetes Care. 2008;31:934–9.
9. Brown SA, Kovatchev BP, Raghinaru D, Lum JW, Buckingham BA, Kudva YC, et al. Six-month randomized, multicenter trial of closed-loop control in type 1 diabetes. N Engl J Med. 2019;381:1707–17.
10. Breton MD, Kanapka LG, Beck RW, Ekhlaspour L, Forlenza GP, Cengiz E, et al. A randomized trial of closed-loop control inchildren with type 1 diabetes. N Engl J Med. 2020;383:836–45.

11. Brown SA, Forlenza GP, Bode BW, Pinsker JE, Levy CJ, Criego AB, at al. Multicenter trial of a tubeless, on-body automated insulin delivery system with customizable glycemic targets in pediatric and adult participants with type 1 diabetes. Diabetes Care. 2021;44:1630–40.
12. Collyns OJ, Meier RA, Betts ZL, Chan DSH, Frampton C, Frewen CM, et al. Improved glycemic outcomes with medtronic minimed advanced hybrid closed-loop delivery: results from a randomized crossover trial comparing automated insulin delivery with predictive low glucose suspend in people with type 1 diabetes. Diabetes Care. 2021;44:969–75.
13. Fuchs J, Allen JM, Boughton CK, Wilinska ME, Thankamony A, de Beaufort C, et al. Assessing the efficacy, safety and utility of closed-loop insulin delivery compared with sensor-augmented pump therapy in very young children with type 1 diabetes (KidsAP02 study): an open-label, multicentre, multinational, randomised cross-over study protocol. BMJ Open. 2021;11(2):e042790.
14. Kovatchev B. A century of diabetes technology: signals, models, and artificial pancreas control. Trends Endocrinol Metab. 2019;30:432–44.
15. El-Khatib FH, Russell SJ, Magyar KL, Sinha M, McKeon K, Nathan DM, et al. Autonomous and continuous adaptation of a bihormonal bionic pancreas in adults and adolescents with type 1 diabetes. J Clin Endocrinol Metab. 2014;99:1701–11.
16. Russell SJ, El-Khatib FH, Sinha M, Magyar KL, McKeon K, Goergen LG, et al. Outpatient glycemic control with a bionic pancreas in type 1 diabetes. N Engl J Med. 2014;371:313–25.
17. El-Khatib FH, Balliro C, Hillard MA, Magyar KL, Ekhlaspour L, Sinha M, et al. Home use of a bihormonal bionic pancreas versus insulin pump therapy in adults with type 1 diabetes: a multicentre randomised crossover trial. Lancet. 2017;389:369–80.
18. Haidar A, Tsoukas MA, Bernier-Twardy S, Yale JF, Rutkowski J, et al. A Novel Dual-Hormone Insulin-and-Pramlintide Artificial Pancreas for Type 1 Diabetes: A Randomized Controlled Crossover Trial. Diabetes Care. 2020;43:597–606.
19. Bergenstal RM, Klonoff DC, Garg SK, Bode BW, Meredith M, Slover RH, et al. Threshold-based insulin-pump interruption for reduction of hypoglycemia. N Engl J Med. 2013;369:224–32.
20. Battelino T, Nimri R, Dovc K, Phillip M, Bratina N. Prevention of hypoglycemia with predictive low glucose insulin suspension in children with type 1 diabetes: a randomized controlled trial. Diabetes Care. 2017;40:764–70.
21. Bergenstal R, Garg S, Weinzimer SA, Buckingham BA, Bode BW, Tamborlane WV, et al. Safety of a hybrid closed-loop insulin delivery system in patients with type 1 diabetes. JAMA. 2016;316:1407–8.
22. Boughton CK, Hartnell S, Thabit H, Poettler T, Herzig D, Wilinska ME, et al. Hybrid closed-loop glucose control with faster insulin aspart compared with standard insulin aspart in adults with type 1 diabetes: a double-blind, multicentre, multinational, randomized, crossover study. Diabetes Obes Metab. 2021;23:1389–96.
23. Garcia-Tirado J, Diaz JL, Esquivel-Zuniga R, Koravi CLK, Corbett JP, Dawson M, et al. Advanced closed-loop control system improves postprandial glycemic control compared with a hybrid closed-loop system following unannounced meal. Diabetes Care. 2021:dc210932. https://doi.org/10.2337/dc21-0932. Online ahead of print.
24. Atkinson MA, Eisenbarth GS, Michels AW. Type 1 diabetes. Lancet. 2014;383:69–82.
25. Atkinson MA, Roep BO, Posgai A, Wheeler DCS, Peakman M. The challenge of modulating β-cell autoimmunity in type 1 diabetes. Lancet Diabetes Endocrinol. 2019;7:52–64.
26. Roep BO, Wheeler DCS, Peakman M. Antigen-based immune modulation therapy for type 1 diabetes: the era of precision medicine. Lancet Diabetes Endocrinol. 2019;7:65–74.
27. Jacobsen LM, Schatz DA. Insulin immunotherapy for pretype 1 diabetes. Curr Opin Endocrinol Diabetes Obes. 2021;28:390–6.
28. Herold KC, Bundy BN, Long SA, Bluestone JA, DiMeglio LA, Dufort MJ, et al. An anti-CD3 antibody, teplizumab, in relatives at risk for type 1 diabetes. N Engl J Med. 2019;381:603–13.
29. Sims EK, Bundy BN, Stier K, Serti E, Lim N, Long SA, et al. Teplizumab improves and stabilizes beta cell function in antibody-positive high-risk individuals. Sci Transl Med. 2021;13(583):eabc8980.

30. Feutren G, Assan R, Karsenty G, Du Rostu H, Sirmai J, Papoz L, et al. Cyclosporin increases the rate and length of remissions in insulin dependent diabetes of recent onset. Results of a multicentre double-blind trial. Lancet. 1986;2:119–24.
31. The Canadian-European Randomized Control Trial Group. Cyclosporin-induced remission of IDDM after early intervention. Association of 1 yr of cyclosporin treatment with enhanced insulin secretion. Diabetes. 1988;37:1574–82.
32. Silverstein J, Maclaren N, Riley W, Spillar R, Radjenovic D, Johnson S. Immunosuppression with azathioprine and prednisone in recent-onset insulin-dependent diabetes mellitus. N Engl J Med. 1988;319:599–604.
33. Herold KC, Hagopian W, Auger JA, Poumian-Ruiz E, Taylor L, Donaldson D, et al. Anti-CD3 monoclonal antibody in new-onset type 1 diabetes mellitus. N Engl J Med. 2002;346:1692–8.
34. Keymeulen B, Vandemeulebroucke E, Ziegler AG, Mathieu C, Kaufman L, Hale G, et al. Insulin needs after CD3-antibody therapy in new-onset type 1 diabetes. N Engl J Med. 2005;352:2598–608.
35. Herold KC, Gitelman SE, Ehlers MR, Gottlieb PA, Greenbaum CJ, Hagopian W, et al. Teplizumab (anti-CD3 mAb) treatment preserves C-peptide responses in patients with new-onset type 1 diabetes in a randomized controlled trial: Metabolic and immunologic features at baseline identify a subgroup of responders. Diabetes. 2013;62:3766–74.
36. Pescovitz MD, Greenbaum CJ, Krause-Steinrauf H, Becker DJ, Gitelman SE, Goland R, et al. Rituximab, B-lymphocyte depletion and preservation of beta-cell function. N Engl J Med. 2009;361:2143–52.
37. Orban T, Bundy B, Becker DJ, DiMeglio LA, Gitelman SE, Goland R, et al. Co-stimulation modulation with abatacept in patients with recent-onset type 1 diabetes: a randomised double-blind. Placebo-Controlled Trial Lancet. 2011;378:412–9.
38. Rigby MR, DiMeglio LA, Rendell MS, Felner EI, Dostou JM, Gitelman SE, et al. Targeting of memory T cells with alefacept in new-onset type 1 diabetes (T1DAL study): 12 month results of a randomised, double-blind, placebo-controlled phase 2 trial. Lancet Diabetes Endocrinol. 2013;1:284–94.
39. Haller MJ, Long SA, Blanchfield JL, Schatz DA, Skyler JS, Krischer JP, et al. Low-dose anti-thymocyte globulin preserves C-peptide and reduces A1c in new onset type 1 diabetes: two year clinical trial data. Diabetes. 2019;68:1267–76.
40. von Herrath M, Bain SC, Bode B, Clausen JO, Coppieters K, Gaysina L, et al. Anti-interleukin-21 antibody and liraglutide for the preservation of β-cell function in adults with recent-onset type 1 diabetes: a randomised, double-blind, placebo-controlled, phase 2 trial. Lancet Diabetes Endocrinol. 2021;9:212–24.
41. Quattrin T, Haller MJ, Steck AK, Felner EI, Li Y, Xia Y, et al. Golimumab and beta-cell function in youth with new-onset type 1 diabetes. N Engl J Med. 2020;383:2007–17.
42. Gitelman SE, Bundy BN, Ferrannini E, Lim N, Blanchfield JL, DiMeglio LA, et al. Imatinib therapy for patients with recent-onset type 1 diabetes: a randomised, double blind, multicentre, placebo controlled phase 2 trial. Lancet Diabetes Endocrinol. 2021;9:502–14.
43. Ziegler AG, Danne T, Dunger DB, Berner R, Puff R, Kiess W, et al. Primary prevention of beta-cell autoimmunity and type 1 diabetes - The Global Platform for the Prevention of Autoimmune Diabetes (GPPAD) perspectives. Mol Metab. 2016;5:255–62.
44. Smilek DE, Ehlers ME, Nepom GT. Restoring the balance: immunotherapeutic combinations for autoimmune disease. Dis Model Mech. 2014;7:503–13.
45. Skyler JS. The prevention & reversal of type 1 diabetes – past challenges & future opportunities. Diabetes Care. 2015;38:997–1007.
46. Gruessner AC, Gruessner RW. Long-term outcome after pancreas transplantation: a registry analysis. Curr Opin Organ Transplant. 2016;21:377–85.
47. Hering BJ, Clarke WR, Bridges ND, Eggerman TL, Alejandro R, Bellin MD, et al. Phase 3 trial of transplantation of human islets in type 1 diabetes complicated by severe hypoglycemia. Diabetes Care. 2016;39:1230–40.

48. Vantyghem MC, Chetboun M, Gmyr V, Jannin A, Espiard S, Le Mapihan K, et al. Ten-year outcome of islet alone or islet after kidney transplantation in type 1 diabetes: a prospective parallel-arm cohort study. Diabetes Care. 2019;42:2042–9.
49. Ryan EA, Shandro T, Green K, Paty BW, Senior PA, Bigam D, et al. Assessment of the severity of hypoglycemia and glycemic lability in type 1 diabetic subjects undergoing islet transplantation. Diabetes. 2004;53:955–62.
50. Ricordi C, Lacy PE, Finke EH, Olack BJ, Sharp DW. Automated method for isolation of human pancreatic islets. Diabetes. 1988;37:413–20.
51. Baidal DA, Ricordi C, Berman DM, Alvarez A, Padilla N, Ciancio G, et al. Bioengineering of an intraabdominal endocrine pancreas. N Engl J Med. 2017;376:1887–9.
52. Kandaswamy R, Stock PG, Miller J, Skeans MA, White J, Wainright J, et al. OPTN/SRTR 2019 annual data report: pancreas. Am J Transplant. 2021;21(Suppl 2):138–207.
53. Vendrame F, Pileggi A, Laughlin E, Allende G, Martin-Pagola A, Molano RD, et al. Recurrence of type 1 diabetes after simultaneous pancreas-kidney transplantation, despite immunosuppression, is associated with autoantibodies and pathogenic autoreactive CD4 T-cells. Diabetes. 2010;59:947–57.
54. Burke GW 3rd, Vendrame F, Pileggi A, Ciancio G, Reijonen H, Pugliese A. Recurrence of autoimmunity following pancreas transplantation. Curr Diab Rep. 2011;11:413–9.
55. Ludwig B, Ludwig S, Steffen A, Knauf Y, Zimerman B, Heinke S, et al. Favorable outcome of experimental islet xenotransplantation without immunosuppression in a nonhuman primate model of diabetes. Proc Natl Acad Sci U S A. 2017;114:11745–50.
56. Niu D, Wei HJ, Lin L, George H, Wang T, Lee IH, et al. Inactivation of porcine endogenous retrovirus in pigs using CRISPR-Cas9. Science. 2017;357:1303–7.
57. D'Amour KA, Bang AG, Eliazer S, Kelly OG, Agulnick AD, Smart NG, et al. Production of pancreatic hormone-expressing endocrine cells from human embryonic stem cells. Nat Biotechnol. 2006;24:1392–401.
58. Schulz TC, Young HY, Agulnick AD, Babin MJ, Baetge EE, Bang AG, et al. A scalable system for production of functional pancreatic progenitors from human embryonic stem cells. PLoS One. 2012;7(5):e37004.
59. Pagliuca FW, Millam JR, Gürtler M, Segel M, Van Devort A, Ryu JH, et al. Generation of functional human pancreatic beta cells in vitro. Cell. 2014;159:428–39.
60. Sneddon JB, Qizhi T, Stock P, Bluestone JA, Roy D, Desai T, et al. Stem cell therapies for treating diabetes: progress and remaining challenges. Cell Stem Cell. 2018;6:810–23.
61. Meivar-Levy I, Ferber S. Liver to pancreas transdifferentiation. Curr Diab Rep. 2019;19:76.
62. Pepper AR, Bruni A, Pawlick R, O'Gorman D, Kin T, Thiesen A, et al. Posttransplant characterization of long term functional hESC-derived pancreatic endoderm grafts. Diabetes. 2019;68:953–62.
63. ClinicalTrials.Gov NCT04786262. A safety, tolerability, & efficacy study of VX-880 in participants with type 1 diabetes. Accessed 1 Sept, 2021.
64. Desai TA, Tang Q. Islet encapsulation therapy - racing towards the finish line? Nat Rev Endocrinol. 2018;14:630–2.
65. Stock AA, Manzoli V, De Toni T, Abreu MM, Poh YC, Ye L, et al. Conformal coating of stem cell-derived islets for beta cell replacement in type 1 diabetes. Stem Cell Reports. 2020;14:91–104.
66. Parent AV, Faleo G, Chavez J, Saxton M, Berrios DI, Kerper NR, et al. Selective deletion of human leukocyte antigens protects stem cell-derived islets from immune rejection. Cell Rep. 2021;36:109538.
67. Zhou Q, Melton DA. Pancreas Regeneration. Nature. 2018;557:351–8.
68. Wang P, Karakose E, Choleva L, Kumar K, DeVita RJ, Garcia-Ocaña A, et al. Human beta cell regenerative drug therapy for diabetes: past achievements and future challenges. Front Endocrinol. 2021;12:671946.
69. Skyler JS. Hope versus hype: where are we in type 1 diabetes? Diabetologia. 2018;61:509–16.

Index

R. Basu (ed.), *Precision Medicine in Diabetes*,
https://doi.org/10.1007/978-3-030-98927-9

The manufacturer's authorised representative in the EU is Springer Nature Customer Service Centre GmbH, Europaplatz 3, 69115 Heidelberg, Germany. If you have any concerns regarding our products, please contact ProductSafety@springernature.com

Printed and bound by CPI Group (UK) Ltd, Croydon, CR0 4YY
15/07/2026
02167636-0001